Adolescent Cardiac Issues

Editors

POOJA GUPTA
RICHARD HUMES

PEDIATRIC CLINICS
OF NORTH AMERICA

www.pediatric.theclinics.com

Consulting Editor
BONITA F. STANTON

February 2014 • Volume 61 • Number 1

ELSEVIER

1600 John F. Kennedy Boulevard • Suite 1800 • Philadelphia, Pennsylvania, 19103-2899

http://www.theclinics.com

THE PEDIATRIC CLINICS OF NORTH AMERICA Volume 61, Number 1
February 2014 ISSN 0031-3955, ISBN-13: 978-0-323-26676-5

Editor: Kerry Holland
Developmental Editor: Casey Jackson

The Pediatric Clinics of North America (ISSN 0031-3955) is published bimonthly by Elsevier Inc., 360 Park Avenue South, New York, NY 10010-1710. Months of issue are February, April, June, August, October, and December. Periodicals postage paid at New York, NY and additional mailing offices. Subscription prices are $200.00 per year (US individuals), $493.00 per year (US institutions), $270.00 per year (Canadian individuals), $657.00 per year (Canadian institutions), $325.00 per year (international individuals), $657.00 per year (international institutions), $100.00 per year (US students and residents), and $165.00 per year (international and Canadian residents and students). To receive students/resident rare, orders must be accompanied by name of affiliated institution, date of term, and the signature of program/residency coordinator on institution letterhead. Orders will be billed at individual rate until proof of status is received. Foreign air speed delivery is included in all *Clinics* subscription prices. All prices are subject to change without notice. **POSTMASTER:** Send address changes to *The Pediatric Clinics of North America*, Elsevier Health Sciences Division, Subscription Customer Service, 3251 Riverport Lane, Maryland Heights, MO 63043. **Customer Service: 1-800-654-2452 (US and Canada). From outside of the US and Canada: 1-314-447-8871. Fax: 1-314-447-8029. For print support, E-mail: JournalsCustomerService-usa@elsevier.com. For online support, E-mail: JournalsOnlineSupport-usa@elsevier.com.**

Reprints. For copies of 100 or more, of articles in this publication, please contact the Commercial Reprints Department, Elsevier Inc., 360 Park Avenue South, New York, NY 10010-1710. Tel.: 212-633-3874; Fax: 212-633-3820; E-mail: reprints@elsevier.com.

The Pediatric Clinics of North America is also published in Spanish by McGraw-Hill Inter-americana Editores S.A., Mexico City, Mexico; in Portuguese by Riechmann and Affonso Editores, Rua Comandante Coelho 1085, CEP 21250, Rio de Janeiro, Brazil; and in Greek by Althayia SA, Athens, Greece.

The Pediatric Clinics of North America is covered in *MEDLINE/PubMed (Index Medicus), Excerpta Medica, Current Contents, Current Contents/Clinical Medicine, Science Citation Index, ASCA, ISI/BIOMED,* and *BIOSIS.*

Printed and bound by CPI Group (UK) Ltd, Croydon, CR0 4YY

Transferred to digital print 2013

PROGRAM OBJECTIVE

The goal of the *Pediatric Clinics of North America* is to keep practicing physicians and residents up to date with current clinical practice in pediatrics by providing timely articles reviewing the state-of-the-art in patient care.

TARGET AUDIENCE

All practicing pediatricians, physicians and healthcare professionals who provide patient care to pediatric patients.

LEARNING OBJECTIVES

Upon completion of this activity, participants will be able to:
1. Review cardiomyopathies encountered commonly in the teenage years.
2. Discuss a pediatric approach to family history of cardiovascular disease.
3. Recognize obesity and cardiovascular risk factors in childhood and adolescence.

ACCREDITATION

The Elsevier Office of Continuing Medical Education (EOCME) is accredited by the Accreditation Council for Continuing Medical Education (ACCME) to provide continuing medical education for physicians.

The EOCME designates thisenduringmaterial for a maximum of 15 *AMA PRA Category 1 Credit*(s)™. Physicians should claim only the credit commensurate with the extent of their participation in the activity.

All other health care professionals requesting continuing education credit for this enduring material will be issued a certificate of participation.

DISCLOSURE OF CONFLICTS OF INTEREST

The EOCME assesses conflict of interest with its instructors, faculty, planners, and other individuals who are in a position to control the content of CME activities. All relevant conflicts of interest that are identified are thoroughly vetted by EOCME for fair balance, scientific objectivity, and patient care recommendations. EOCME is committed to providing its learners with CME activities that promote improvements or quality in healthcare and not a specific proprietary business or a commercial interest.

The planning committee, staff, authors and editors listed below have identified no financial relationships or relationships to products or devices they or their spouse/life partner have with commercial interest related to the content of this CME activity:

Elizabeth Anyaegbu, MD; Preetha Balakrishnan, MD; Jennifer M. Blake, MD; Demetrios Demetriades, MD; Vikas Dharnidharka, MD, MPH; James Galas, MD; Pooja Gupta, MD; Robert Hinton, MD; Kerry Holland; Rick Humes, MD; Brynne Hunter; Peter P. Karpawich, Msc, MD, FAAP, FACC, FHRS; Peter Koenig, MD; Indu Kumari; Sandy Lavery; Jill McNair; Erin Miller, MS, CGC; Ronak J. Naik, MD, DNB; Lindsay Parnell; Michael Pettersen, MD; Thomas A. Pilcher, MD; Elizabeth Saarel, MD; Farshad Sedaghat-Yazdi, MD; Nishant Shah, MD; Harinder R. Singh, MD; Heather A. Sowinski, DO, FAACP; Bonita F. Stanton, MD; Peep Talving, MD, PhD.

The planning committee, staff, authors and editors listed below have identified financial relationships or relationships to products or devices they or their spouse/life partner have with commercial interest related to the content of this CME activity:

UNAPPROVED/OFF-LABEL USE DISCLOSURE

The EOCME requires CME faculty to disclose to the participants:
1. When products or procedures being discussed are off-label, unlabelled, experimental, and/or investigational (not US Food and Drug Administration (FDA) approved); and
2. Any limitations on the information presented, such as data that are preliminary or that represent ongoing research, interim analyses, and/or unsupported opinions. Faculty may discuss information about pharmaceutical agents that is outside of FDA-approved labelling. This information is intended solely for CME and is not intended to promote off-label use of these medications. If you have any questions, contact the medical affairs department of the manufacturer for the most recent prescribing information.

TO ENROLL

To enroll in the *Pediatric Clinics of North America* Continuing Medical Education program, call customer service at 1-800-654-2452 or sign up online at http://www.theclinics.com/home/cme. The CME program is available to subscribers for an additional annual fee of USD 261.

METHOD OF PARTICIPATION

In order to claim credit, participants must complete the following:

1. Complete enrolment as indicated above.
2. Read the activity.
3. Complete the CME Test and Evaluation. Participants must achieve a score of 70% on the test. All CME Tests and Evaluations must be completed online.

CME INQUIRIES/SPECIAL NEEDS

For all CME inquiries or special needs, please contact elsevierCME@elsevier.com.

Contributors

CONSULTING EDITOR

BONITA F. STANTON, MD
Vice Dean for Research and Professor of Pediatrics, School of Medicine, Wayne State University, Detroit, Michigan

EDITORS

POOJA GUPTA, MD
Assistant Professor, Pediatric Cardiology, Children's Hospital of Michigan; Assistant Professor of Pediatrics, Division of Cardiology, The Carman and Ann Adams Department of Pediatrics, Wayne State University School of Medicine, Detroit, Michigan

RICHARD HUMES, MD
Director, Pediatric Cardiology, Children's Hospital of Michigan; Professor of Pediatrics, Wayne State University, Detroit, Michigan

AUTHORS

ELIZABETH I. ANYAEGBU, MD, MSCI
Division of Pediatric Nephrology, Driscoll Children's Hospital; Clinical Assistant Professor of Pediatrics, College of Medicine, Texas A&M University, Corpus Christi, Texas

PREETHA L. BALAKRISHNAN, MD
Assistant Professor of Pediatrics, Division of Cardiology, The Carman and Ann Adams Department of Pediatrics, Wayne State University School of Medicine, Detroit, Michigan

JENNIFER M. BLAKE, MD
Assistant Professor of Pediatrics, Division of Pediatric Cardiology, Children's Hospital of Michigan, Wayne State University School of Medicine, Detroit, Michigan

DEMETRIOS DEMETRIADES, MD, PhD, FACS
Professor of Surgery, Division of Acute Care Surgery (Trauma, Emergency Surgery and Surgical Critical Care), Department of Surgery, Keck School of Medicine, LAC+USC Medical Center, University of Southern California, Los Angeles, California

VIKAS R. DHARNIDHARKA, MD, MPH
Director, Division of Pediatric Nephrology, St Louis Children's Hospital; Associate Professor of Pediatrics, Washington University School of Medicine in St Louis, St Louis, Missouri

JAMES M. GALAS, MD
Assistant Professor of Pediatrics, Division of Pediatric Cardiology, The Carman and Ann Adams Department of Pediatrics, Wayne State University School of Medicine, Detroit, Michigan

POOJA GUPTA, MD
Assistant Professor, Pediatric Cardiology, Children's Hospital of Michigan; Assistant
Professor of Pediatrics, Division of Cardiology, The Carman and Ann Adams Department
of Pediatrics, Wayne State University School of Medicine, Detroit, Michigan

ROBERT B. HINTON, MD
Division of Cardiology, The Heart Institute, Cincinnati Children's Hospital Medical Center,
Cincinnati, Ohio

PETER P. KARPAWICH, MSc, MD, FAAP, FACC, FHRS
Section of Pediatric Cardiology, The Carmen and Ann Adams Department of Pediatrics,
The Children's Hospital of Michigan, School of Medicine, Wayne State University, Detroit,
Michigan

PETER R. KOENIG, MD
Associate Professor of Pediatrics, Department of Cardiology, The Willis J. Potts Heart
Center, Ann and Robert H. Lurie Children's Hospital of Chicago, Feinberg School of
Medicine, Northwestern University, Chicago, Illinois

ERIN M. MILLER, MS, CGC
Division of Cardiology, The Heart Institute; Division of Human Genetics, Cincinnati
Children's Hospital Medical Center, Cincinnati, Ohio

RONAK J. NAIK, MD, DNB, FACC
Division of Cardiology, Department of Pediatrics, Le Bonheur Children's Hospital,
University of Tennessee Health Science Center, Memphis, Tennessee

MICHAEL D. PETTERSEN, MD
Department of Pediatrics, Rocky Mountain Hospital for Children, Denver, Colorado

THOMAS A. PILCHER, MD, MS, FHRS
Assistant Professor of Pediatrics, Division of Pediatric Cardiology, Primary Children's
Medical Center, Director of Electrocardiography and Outpatient Monitoring, University
of Utah, Salt Lake City, Utah

ELIZABETH V. SAAREL, MD, FHRS
Associate Professor of Pediatrics, Division of Pediatric Cardiology, Primary Children's
Medical Center, Director of Pediatric Electrophysiology, University of Utah, Salt Lake City,
Utah

FARSHAD SEDAGHAT-YAZDI, MD
Instructor of Pediatrics, Department of Cardiology, The Willis J. Potts Heart Center, Ann
and Robert H. Lurie Children's Hospital of Chicago, Feinberg School of Medicine,
Northwestern University, Chicago, Illinois

NISHANT C. SHAH, MD
Department of Pediatrics, Penn State Hershey Children's Hospital, Penn State University,
Hershey, Pennsylvania

HARINDER R. SINGH, MD, FHRS, CEPS, CCDS
Division of Cardiology, The Carman and Ann Adams Department of Pediatrics,
Children's Hospital of Michigan, Wayne State University School of Medicine, Detroit,
Michigan

HEATHER SOWINSKI, DO, FAAP
Section of Pediatric Cardiology, The Carmen and Ann Adams Department of Pediatrics, The Children's Hospital of Michigan, School of Medicine, Wayne State University, Detroit, Michigan

PEEP TALVING, MD, PhD, FACS
Assistant Professor of Surgery, Division of Acute Care Surgery (Trauma, Emergency Surgery and Surgical Critical Care), Department of Surgery, Keck School of Medicine, LAC+USC Medical Center, University of Southern California, Los Angeles, California

Contents

The first-time appearance of a murmur in an adolescent can create a substantial amount of anxiety in the parents and the teenager. The appropriate evaluation and diagnosis is very important in decision making regarding sports participation in this population. Accurate identification of the innocent murmurs can obviate the need for echocardiography. Identification of a pathologic murmur may reduce morbidity and, possibly, mortality in critical lesions such as hypertrophic cardiomyopathy. This article discusses the physiology and characteristics of different murmurs and outlines an approach to cardiac murmurs in adolescents.

Chest pain is a frequent symptom and complaint in the teenage population. There are many common, benign causes of chest pain. However, it can create tremendous anxiety in the mind of the patient and family members and sometimes it can be perplexing even for the primary providers especially if there is associated family history of premature coronary artery disease. This article focuses on the evaluation of chest pain and how to differentiate between noncardiac and cardiac causes of chest pain in teenagers.

This article informs the general pediatrician about the diagnosis, evaluation, and treatment of teenage patients with presyncope and loss of consciousness. The focus is on distinguishing noncardiac fainting from life-threatening syncope. Current treatment strategies of vasovagal syncope and postural orthostatic tachycardia syndrome are also outlined.

Use of medications for attention-deficit hyperkinetic disorder and preparticipation sports physical examination has led to an increase in number of electrocardiograms (ECG) performed during adolescence. Interpreting ECGs in children and young adults must take into account the evolutionary changes with age and the benign variants, which are usually not associated with heart disease. It is crucial for primary-care providers to recognize the

common in the United States, encountered frequently in major urban centers. Most patients are dead at the scene and never reach hospital. The incidence of cardiac sequelae in survivors is high, and these patients should be evaluated with early and late echocardiography to detect anatomic or functional cardiac involvement.

cardiovascular disease. As more is learned about the genetic basis of cardiovascular disease, the family history will play an increasingly central role in management. Improved understanding of the causes of pediatric cardiovascular disease promises the opportunity to develop new diagnostic and therapeutic strategies.

Adolescents with congenital heart disease (CHD) are a rapidly growing population with complex medical needs and psychosocial challenges. Identity formation is an important developmental task accomplished during the teenage years. This article reviews different aspects of ongoing care that pertain to teenagers with CHD, with a particular focus on primary care issues and a summary of recommendations from various scientific societies. A successful smooth transition to the adult health care setting should achieve two important goals: to prevent loss of follow-up and to foster and encourage self-care behaviors.

PEDIATRIC CLINICS OF NORTH AMERICA

Foreword

Understanding the Adolescent Heart

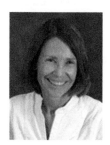

Bonita F. Stanton, MD
Consulting Editor

A great deal is asked of primary care providers taking care of children in the community. Their knowledge base must be vast and their index of suspicion heightened, while not undermining their role in the provision of both preventive care and reassurance. Appropriately, general pediatric training emphasizes critical parts of the history and physical examination during specific age intervals. General pediatric training has long focused on the importance of a detailed and careful cardiac examination among neonates and infants. This emphasis during training provides primary care pediatricians with confidence in their abilities to identify the abnormal heart in a very young child.

Given the epidemiology of the appearance of cardiac disease, an emphasis on the cardiac examination early in life remains appropriate. However, over the last few decades, pediatric health care providers have become more concerned with the cardiac function of adolescents and young adults. The awareness among both the lay audience and the health care practitioner of serious cardiac-related morbidity among adolescents and young adults has risen; in some cases, the actual incidence appears also to have increased. While some of these deaths and near-deaths are occurring in children with previously identified cardiac lesions, many are occurring in children who were (or seemed to have been) healthy, including elite athletes. Whether as part of an adolescent preventative care physical examination or as an adolescent sports physical examination, the pediatrician must assess the heart and determine whether there is any cause for concern and, if so, what additional diagnostic steps must be undertaken. Given the range of underlying conditions and the relative low frequency of any single condition, many pediatric care providers feel uncomfortable assessing the heart among adolescents.

Pediatr Clin N Am 61 (2014) xv–xvi
http://dx.doi.org/10.1016/j.pcl.2013.10.001
0031-3955/14/$ – see front matter © 2014 Elsevier Inc. All rights reserved.

pediatric.theclinics.com

Accordingly, this volume of *Pediatric Clinics of North America*, targeting primary care providers of adolescents, focuses on the adolescent heart and reviews the possible causes of cardiac disease among adolescents as well as their recognition and treatment approaches.

Bonita F. Stanton, MD
School of Medicine
Wayne State University
1261 Scott Hall
540 East Canfield, Suite 1261
Detroit, MI 48201, USA

E-mail address:
bstanton@med.wayne.edu

Preface

Adolescent Cardiac Issues

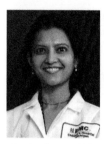 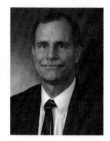

Pooja Gupta, MD   Richard Humes, MD

Editors

Pediatric cardiology has always been focused on the care and management of patients with congenital heart disease. Most cardiologists entered the profession for the opportunity to diagnose and manage this incredibly interesting and diverse set of problems and anomalies. In addition, pediatric cardiology has been driven over the years by the rapidly developing technology in imaging and intervention in both the catheterization laboratory and the operating room. Patients with congenital defects once considered lethal are now living into adolescence and adulthood. There is almost no congenital heart defect for which there is not some possible intervention.

Most congenital heart diseases are evident in early life, presenting with cyanosis, heart murmur, congestive heart failure, or shock. Textbooks in pediatric cardiology are filled overwhelmingly with chapters on the various congenital heart lesions that are encountered, both rare and common. However, practicing pediatric cardiologists will be quick to point out that a significant number of referrals to their practice may be due to symptoms referred to the heart but the majority of them do not involve congenital heart problems. Many of these problems may be perplexing to the general pediatrician and create tremendous anxiety for the patients and families. Heart murmur, chest pain, syncope, and suspected rhythm problems constitute the top four reasons for new outpatient referral to any pediatric cardiology practice. Many of these problems present to the general pediatrician during the teen years and the numbers of referrals reflect the concern and uncertainty that pediatricians have in diagnosing and managing these problems. There are also rare congenital heart problems that can have a lethal outcome and must be addressed in a timely manner. Sudden death in young athletes, even though rare, often receives sensational press coverage.

Reviewing our own statistics at the Children's Hospital of Michigan Cardiology Center for the past two years (2010–2012) reveals that outpatient visits for new patient consultations examined by age groups are as follows: less than 1 year of age, 11%; 1 to 5 years, 23%; 6 to 10 years, 21%; 11 to 18 years, 45%. Retrospective data collected from billing codes, as in this brief survey, may be imprecise. However, it does provide

Pediatr Clin N Am 61 (2014) xvii–xviii
http://dx.doi.org/10.1016/j.pcl.2013.09.022
0031-3955/14/$ – see front matter © 2014 Published by Elsevier Inc.

pediatric.theclinics.com

a snapshot of the usual referral problems encountered by pediatric cardiologists. In our practice, the most common overall reason for referral in all ages was "heart murmur," constituting 26% of total referrals. The second most common were rhythm and rhythm-related problems (inclusive of palpitations, abnormal ECG, and diagnosed premature beats), which constituted 19% of the total.

In the age group of interest for this issue of 11 to 18 years, the most common presenting issues, were rhythm-related (23%) and chest pain (23%), followed by syncope or dizziness (19%), and heart murmur (12%). Congenital heart disease diagnoses encountered in the 11- to 18-year age group comprised only 6.5% of referrals within that age group. It is likely that many of these were not new diagnoses (with a few exceptions), but rather represented transfers to our practice.

Our own outpatient clinical experience reveals that the majority of outpatients referred by pediatricians for pediatric cardiology evaluation are between the ages of 11 and 18. We decided to devote this text to defining the spectrum of cardiac issues and problems commonly encountered during adolescence by pediatricians and other primary caregivers. We have asked the authors to emphasize the role of the pediatrician/primary caregiver in diagnosing and managing these issues, as well as defining when appropriate referral is needed.

Pooja Gupta, MD
Pediatric Cardiology
Children's Hospital of Michigan
3901 Beaubien Boulevard
Pediatric Cardiology, 4th Floor
Carls Building
Detroit, MI 48201, USA

Richard Humes, MD
Pediatric Cardiology
Children's Hospital of Michigan
3901 Beaubien Boulevard
Pediatric Cardiology, 4th Floor
Carls Building
Detroit, MI 48201, USA

E-mail addresses:
pgupta2@dmc.org (P. Gupta)
rhumes@dmc.org (R. Humes)

Teenage Heart Murmurs

Ronak J. Naik, MD, DNB[a], Nishant C. Shah, MD[b],*

KEYWORDS

• Adolescents • Innocent murmur • Pathologic murmur

KEY POINTS

• A heart murmur may be innocent without any pathologic significance or may present as the first or only sign of valvular, congenital, or other structural heart diseases.
• Proper evaluation of murmurs along with history and physical examination should help physicians in deciding the need for further referral.
• Referral to a pediatric cardiologist is recommended when a murmur is suspected to be pathologic or when diagnostic uncertainty remains.
• This article discusses physiologic and clinical aspects of innocent and pathologic murmurs and outlines an approach to cardiac murmurs in adolescents.

INTRODUCTION

Heart murmurs constitute the most common cause of pediatric cardiology referrals.[1,2] Most of these murmurs are innocent; less than 1% of murmurs are a result of congenital heart defects in all pediatric age groups.[2,3] In children and adolescents, as age advances, the number of referrals identifying undiagnosed congenital heart disease decreases. However, the incidence of identifying acquired heart disease, such as mitral valve prolapse (MVP), increases.[4] In certain congenital lesions, such as bicuspid aortic valve, valvular dysfunction may progress as age advances.[5] In a large-scale study involving 17-year-old adolescents, the most prevalent cardiac diagnoses were congenital valvular heart disease; syncope, including neurocardiogenic; MVP; and nonvalvular congenital heart diseases.[6] Therefore, the first-time appearance of a murmur in an adolescent is always a concern. Moreover, finding a murmur creates a substantial amount of anxiety in both parents and teenagers. The appropriate evaluation and diagnosis of a murmur is very important in decision-making regarding sports participation in this population. A vital aspect of cardiovascular examination is an ability to identify different types of murmurs and relate them to other clinical

[a] Division of Cardiology, Department of Pediatrics, Le Bonheur Children's Hospital, University of Tennessee Health Science Center, 50 North Dunlap Avenue, Level 3, Memphis, TN 38103, USA; [b] Department of Pediatrics, Penn State Hershey Children's Hospital, Penn State University, 500 University Drive, Hershey, PA 17033, USA
* Corresponding author.
E-mail address: nshah@hmc.psu.edu

Pediatr Clin N Am 61 (2014) 1–16
http://dx.doi.org/10.1016/j.pcl.2013.09.014
0031-3955/14/$ – see front matter © 2014 Elsevier Inc. All rights reserved.

findings. Accurate identification of the innocent murmurs can obviate the need for echocardiography and provide an opportunity to educate and reassure patients and their family. More importantly, identification of a pathologic murmur allows appropriate management in timely fashion and reduces morbidity and, possibly, mortality in critical lesions such as hypertrophic cardiomyopathy (HCM). This article discusses the physiology and characteristics of murmurs, and outlines an approach to cardiac murmurs in adolescents.

WHAT IS A MURMUR?

An organized movement of molecules in a medium caused by a vibrating body is defined as a sound.[7] Murmurs are the sounds produced by the vibrations caused by turbulence of the blood flow in the heart.[8] The most comprehensive mechanism of murmur origin is the direct impact of the jet-producing vibration. Several other mechanisms have been proposed[9] as producing vessel vibrations, such as vibrations from Bernoulli effect, eddy currents, and bubbles of vapor. The amount of turbulence-causing vibrations and, hence, the intensity of the murmur depends on blood volume and pressure differences (which determine blood flow velocity) across the site, in addition to the size of the orifice.

CARDIAC CYCLE

The classification of heart murmurs is based on their timing. Therefore, knowledge of the timing of the events in the cardiac cycle is crucial for a better understanding of various murmurs. **Fig. 1** shows the phases of the cardiac cycle and its relationship with heart sounds. The relationship of pressure and blood volume between chambers and/or arteries determines characteristic heart sounds and murmurs. Systole is comprised of isovolumetric contraction, rapid ejection, and reduced ejection phases; whereas diastole includes isovolumetric relaxation, early filling (rapid filling), and reduced filling followed by atrial contraction.

Atrial Contraction

The atria contract during the terminal period of diastole. This atrial systole augments ventricular filling just before the onset of the next ventricular contraction.

Isovolumetric Contraction

As ventricular muscle contracts, ventricular pressure increases rapidly, accompanied by closure of the atrioventricular (AV) valves, producing the first heart sound (S1). Clinically, S1 denotes the beginning of systole. During this short period of isovolumic contraction, pressure builds within the ventricle without change in the ventricular volume.

Rapid Ejection Phase

The rapid ejection phase begins with the opening of semilunar valves. During this period, the ventricles eject blood into the aorta and pulmonary artery. Approximately two-thirds of the blood in the ventricles is ejected during the rapid ejection phase.

Reduced Ejection Phase

During the reduced ejection phase, a lesser volume is pumped out of the ventricles. As ventricular contraction ceases, pressure drops in the ventricles leading to closure of the semilunar valves producing the second heart sound (S2). Clinically, S2 denotes the end of systole.

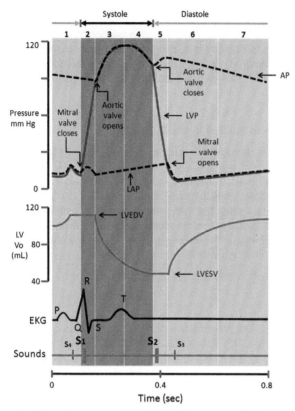

Fig. 1. Cardiac cycle. AP, aortic pressure; LAP, left atrial pressure; LVEDV, left ventricular end-diastolic volume; LVESV, left ventricular end-systolic volume; LVP, left ventricular pressure; S1, first heart sound; S2, second heart sound; S3, third heart sound; S4, fourth heart sound; 1, atrial contraction; 2, isovolumetric contraction; 3, rapid ejection phase; 4, reduced ejection phase; 5 isovolumetric relaxation; 6, rapid filling phase; 7, reduced filling phase.

Isovolumetric Relaxation

During isovolumetric relaxation, pressure decreases rapidly in the ventricles without a change in the volume. When the ventricular pressure drops below the atrial pressure, the AV valves open, ending the isovolumetric relaxation phase.

Rapid Filling Phase

The rapid inflow phase occurs immediately after the opening of the AV valves. The blood accumulated in the atria during systole rushes into the ventricles. Most ventricular filling occurs during this phase.

Reduced Filling Phase

During the reduced filling phase, venous blood returning from the body continues to flow through the atria into the ventricles at a slower rate.

CHARACTERISTICS OF MURMUR

Each murmur should be determined and described based on the characteristics listed later. It is crucial to identify these characteristics for proper diagnosis of murmurs.

Timing and Duration

Murmurs are classified based on their timing in relation to cardiac cycle (ie, systole or diastole). Duration is the length of a murmur from beginning to end. Compared with infants and young children, timings and duration can be defined more precisely in adolescents due to their slower heart rate and better cooperation.

Intensity

Intensity is graded with the Levine grading system[10]:

Grade I: very faint, heard with intense concentration, may not be heard in all positions

Grade II: faint, but heard immediately and in all positions

Grade III: intermediate intensity, easily heard

Grade IV: loud, with a palpable thrill (murmurs with a thrill are always abnormal)

Grade V: very loud, heard with stethoscope partly off the chest, with a palpable thrill

Grade VI: loudest, heard with stethoscope just above the precordium completely off the chest, with a palpable thrill.

Of note, murmurs of grades IV to VI have a palpable thrill.

Location

In classic auscultation, the precordium is divided into four areas[11]: (1) mitral, located at the cardiac apex in the fifth intercostal space (ICS) along the midclavicular line; (2) tricuspid, located in the left fourth or fifth ICS along the left sternal border; (3) pulmonary, located in the left second ICS near the left sternal border; and (4) aortic, located in the right second ICS along the right sternal border. In addition to these areas, auscultation of the precordium in between these areas is very important to avoid missing pathologic murmurs. For example, the murmur of a small, muscular ventricular septal defect may be heard best in between pulmonary and tricuspid areas. Similarly, the murmur of a coronary fistulae is heard best at the lower right sternal border. In dextrocardia, heart sounds and murmurs are better heard over the right precordium. After auscultating the entire precordium, an area with the highest intensity of murmur should be identified carefully to localize the origin of a murmur. Loud murmurs may be heard in multiple areas. However, the "location" of a murmur describes the area where it is the loudest.

Configuration

The descriptor "configuration" indicates a change in the murmur intensity during different phases of cardiac cycle. Various configurations of murmurs include

1. Crescendo: increasing intensity from beginning to end
2. Decrescendo: decreasing intensity from beginning to end
3. Crescendo-decrescendo: increasing and then decreasing intensity
4. Decrescendo-crescendo: decreasing and then increasing intensity
5. Plateau: constant intensity.

Quality

The tonal qualities of murmurs often have somewhat subjective descriptions, which may be characterized as harsh, blowing, or musical. In general, a blowing quality is thought to be specific for regurgitant murmurs.

Pitch

The pitch can be low, medium, or high. Pitch often reflects the pressure gradient across the site of murmur origin, with higher pitches usually corresponding to higher gradients.

Quality and pitch are often combined when describing murmurs.

Radiation

Murmurs usually radiate in the direction of the blood flow. Additional areas should be auscultated for complete evaluation of murmurs. The typical areas for describing radiation are the back or the neck. For example, in mitral regurgitation, the murmur radiates to axilla; murmurs from the pulmonary valve or arteries radiate to the back; and murmurs from aortic valve and left ventricle radiate to the neck.

MURMUR CLASSIFICATION

Murmurs are classified into two major categories based on their timing: systolic and diastolic. **Fig. 2** is a schematic presentation of various murmurs. Murmurs may be pathologic or innocent based on their cause. Common pathologic murmurs produced by various congenital and acquired heart diseases presenting in teenage are summarized in **Box 1**. See later discussion on innocent murmurs.

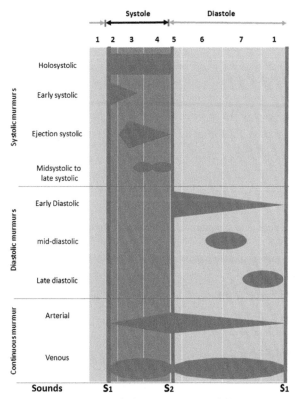

Fig. 2. Murmurs based on timing and duration. 1, atrial contraction; 2, isovolumetric contraction; 3, rapid ejection phase; 4, reduced ejection phase; 5 isovolumetric relaxation; 6, rapid filling phase; 7, reduced filling phase.

Box 1
Pathologic murmurs in adolescents

SYSTOLIC MURMURS

Holosystolic (pansystolic)

- Mitral regurgitation (MR)
  - Congenital: cleft mitral valve, postsurgical (after AV canal defect repair)
  - Acquired: rheumatic carditis, Infective endocarditis, Kawasaki disease
  - Functional: left ventricular dysfunction, annular dilatation
- Tricuspid regurgitation (TR)
  - Congenital: Ebstein anomaly, congenitally corrected transposition of great arteries
  - Acquired: infective endocarditis, trauma
  - Functional: Eisenmenger syndrome, pulmonary hypertension, annular dilatation
- Left-to-right shunt from ventricular septal defect (VSD)

Early systolic

- Most likely from small muscular VSD in adolescents

Ejection systolic (midsystolic)

- Aortic
  - Obstructive
    - Congenital-bicuspid aortic valve, congenitally dysplastic aortic valve, supravalvular aortic stenosis, coarctation of the aorta
    - Acquired-discrete, tunnel-type subaortic membrane, hypertrophic cardiomyopathy, rheumatic heart disease
  - Increased flow
    - Severe aortic regurgitation (AR)
    - Large patent ductus arteriosus (PDA), systemic arteriovenous malformation
    - Complete heart block
    - Hyperkinetic state
- Pulmonary
  - Obstructive
    - Congenital-pulmonic valve stenosis, pulmonary artery stenosis, branch stenosis, double chamber right ventricle in presence of membranous VSD
    - Functional-compression in pectus excavatum, kyphoscoliosis
  - Increased flow
    - Atrial septal defect (ASD)
    - Anomalous pulmonary venous return
    - Severe pulmonary regurgitation
    - Hyperkinetic state

Midsystolic to late systolic

- Mitral-MVP, HCM
- Tricuspid-tricuspid valve prolapse

(continued on next page)

Box 1 (*continued*)

DIASTOLIC MURMURS

Early diastolic

- AR—high-pitched due to higher difference between aortic and left ventricular diastolic pressures
  - Congenital: bicuspid valve, after valvuloplasty, after Ross procedure, aortic cusp prolapse in presence of membranous VSD and subaortic membrane
  - Acquired: rheumatic, infective endocarditis
  - Functional: dilation of annulus—Marfan syndrome, connective tissue disease
- Pulmonic regurgitation—medium to low pitch due to lower difference between pulmonary artery and right ventricular diastolic pressure
  - Congenital; after valvulotomy, after valvuloplasty, after transannular patch in tetralogy of Fallot
  - Acquired: endocarditis, rheumatic heart disease, carcinoid
  - Functional: dilatation of annulus—Marfan syndrome, connective tissue disease

Mid-diastolic

- Mitral
  - Mitral stenosis
    - Congenital: dysplastic mitral valve, parachute mitral valve
    - Acquired: rheumatic heart disease
    - Functional: left atrial myxoma
  - Carey Coombs murmur (mid-diastolic apical murmur in acute rheumatic fever)
  - Increased flow across nonstenotic mitral valve (eg, MR, VSD, PDA, high-output states, complete heart block)
  - Severe or eccentric AR (Austin Flint murmur)
- Tricuspid
  - Tricuspid stenosis—congenital after repair
  - Increased flow across nonstenotic tricuspid valve (eg, TR, ASD, and anomalous pulmonary venous return)
  - Right atrial myxoma

Late diastolic

- Presystolic accentuation of true mitral stenosis murmur

CONTINUOUS MURMURS

- Arterial:
  - Aortopulmonary shunts such as PDA, surgical shunts, aortopulmonary window
  - Arteriovenous fistula, coronary fistula
  - Ruptured sinus of Valsalva aneurysm
  - Turbulent flow in arteries
    - Anomalous left coronary artery
    - Proximal coronary artery stenosis
    - Coarctation of aorta

(*continued on next page*)

Box 1 (*continued*)

- ■ Severe branch pulmonary artery stenosis
- ■ Bronchial collateral circulation
- • Venous:
  - ○ Turbulent flow in veins—obstructed total anomalous pulmonary venous return

Adapted from Fang JC, O.Gara PT. The history and physical examination: an evidence-based approach. In: Braunwald E, Bonow RO, editors. Braunwald's heart disease: a textbook of cardiovascular medicine. 9th edition. Philadelphia: Saunders; 2012; with permission.

Systolic Murmurs

- • Early systolic murmurs coincide with S1 and start during the isovolumetric contraction phase. They extend up to midsystole or late systole and terminate before the end of the ejection period. In the adolescent age group, these likely arise from small muscular ventricular septal defects.
- • Ejection systolic (midsystolic) murmurs start immediately after opening of semilunar valves. Remember that these murmurs start after a brief murmur-free period of isovolumetric contraction and do not coincide with S1. The intensity of these murmurs increase during the rapid ejection phase and decrease during the reduced ejection phase giving a crescendo-decrescendo, or diamond-shaped characteristic. Most of the innocent murmurs fall in this category. Ventricular outflow tract obstructions also produce this type of murmur.
- • Midsystolic to late systolic murmurs start later in systole and are often preceded by a midsystolic click from mitral or tricuspid valve prolapse.
- • Holosystolic (pansystolic) murmurs start with S1 and extend throughout systole with more or less same intensity. These murmurs continue through S2 resulting into muffled S2 on examination. Holosystolic murmurs, presenting for the first time during adolescence, are frequently due to mitral or tricuspid valve regurgitation.

Diastolic Murmurs

- • Early diastolic murmurs begin immediately after S2 (in the period of isovolumetric relaxation), end variably during diastole, and are of decreasing intensity. Aortic valve regurgitation is typical for this timing.
- • Mid-diastolic murmurs start when the AV valves open. These murmurs coincide with the rapid filling phase of diastole. Usually they are low-pitched, rumbling noises and heard best with the bell of the stethoscope. Remember that these murmurs start after a brief murmur-free period of isovolumetric relaxation and do not coincide with S2. These murmurs, though rare in teens, are often due to AV valve stenosis. If first heard in adolescence, they may reflect acquired heart disease such as seen after rheumatic carditis.
- • Late diastolic murmurs occur during the period of atrial contraction in diastole. The potential origins are similar to mid-diastolic murmurs.

Continuous Murmurs

- • Continuous murmurs begin in systole and extend into diastole. They can be arterial or venous in origin, although in the teenage group they are more likely arterial. Some innocent murmurs may also be continuous (see later discussion).

RESPONSE TO THE MANEUVERS

Various maneuvers can change the intensity of specific murmurs in a predictable way. This predictable change can be used to the physician's advantage in confirming the origin of the murmur. Once a murmur is identified, relevant maneuvers should be routinely performed in the clinical practice to differentiate various murmurs.

Respiration

Murmurs arising from right-sided cardiac structures get louder during inspiration, whereas the intensity of left-sided murmurs increase during expiration.

Valsalva Maneuver

A Valsalva maneuver increases the intrathoracic pressure resulting in decreased pre-load. Thus, most murmurs will decrease in length and/or intensity with two exceptions. In HCM, Valsalva maneuver leads to reduction in ventricular end-diastolic volume and stroke volume. This causes a worsening of the left ventricular outflow tract narrowing and obstruction, resulting in a louder murmur. The second exception is MVP, in which reduction in preload leads to early prolapse of mitral valve leaflets. With early prolapse, the systolic click moves earlier in systole and the murmur of mitral valve insufficiency becomes longer and often louder.

Exercise

Isotonic and isometric (handgrip) exercises increase stroke volume and, therefore, increase the intensity of most murmurs.

Positional Changes

1. Supine to standing or supine to sitting. Sitting to standing position change reduces the preload due to the effect of gravity. It has a similar effect when compared with the Valsalva maneuver. Most murmurs will diminish in their intensity except the murmurs of HCM and MVP. A venous hum murmur, although rare in this age group, is more prominent in upright position and disappears in supine position.
2. Standing to squatting. Brisk squatting increases venous return to the heart. This re-sults in an increase in preload, ventricular end-diastolic volume, and stroke volume. Furthermore, compression of distal arteries and arterioles by muscle contraction increases the afterload. Together, these increase the intensity of regurgitant mur-murs. However, in HCM[12] and MVP, murmurs usually become softer and may disappear. This produces the exact opposite effect when compared with Valsalva maneuver. Passive leg raises usually have an effect similar to brisk squatting.
3. Lateral decubitus position. With this maneuver, the apex of the heart gets closure to the chest wall. Pathologic murmurs of the mitral valve become louder with this maneuver.
4. Sitting forward and exhaling completely. This decreases the heart rate and increases the stroke volume. Aortic valve murmurs are accentuated with this maneuver.

Premature Ventricular Contraction

Stroke volume increases during the subsequent beat after a premature ventricular contraction. Murmurs from aortic or pulmonary stenosis increase in intensity, whereas systolic murmurs of AV valve insufficiency generally do not change (except the murmur of MVP, which becomes shorter).

Table 1
Innocent murmurs

Name	Description	Mechanism	Change With Maneuvers	Mimics

Still murmur (infancy to adolescence, most common 2–6 y)	• Vibratory, musical
	• Grade I to III
	• Midsystolic
	• Low to medium pitch
	• Diamond shape
	• Located at left lower sternal border
	• Radiating to apex
		• Exaggerated vibrations from ventricular contractions[22]
		• Left ventricular false tendon[23]
		• Physiologic narrowing of the left ventricular outflow tract[24] and ↑ aortic velocity[25]
			• Louder in supine position, hyperdynamic cardiac states
			• Becomes softer on standing and on inspiration
				• Ventricular septal defect
				  ○ Harsh
				  ○ Holosystolic

Pulmonary flow murmurs (all ages, particularly 8–14 y)	• Harsh quality
	• Grade II–III
	• Ejection systolic
	• Low-medium pitch
	• Diamond shaped
	• Located between left 2nd and 3rd ICS near sternal border
	• Radiates to back
		• Turbulence in blood flow through pulmonary outflow	• Loudest with inspiration and
			• In supine position
			• Decreases on standing
			• Exaggerated by pectus excavatum, kyphoscoliosis
				• Atrial septal defect
				  ○ Wide fix split S2
				• Pulmonary stenosis
				  ○ With click
				  ○ Harsh
				  ○ Mid–high pitch

Supraclavicular or brachiocephalic systolic murmur (children and young adults)	• Harsh, brief
	• First 2/3 of systole
	• Low-medium pitched
	• Crescendo-decrescendo
	• Best heart above clavicle
	• Radiates to neck
		• Turbulence from blood flow from aorta to brachiocephalic and head-neck vessels[26]	• Loudest in supine position; decreases on hyperextension of neck[27]	• Bicuspid aortic valve/aortic stenosis
				  ○ Click present
				  ○ Harsh
				  ○ Best in aortic area
				  ○ >Grade III

Murmur	Characteristics	Mechanism	Conditions/Maneuvers	Differential
Aortic systolic murmur (most common in adolescent age)	• Systolic ejection murmur • Harsh located in aortic area	• Increased cardiac output	• Audible in hyperdynamic conditions	• Mild aortic stenosis ○ Audible regardless hyperdynamic conditions ○ Click may be present
Venous hum (3–8 y)	• Continuous murmur accentuated in diastole • Roaring or whining quality • Best heard at lower neck, lateral to sternocleidomastoid • Louder on right side • Radiates to upper chest and neck	• Turbulence of the flow at the confluence of jugular vein with subclavian vein as it enters the superior vena cava[28]	• Loudest in sitting position patient looking away from examiner • Turning neck toward murmur or compression of jugular veins with thumbs diminishes it • Disappears in supine position	• Patent ductus arteriosus ○ No change with position ○ Harsh ○ Left ventricular heave may be present
Mammary arterial souffle (In late pregnancy or lactating female; rarely in adolescence)	• Systolic murmur that extends in to diastole • High-pitched • Located at the anterior chest near breasts	• Turbulence from the enlarged blood vessels of the chest, arterial in origin[29]	• Varies day to day • Firm pressure with stethoscope abolishes it	• Patent ductus arteriosus ○ No change with position ○ Harsh ○ Left ventricular heave may be present • Arteriovenous malformation ○ Continuous ○ Ventricular enlargement

INNOCENT MURMURS

Innocent murmurs are produced by the blood flow in a structurally normal heart. They are also referred to as physiologic, benign, innocuous, or functional murmurs. Murmurs with a thrill, diastolic murmurs, or the presence of abnormal findings such as click usually suggest a pathologic murmur.[13–15] Common innocent murmurs found in teenagers are described in **Table 1**. Innocent murmurs typically have following characteristics:

- Usually occur in systole (ejection systolic) or continuous; never diastolic
- Soft, grade III or less; never associated with thrill
- Pitch is low to medium
- Short duration and vary with respiration and body position
- No associated gallops or clicks
- Present in otherwise asymptomatic patients.

Key message

- Innocent murmur occurs in a structurally normal heart
- Primary health care providers should be familiar with the common types of innocent murmur and the characteristics of innocent murmur
- Reassurance and patient education in terms of no activity restriction and no endocarditis prophylaxis is crucial.

APPROACH TO A TEENAGER WITH A MURMUR

For evaluation of murmurs in this age group, the physician must obtain a detailed history focusing on symptoms of cardiac origin, a family history of life-threatening cardiac conditions, vital signs, an assessment of peripheral pulses, and a systematic precordial auscultatory examination. Clinicians should make every effort to differentiate between innocent and pathologic murmurs. **Fig. 3** shows an approach to cardiac murmurs. Typical features of the innocent murmurs described in this article combined with this simplified approach should help a clinician decide the need for pediatric cardiology referral.

"NEW" CONGENITAL HEART DISEASE IN TEENAGE YEARS

Most congenital heart defects are diagnosed in first few years of life, long before the teenage years.[16] Those defects that are missed generally due to their asymptomatic nature and subtle physical and auscultatory findings may get diagnosed in teenage years. Two particular defects that are the most frequently encountered and most frequently missed deserve specific discussion. These include bicuspid aortic valve and atrial septal defect.

Congenital bicuspid aortic valve is considered the most common congenital heart malformation.[17] It constitutes a substantial proportion of aortic valve disease seen in adulthood.[18] Many bicuspid aortic valves will function normally during the pediatric years and there may be no murmur or murmurs of grade I only. The characteristic finding to listen specifically for is an ejection click, best heard at the apex. The "click" may give the examiner the impression that the S1 has two components—an unusual finding in the apical location, which demands further evaluation with either cardiology consultation or echocardiography.

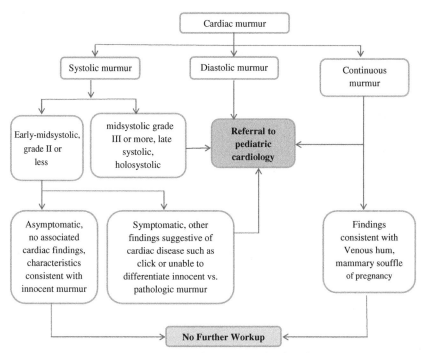

Fig. 3. Approach to evaluate a murmur. (*Adapted* and *Modified from* Bonow RO, Carabello BA, Chatterjee K, et al. 2008 Focused update incorporated into the ACC/AHA 2006 guidelines for the management of patients with valvular heart disease: a report of the American College of Cardiology/American Heart Association Task Force on Practice Guidelines (Writing Committee to Revise the 1998 Guidelines for the Management of Patients With Valvular Heart Disease): endorsed by the Society of Cardiovascular Anesthesiologists, Society for Cardiovascular Angiography and Interventions, and Society of Thoracic Surgeons. Circulation 2008;118(15):e523–661; with permission.)

Atrial septal defects constitute about 8% to 10% of all congenital heart defects[17] and these are considered the most common congenital defects escaping detection until adulthood.[19] Atrial septal defects are the second-most common prevalent congenital lesion in adulthood after bicuspid aortic valve.[20] The characteristic murmur is a soft, systolic ejection murmur over the pulmonic area combined with wide, fixed splitting of S2. Careful and specific attention by the primary caregiver for these findings, particularly the wide and fixed split S2, may lead to greater detection of this defect.

Key message
• New diagnosis of congenital heart defect during adolescence is infrequent
• Two specific defects likely missed until this age are atrial septal defect and bicuspid aortic valve
• Abnormal auscultatory findings of wide and fixed splitting of second heart sound or an ejection systolic click may be the clue to their diagnosis
• It is important for primary providers to differentiate between innocent and pathologic murmurs and refer the patient for cardiology consultation or echocardiogram.

RECOMMENDATIONS FOR PERFORMING ECHOCARDIOGRAPHY IN PATIENTS WITH HEART MURMURS

The following are the recommendations for performing echocardiography in patients with heart murmurs (level of evidence: C).[21]

Class I

1. Echocardiography is recommended for
   a. Asymptomatic patients with diastolic murmurs, continuous murmurs, holosystolic murmurs, late systolic murmurs, murmurs associated with ejection clicks, or murmurs that radiate to the neck or back
   b. Patients with heart murmurs and symptoms or signs of heart failure, myocardial ischemia or infarction, syncope, thromboembolism, infective endocarditis, or other clinical evidence of structural heart disease
   c. Asymptomatic patients who have grade III or louder mid-peaking systolic murmurs (Innocent murmurs can be up to grade III; however, it may be difficult to differentiate grade III innocent murmurs from pathologic murmurs based on clinical examination only).

Class IIa

1. Echocardiography can be useful for
   a. Asymptomatic patients with murmurs associated with other abnormal cardiac physical findings or murmurs associated with an abnormal ECG or chest radiograph
   b. Patients whose symptoms and/or signs are likely noncardiac in origin but in whom a cardiac basis cannot be excluded by standard evaluation.

Class III

1. Echocardiography is not recommended for patients who have a grade II or softer mid-systolic murmur identified as innocent or functional by an experienced observer.

SUMMARY

A murmur is characterized by its intensity (grade), timing, configuration, and location. The most common causes of ejection-systolic murmurs are benign (innocent) murmurs. These physiologic murmurs need to be distinguished from the abnormal mid-systolic murmurs in patients with fixed or dynamic outflow tract obstruction. Innocent murmurs are always considered in the context of a normal history and physical examination. Once an innocent murmur is diagnosed, proper explanation is important to alleviate teenagers' and parental anxiety. Documents written in simple language about innocent murmurs can be used for better education. Nevertheless, pediatric cardiology referral is indicated when murmur seems to be pathologic in origin or when uncertainty exists.

REFERENCES

1. McCrindle BW, Shaffer KM, Kan JS, et al. Factors prompting referral for cardiology evaluation of heart murmurs in children. Arch Pediatr Adolesc Med 1995; 149(11):1277–9.
2. Biancaniello T. Innocent murmurs. Circulation 2005;111(3):e20–2.
3. Hurrell DG, Bachman JW, Feldt RH. How to evaluate murmurs in children. Postgrad Med 1989;86(2):239–41, 243.

4. Newburger JW, Alexander ME, Fulton DR. Chapter 22- Innocent heart murmurs, syncope and chest pain. Exhibit 22-1. Nadas' pediatric cardiology. 2nd edition. Philadelphia: Saunders; 2006. p. 358.
5. Ward C. Clinical significance of the bicuspid aortic valve. Heart 2000;83(1):81–5.
6. Bar-Dayan Y, Elishkevits K, Goldstein L, et al. The prevalence of common cardiovascular diseases among 17-year-old Israeli conscripts. Cardiology 2005;104(1): 6–9.
7. Stevens SS, Warshofsky F. Time-life books. Sound and hearing. Revised edition. Alexandria (VA); Morristown (NJ): Time-Life Books; School and Library Distribution by Silver Burdett Co; 1980.
8. Smythe JF, Teixeira OH, Vlad P, et al. Initial evaluation of heart murmurs: are laboratory tests necessary? Pediatrics 1990;86(4):497–500.
9. Nichols WW, O'Rourke MF, McDonald DA. McDonald's blood flow in arteries: theoretic, experimental and clinical principles. 3rd edition. Philadelphia: Lea & Febiger; 1990.
10. Silverman ME, Wooley CF, Samuel A. Levine and the history of grading systolic murmurs. Am J Cardiol 2008;102(8):1107–10.
11. Bickley LS, Szilagyi PG, Bates B. Bates' guide to physical examination and history taking. 9th edition. Philadelphia: Lippincott Williams & Wilkins; 2007.
12. Nellen M, Gotsman MS, Vogelpoel L, et al. Effects of prompt squatting on the systolic murmur in idiopathic hypertrophic obstructive cardiomyopathy. Br Med J 1967;3(5558):140–3.
13. Mackie AS, Jutras LC, Dancea AB, et al. Can cardiologists distinguish innocent from pathologic murmurs in neonates? J Pediatr 2009;154(1):50–4.e51.
14. McCrindle BW, Shaffer KM, Kan JS, et al. Cardinal clinical signs in the differentiation of heart murmurs in children. Arch Pediatr Adolesc Med 1996;150(2):169–74.
15. Nadas AS. Approach to diagnosis of congenital heart disease without recourse to special tests. Circulation 1959;20:602–5.
16. Hoffman JI. Incidence of congenital heart disease: I. Postnatal incidence. Pediatr Cardiol 1995;16(3):103–13.
17. Hoffman JI, Kaplan S. The incidence of congenital heart disease. J Am Coll Cardiol 2002;39(12):1890–900.
18. Roberts WC, Ko JM. Frequency by decades of unicuspid, bicuspid, and tricuspid aortic valves in adults having isolated aortic valve replacement for aortic stenosis, with or without associated aortic regurgitation. Circulation 2005;111(7):920–5.
19. deLeon AC Jr. Atrial septal defect in the adult. Curr Probl Cardiol 1976;1(9):2–60.
20. Zaidi AN, Daniels CJ. Chapter 68-Adolescents and adults with congenital heart disease. Moss and Adams' heart disease in infants, children, and adolescents: including the fetus and young adult. 8th edition. Philadelphia: Wolters Kluwer Health/Lippincott Williams & Wilkins; 2013. p. 1472.
21. Bonow RO, Carabello BA, Chatterjee K, et al. 2008 Focused update incorporated into the ACC/AHA 2006 guidelines for the management of patients with valvular heart disease: a report of the American College of Cardiology/American Heart Association Task Force on Practice Guidelines (Writing Committee to Revise the 1998 Guidelines for the Management of Patients With Valvular Heart Disease): endorsed by the Society of Cardiovascular Anesthesiologists, Society for Cardiovascular Angiography and Interventions, and Society of Thoracic Surgeons. Circulation 2008;118(15):e523–661.
22. Harris TN, Friedman S, Tuncali MT, et al. Comparison of innocent cardiac murmurs of childhood with cardiac murmurs in high output states. Pediatrics 1964; 33:341–56.

23. Perry LW, Ruckman RN, Shapiro SR, et al. Left ventricular false tendons in children: prevalence as detected by 2-dimensional echocardiography and clinical significance. Am J Cardiol 1983;52(10):1264–6.
24. Stein PD, Sabbah HN. Aortic origin of innocent murmurs. Am J Cardiol 1977; 39(5):665–71.
25. Schwartz ML, Goldberg SJ, Wilson N, et al. Relation of Still's murmur, small aortic diameter and high aortic velocity. Am J Cardiol 1986;57(15):1344–8.
26. Kawabori I, Stevenson JG, Dooley TK, et al. The significance of carotid bruits in children: transmitted murmur or vascular origin, studies by pulsed Doppler ultrasound. Am Heart J 1979;98(2):160–7.
27. Nelson WP, Hall RJ. The innocent supraclavicular arterial bruit–utility of shoulder maneuvers in its recognition. N Engl J Med 1968;278(14):778.
28. Cutforth R, Wiseman J, Sutherland RD. The genesis of the cervical venous hum. Am Heart J 1970;80(4):488–92.
29. Tabatznik B, Randall TW, Hersch C. The mammary souffle of pregnancy and lactation. Circulation 1960;22:1069–73.

A Teen with Chest Pain

Jennifer M. Blake, MD

KEYWORDS

- Chest pain • Cardiac • Noncardiac • Teen • Adolescent

KEY POINTS

- Chest pain in teens is most commonly noncardiac and musculoskeletal in nature.
- Chest pain from a cardiac cause is rare in teenagers.
- A thorough history and physical examination are typically the only evaluation required for assessment of chest pain.
- Patients with a history of repaired congenital heart disease, Kawasaki disease with coronary artery aneurysms, certain connective tissue disorders, symptoms of exertional chest pain, or association with syncope should be referred to a pediatric cardiologist for further evaluation.

INTRODUCTION: NATURE OF CHEST PAIN

Chest pain is a commonly encountered symptom in the outpatient setting as well as the emergency room. The onset of chest pain in adults usually necessitates prompt cardiac evaluation because coronary vascular disease, while potentially life-threatening, can be managed and treated successfully if detected in a timely fashion. When this symptom is seen in the teenage population, teenagers and their parents are typically concerned about cardiac causes for the pain. Fortunately, chest pain in the teenage population is most commonly benign.[1–8] Media coverage of rare and unfortunate events of sudden cardiac death only contributes to teen and parental anxiety about chest pain complaints. Chest pain has been associated with higher health care utilization in children with noncardiac chest pain particularly if the parent or child has increased psychological stress.[9] These factors all add to the challenge for the medical professional who is evaluating the teenage patient with chest pain.

Chest pain has previously been reported to account for 0.29% of patient chief complaints to the emergency room in a prospective trial by Driscoll and colleagues.[1] In more recent studies, chest pain accounted for 5.2% of all cardiology consultations[10]

Disclosures: The author has no conflict of interst to disclose.
Division of Pediatric Cardiology, Children's Hospital of Michigan, Wayne State University, School of Medicine, 3901 Beaubien, Detroit, MI 48201-2119, USA
E-mail address: jblake2@dmc.org

and 15% of all outpatient visits at a large, tertiary center pediatric cardiology practice.[11] However, less than 5% of chest pain complaints are associated with a cardiac condition.[12,13] Although media attention to these episodes in the community gives the sense that these episodes occur on a more frequent basis, several studies have shown that the incidence of sudden cardiac death in teens is fortunately rare.[12–14] Most recently, Roberts and Stovitz[15] reported an incidence of sudden cardiac death in adolescents as 0.24 per 100,000 athlete-years over the last 19 years in Minnesota. Chest pain in teens is most commonly divided into noncardiac and cardiac causes.

Key message

- Chest pain is a common complaint seen in primary care office, emergency room, and pediatric cardiology practice
- Chest pain in adolescents is most commonly benign
- Chest pain in this age group is perceived as cardiac by parents and patients and associated with tremendous anxiety
- Less than 5% of the chest pain is cardiac in origin

NONCARDIAC CHEST PAIN

Musculoskeletal chest pain is a very common type of noncardiac chest pain with reported prevalence anywhere from 15% to 31%.[12,13] Several types of musculoskeletal chest pain are seen in teenagers (**Box 1**).

COSTOCHONDRITIS OR COSTOSTERNAL SYNDROME

Costochondritis or costosternal syndrome typically presents as a sharp, stabbing pain along 2 or more contiguous costochondral joints. Deep breathing usually exacerbates the pain and this pain usually lasts just a few seconds to a few minutes. Signs of joint inflammation are absent, but palpation of the chest over the area reproduces the pain.

TIETZE SYNDROME

Tietze syndrome is most often seen in teens and adults. There is frequently a history of recent upper respiratory infection. Excessive coughing is thought to be a possible mechanism. There is localized inflammation of a single costochondral joint with the second and third ribs most often involved. Signs of inflammation, such as warmth, swelling, and tenderness, are found at the specific costochondral, costosternal, or sternoclavicular joint involved. Signs of inflammation are what helps differentiate this from costochondritis.

TRAUMA AND MUSCLE STRAIN

Trauma and muscle strain are particularly common in teenagers who are active in sports and are prone to chest wall trauma or muscle strain. Skeletal trauma in one series was the cause of chest pain in 2% of teenagers and children.[12] If trauma is the underlying cause, there may be inflammation or signs of injury at the site of pain. In cases where the history of trauma is significant, signs or symptoms of hemopericardium and myocardial contusion should be evaluated. Weight training or history of heavy lifting is often underreported unless specifically asked in cases where muscle strain is suspected to be the source of the chest pain.

Box 1
Common causes of chest pain in teenagers

- Noncardiac causes
  - Musculoskeletal
    - Costochondritis
    - Idiopathic
    - Tietze syndrome
    - Trauma and muscle strain
    - Slipping rib syndrome
    - Scoliosis
  - Chronic cough
  - Asthma
  - Pneumonia
  - Pneumothorax/pneumomediastinum
  - Pulmonary embolism
  - Gastroesophageal reflux disease
  - Gastritis
  - Esophagitis
  - Psychogenic
  - Breast disease, gynecomastia
  - Herpes zoster
  - Sickle cell disease (acute chest syndrome or vaso-occlusive crisis)
- Cardiac causes
  - Arrhythmia—supraventricular tachycardia, ventricular tachycardia
  - Pericarditis—infectious, noninfectious or autoimmune, postpericardiotomy syndrome
  - Left ventricular outflow tract obstruction—aortic stenosis, subaortic stenosis, supravalvar aortic stenosis
  - Anomalous origin of the coronary artery
  - Kawasaki disease
  - Coronary artery vasospasm
  - Hyperlipidemia or family history of early coronary artery disease
  - Cocaine use
  - Other—cardiac device or stent complications, aortic dissection, ruptured aortic aneurysm, pulmonary hypertension

---

IDIOPATHIC CHEST-WALL PAIN

Idiopathic chest pain typically is located over the midsternum or inframammary area and is sharp, lasting only a few seconds to minutes, and is exacerbated by deep inspiration. Palpation over the sternum or rib cage may elicit pain.

Slipping rib syndrome is seen infrequently and involves intense pain in the lower chest or upper abdominal area. The 8th, 9th, and 10th ribs are attached to each other and not directly to the sternum. Trauma or dislocation in this area can lead to this condition and can be diagnosed by a positive "hooking maneuver" whereby the examiner pulls on the inferior rib margin, which pulls the lower rib cage out.

PULMONARY

A pulmonary cause is also a common cause of chest pain. Asthma represents the most common pulmonary cause of chest pain. Seventy-three percent of children with chest pain were found to have evidence of asthma in a study by Weins and colleagues.[16] Infections of the bronchial tree or lungs, such as pneumonia, bronchitis, empyema, pleural effusion, or pleurisy, can cause acute chest pain. Pulmonary embolism can also be associated with chest pain and may be suspected in teens presenting with hypoxia and a predisposition to thrombosis.

GASTROINTESTINAL

Gastrointestinal causes can also account for a certain percentage of teenagers with chest pain. Evangelista and colleagues[17] reported a prevalence of gastrointestinal causes for chest pain as high as 8%. Gastroesophageal reflux disease, peptic ulcer disease, esophagitis, gastritis, and cholecystitis may present as chest pain. More rarely, ingestion of caustic substances, foreign body, or an esophageal stricture may present as chest pain.

PSYCHOGENIC

Psychogenic chest pain is typically caused by anxiety or a history of a recent stressful event. Often, psychogenic chest pain is associated with other somatic complaints such as abdominal pain or headache. Psychosocial factors have been attributed to the development and maintenance of chest pain as defined by Gilleland and colleagues.[18] Psychogenic chest pain has also been demonstrated in other somatic complaints such as abdominal pain and headache.[19–21]

MISCELLANEOUS

There are various other causes of chest pain that can be placed in this category. Chest pain from breast-related causes can be seen in postmenarche teen girls in association with mastitis, fibrocystic disease, or pregnancy. In teen boys, gynecomastia may occasionally cause unilateral or bilateral chest pain. Herpes zoster infection may initially present with pain or paresthesia in a dermatomal pattern, be extremely painful and uncomfortable, and precede the rash by several days. Scoliosis or other deformities can cause chest pain because of nerve compression or abnormal posture and positioning or stretching of the chest wall.

Key message

- Musculoskeletal chest pain is extremely common in this age group
- Associated symptoms may suggest a pulmonary, gastrointestinal cause for the chest pain
- Psychogenic chest pain is a diagnosis of exclusion and may be seen with other somatic symptoms such as headaches and abdominal pain

CARDIAC CHEST PAIN

Actual cardiac causes of chest pain are rare. However, there are several cardiac diagnoses for which chest pain can be one of several presenting symptoms.

Inflammatory

Pericarditis, whether present with or without a pericardial effusion, is typically infectious in origin. Pain can be associated with pericarditis, but there are often other symptoms present as well. Patients usually have fever and may have a friction rub on examination. The pain is typically retrosternal and can radiate to the left shoulder. The pain tends to be more constant and unrelenting than the noncardiac chest pain. It worsens with deep breathing and lying in the supine position. Sitting up and leaning forward tends to alleviate the pain.

Tachyarrhythmia

Supraventricular tachycardia, particularly in younger patients, may be reported as chest pain. However, there are other symptoms such as a feeling of the heart "pounding," nausea, dizziness, or fatigue. There should be no symptoms in between these episodes. In studies focusing on patients presenting to a pediatric cardiologist, Kadun and colleagues[22] found that supraventricular tachycardia or palpitations interpreted as chest pain was the most common presentation in young, school-aged children and some teenagers presenting for palpitations. The chest pain, however, was usually also associated with other symptoms such as nausea and/or vomiting along with the episodes. Isolated premature ventricular contractions and ventricular tachycardia have a rare association with chest pain. Ventricular tachycardia usually has symptoms of palpitations, exercise intolerance, and/or syncope. Patients with a history of cardiac disease and surgical repair such as d-transposition of the great arteries with a Mustard or Senning repair are at risk of intra-atrial reentry arrhythmias. Teenagers with single-ventricle physiology who have undergone Fontan palliation are also at risk for intra-atrial reentry arrhythmias, which may present with chest pain but more likely with palpitations.[8]

Left Ventricular Outflow Tract Obstruction

Left ventricular outflow tract obstruction (aortic valve, subaortic area, or supra-aortic area) and coarctation of the aorta may have complaints of chest pain, but will usually also have other symptoms, such as dizziness, fatigue, and/or syncope with exertion. Severe aortic obstruction increases the likelihood of chest pain. The physical examination will have a harsh, systolic ejection murmur, which radiates into the neck. The most common cause of sudden cardiac death in this age group is hypertrophic cardiomyopathy. However, chest pain is actually an unusual symptom.[8,22] Sudden death, likely from ventricular arrhythmia, is a frequent initial presentation in teenagers with hypertrophic cardiomyopathy. Syncope is more often the presenting complaint compared with chest pain, and a family history for unexplained sudden death should raise suspicion for this diagnosis. However, many cases are de novo so the family history may not always be helpful. A systolic murmur may be heard on examination over the left ventricular outflow tract, which should increase in intensity with standing or Valsalva maneuver.

Kawasaki Disease

Coronary artery stenosis is a well-known long-term complication for those who had a history of coronary artery aneurysms due to Kawasaki disease. After the inflammatory phase, the healing coronary aneurysms can lead to areas of stenosis. It is also known that, due to these areas of stenosis, there may be decreased reserve for myocardial perfusion. The aneurysms themselves can cause decreased flow and thrombosis, which affects myocardial perfusion even further. Chest pain in a teenager with a history of coronary artery complications from Kawasaki disease usually is exertional in nature and should prompt a thorough evaluation for myocardial ischemia. Known risk factors that contribute to the likelihood of developing coronary aneurysms, coronary stenosis, or obstruction include male gender and onset at an early age (<6 months) or at an older age (>5 years).[23]

Coronary Artery Anomalies

Congenital anomalies of the coronary arteries can also lead to an increased risk of myocardial ischemia, which may present with anginal chest pain. After hypertophic cardiomyopathy, they are the second most common reason for sudden cardiac death in teenagers. Chest pain is not the typical presenting symptom. Teenagers with these coronary anomalies may have sudden death as the first symptom. For those that do present with chest pain, it is most often associated with exertion. Chest pain related to ischemia is usually described by patients as a crushing tightness, pressure, burning, or fullness in the chest. These patients often are diaphoretic, nauseous, and/or dyspneic. They may also present with syncope. A typical example in this category is the left main coronary artery or left anterior descending coronary artery arising from the right sinus of Valsalva or from the right coronary artery. The left main coronary artery or left anterior descending coronary artery then typically courses between the aorta and pulmonary artery, which leads to compression of the coronary artery during exertion, resulting in myocardial ischemia and/or ventricular arrhythmia and sudden death in a teen.

Coronary vasospasm is known to be associated with atherosclerotic coronary artery disease in adults. There are case reports[24–26] of ischemia presumed to be secondary to coronary vasospasm in the literature in teenagers with no known risk factors. Cocaine abuse during adolescence can also present with chest pain due to coronary vasospasm and evidence of myocardial ischemia. Additional symptoms may include combativeness or confusion and the drug screen will be positive.

Teenagers with a family history significant for hyperlipidemia and early coronary artery disease are also at an increased risk for lipid abnormalities and myocardial ischemia.

Some teenagers with repaired congenital heart disease may experience chest pain. Patients at an increased risk for coronary complications are those who have undergone manipulation of their coronary arteries during their initial surgical repair as seen in the arterial switch operation for d-transposition of the great arteries and the Ross procedure. Both of these surgical procedures require reimplantation of the coronary arteries, which puts these patients at an increased risk for developing coronary artery ostial stenoses.

Connective Tissue Disorders

Although rare in this age group, teenagers with Marfan syndrome may present with sudden onset of severe chest pain along with back pain due to a dissecting aortic aneurysm. Teenage girls with Turner syndrome are also at risk of aortic root dissection, which is associated with sudden, intense chest pain. The other associated connective tissue disease with cardiac implications for chest pain is Ehlers-Danlos syndrome type IV. These patients may experience acute aortic dissection and may complain of chest pain that is mid sternal and radiates to the back. Pain associated with dissection is typically severe and may be described as a "tearing" quality. Patients with any one of these syndromes complaining of chest pain with these qualities should have a workup (cross-sectional imaging, CT or MRI) to rule out aortic dissection immediately because of the life-threatening implications.

Mitral Valve Prolapse

Chest pain associated with palpitations, dizziness, and panic attacks have been seen in patients with mitral valve prolapse. However, Bisset and colleagues[27] reported only 18% of patients with mitral valve prolapse in their study group presented with complaints of atypical chest pain. Mitral valve prolapse can also be seen in individuals with connective tissue disorders.

Key message

- Cardiac cause for chest pain in this age group is extremely rare but clinical implications can be serious
- A thorough history and physical examination can be helpful in ruling out a cardiac cause

---

PATIENT HISTORY

Even though cardiac causes of chest pain are rare, it is important to perform a thorough history and physical examination to rule out the possibility of underlying disease. A comprehensive history and physical examination are the most helpful elements in evaluation of chest pain (**Box 2**).

Within the patient history, a description of the pain in the patient's own words, severity of the pain, associated symptoms, aggravating, precipitating, and alleviating factors are important to describe. The acuteness or chronicity of the pain is also helpful. Acute pain can be associated with trauma, asthma, pulmonary embolism, and cardiac causes such as aortic dissection or ischemia due to coronary anomalies. Chronic, recurrent pain is most often likely due to noncardiac causes, such as pain from musculoskeletal, gastrointestinal, or psychogenic causes.

Pain location may also aid the practitioner in assessing the underlying cause. Pain that is localized is typically chest wall or pleuritic pain. Pain that is diffuse can be from underlying diseases of the lungs or heart. Whether and where the pain radiates may also be helpful to pinpoint a specific cause. An example would be pain that radiates to the neck, jaw, upper extremity, or shoulder is commonly associated with myocardial ischemia. Chest pain that radiates to the left shoulder can be seen in patients with pericarditis. Pain due to aortic dissection may radiate to the back or interscapular space.

Aggravating and/or precipitating factors are also very useful in aiding diagnosis. Pain exacerbated by deep breathing, change in body position, or with specific movements is typically musculoskeletal. Pain brought on by exertion or associated with dyspnea should prompt a search for a cardiac or respiratory cause. A recent history of respiratory illness and fever makes the diagnosis of an infectious cause leading to pericarditis or pneumonia likely. Patients with arrhythmia often complain of chest discomfort, but usually in association with palpitations. If complaints of vomiting or regurgitation are present with the chest pain and the pain worsens with eating or swallowing, the patient may have a gastrointestinal cause. Chest pain in association with various other symptoms like abdominal pain, headache, or limb pain makes a psychogenic cause most likely. Lightheadedness and paresthesias are often seen during panic attacks and/or hyperventilation episodes.

Box 2
History

- Chest pain description
  - Onset, duration, location, quality, severity, and radiation
  - Precipitating, aggravating, or alleviating factors
- Other elements of history
  - Associated symptoms
  - Trauma
  - Drug abuse
  - Presence of psychological stressors
  - Recent weight training or heavy lifting
- Past medical history
  - Cardiac disease, Kawasaki disease, hypercholesterolemia
  - Asthma, recent respiratory illness
  - Autoimmune disease
  - Sickle cell disease
  - Other chronic diseases
- Surgical history
  - Any previous chest or abdominal surgery
- Family history
  - Cardiomyopathy
  - Sudden cardiac death
  - Arrhythmia
  - Dyslipidemia
  - Premature coronary artery disease
- Genetic diseases
  - Marfan syndrome
  - Turner syndrome
  - Ehlers-Danlos syndrome, type IV

A history of asthma may suggest chest pain due to the underlying condition. Also, association of chest pain with difficulty in breathing, and cough temporally related to exercise, raises concern for exercise-induced asthma. A recent history of trauma, weight lifting, or a muscular trauma is the likely cause for the pain in teens involved in sports. Illicit drugs such as cocaine and other sympathomimetics are strong vaso-constrictors and can cause coronary vasospasm and vasoconstriction, which leads to pain from myocardial ischemia. It is crucial for health care providers to elicit a drug history and this might require a private interview with the adolescent.

It is also important to know about any history of cardiac diseases in the teen's past such as Kawasaki disease or d-transposition of the great arteries with an arterial switch operation. These patients could have coronary ostial stenosis leading to myocardial ischemia and pain. Patients who have undergone a recent cardiac catheterization and device placement for an atrial septal defect or stent placements may have pain if there is device embolization leading to impingement on other cardiac structures. Patients with coronary vasculopathy from cardiac transplantation, primary coronary anomalies, or coronary artery stenosis in association with familial hypercholesterolemia may have anginal chest pain. History of sickle cell disease or other chronic conditions may be important as patients may experience chest pain caused by complications of their underlying chronic disease. Sickle cell patients may experience chest pain during acute chest syndrome and patients with autoimmune disorders such as Crohn disease or systemic lupus erythematous may develop pericarditis with or without pericardial effusions and may complain of chest pain.

Familial genetic or connective tissue disorders are also important to elucidate because these can be associated with conditions that cause chest pain (Marfan, Turner, or Ehlers-Danlos syndrome type IV).

Key message

- The description of the pain, exact location, and associated activity is key to the diagnosis
- Recent initiation of weight training or heavy lifting is underreported by teenagers
- Chronic pain ongoing for several years suggests a benign nature
- Private interview with a teen may be warranted in cases of suspected drug abuse

---

PHYSICAL EXAMINATION

Vital signs and anthropometric measurements should be obtained during the comprehensive examination. Certain vital signs, anthropometric measurements, and/or clinical examination abnormalities may help direct the provider to further evaluations or testing (**Box 3**).

A teen with a very tall stature may need evaluation for Marfan syndrome. Tachypnea and fever may raise concern for a respiratory illness. Tachypnea and fever may also be associated with pericarditis (with or without effusion) if accompanied with tachycardia. In this situation, chest pain worsens with lying down and is relieved by sitting and leaning forward. Hypotension with evidence of jugular venous distention may indicate systolic or diastolic ventricular dysfunction, which would raise concerns for myocarditis or cardiomyopathy. Evidence of dysmorphism raises concern for a genetic disorder. The chest needs to be inspected thoroughly, looking for any chest wall or bony abnormalities, pectus excavatum or carinatum, scoliosis, or surgical scars. Thelarche in teen girls or gynecomastia in teen boys is not an uncommon source of chest pain.

On palpation of the chest, reproducible chest tenderness similar to the experienced pain is a very important and reassuring sign, effectively ruling out a primary cardiac cause. Rales or wheezing on chest auscultation might raise concerns for a pneumonic process or a hyperreactive bronchial airway (asthma, exercise-induced asthma).

A detailed cardiac examination is very important to look for potential cardiac causes of chest pain. Palpation of the chest is performed for thrills (obstructive lesions) or heaves (increased right ventricular impulse seen in pulmonary hypertension). Attention should also be paid to the examination of the heart sounds. Distant or muffled heart sounds are suspicious for a pericardial effusion. When the fluid accumulation in the pericardial cavity is in the mild to moderate range, a pericardial rub may be heard. Myocarditis often has evidence of a gallop rhythm and may have a mitral regurgitation murmur. Fixed left ventricular outflow tract obstruction from supravalvar, valvar, or subvalvar aortic stenosis and obstructive hypertrophic cardiomyopathy usually

---

Box 3
Physical examination

- Vital signs
  - Height, weight, body mass index, heart rate, blood pressure (lower extremity blood pressure with hypertension), respiratory rate
- General inspection
  - Dysmorphic features
- Chest inspection
  - Chest wall abnormalities (pectus excavatum or carinatum)
  - Scoliosis
  - Signs of trauma, healed surgical scars
  - Reproducible chest wall tenderness on palpation
- Cardiac
  - Hyperdynamic precordium
  - Distant heart sounds, abnormally loud second heart sound
  - Murmur (+/−), systolic click (+/−), gallop (+/−)
  - Upper extremity (right arm) hypertension (greater than 20 mm Hg difference between upper and lower limb blood pressure)
  - Decreased femoral pulse

---

presents with a harsh, mid-systolic ejection type of murmur. An ejection systolic click may be heard in aortic stenosis. Patients with mitral valve prolapse typically have a mid-systolic click and an apical mid to late systolic honking murmur. If a continuous murmur is heard, a coronary fistula may be present. Patients with coarctation of the aorta will have weak femoral pulses and upper limb hypertension (blood pressure ideally obtained from the right arm). In some coarctation patients, a continuous murmur over the back in the lower scapular margin may suggest the presence of extensive collateral arteries. Congestive heart failure should be suspected if hepatomegaly, ascites, and peripheral edema are present.

Key message

- Reproducible chest wall tenderness is the single most important examination finding in the evaluation of a teenager with chest pain, yet is commonly missed

---

IMAGING AND ADDITIONAL TESTING

Many teenagers who present with chest pain have a normal history and physical examination, and in that case, no further evaluation or testing is required. If there are any positive elements in their history or physical examination as described above, further testing should be performed accordingly. In patients with benign causes of chest pain, reassurance to the both the teenager and the parents that this pain is not cardiac and that the cardiac examination is normal is usually all that is required. Families should also be educated that these chest pain episodes may be recurrent but it does not imply heart disease. Several studies[5,7,8] have shown that additional or routine testing is not required. Follow-up in these patients[28] has shown that those who had previously been evaluated for chest pain do not present later with concerning pathologic abnormality.

Patients with chest pain related to other disease processes like asthma or gastroesophageal reflux disease should be referred to the appropriate specialists as deemed necessary. Most cases of teenage chest pain do not require cardiology referral and can be managed by the primary providers. However, in patients with chest pain that occurs with exertion, palpitations, exertional syncope, or in those with known cardiac disease, the chest pain episodes should be evaluated by a pediatric cardiologist.

Key message

- Most adolescents with chest pain do not require any additional testing
- Only those with chest pain associated with activity, syncope, palpitations, abnormal cardiac examination, or those with known cardiac disease require referral to cardiology

---

SUMMARY

Chest pain in the teenage population is seen frequently, but is typically benign. A thorough history and physical examination should provide enough information to confirm or rule out suspicions for cardiac disease. Time spent in counseling and reassurance of the teenager and parents in regards to the benign nature of their chest pain is most important. In those individuals who have symptoms with exertion, additional associated symptoms, or an abnormal cardiac examination require referral to a pediatric cardiologist.

REFERENCES

1. Driscoll DJ, Glicklich LB, Gallen WJ. Chest pain in children: a prospective study. Pediatrics 1976;57(5):648–51.
2. Danduran MJ, Earing MG, Sheridan DC, et al. Chest pain: characteristics of children/adolescents. Pediatr Cardiol 2008;29:775–81.
3. Friedman KG, Kane DA, Rathod RH, et al. Management of pediatric chest pain using a standardized assessment and management plan. Pediatrics 2011;128: 239–45.
4. Verghese GR, Friedman KG, Rathod RH, et al. Resource utilization reduction for evaluation of chest pain in pediatrics using a novel Standardized Clinical Assessment and Management Plan (SCAMP). J Am Heart Assoc 2012;1(2).
5. Sert A, Aypar E, Odabas D, et al. Clinical characteristics and causes of chest pain in 380 children referred to a paediatric cardiology unit. Cardiol Young 2013;23:361–7.
6. Selbst SM, Ruddy RM, Clark BJ, et al. Pediatric chest pain: a prospective study. Pediatrics 1988;82(3):319–23.
7. Thull-Freeman J. Evaluation of chest pain in the pediatric patient. Med Clin North Am 2010;94:327–47.
8. Reddy SR, Singh HR. Chest pain in children and adolescents. Pediatr Rev 2010; 31(1):e1–9.
9. Loiselle KA, Lee JL, Gilleland J, et al. Factors associated with healthcare utilization among children with noncardiac chest pain and innocent heart murmurs. J Pediatr Psychol 2012;37(7):817–25.
10. Geggel RL. Conditions leading to pediatric cardiology consultation in a tertiary academic hospital. Pediatrics 2004;114:409–17.

11. Friedman KG, Alexander ME. Chest pain and syncope in children: a practical approach to the diagnosis of cardiac disease. J Pediatr 2013;163(3):896–901.e3.
12. Berger S, Kugler JD, Thomas JA, et al. Sudden cardiac death in children and adolescents; introduction and overview. Pediatr Clin North Am 2004;51:1201–9.
13. Cava JR, Danduran MJ, Fedderly RT, et al. Exercise recommendations and risk factors for sudden cardiac death. Pediatr Clin North Am 2004;51:1401–20.
14. Maron BJ, Thompson PD, Ackerman MJ, et al. Recommendations and considerations related to preparticipation screening for cardiovascular abnormalities in competitive athletes: 2007 update a scientific statement from the american heart association council on nutrition, physical activity, and metabolism—endorsed by the American College of Cardiology Foundation. Circulation 2007;115(12): 1643–55.
15. Roberts WO, Stovitz SD. Incidence of sudden cardiac death in Minnesota high school athletes 1993-2012 screened with a standardized preparticipation evaluation. J Am Coll Cardiol 2013;62(14):1298–301.
16. Weins L, Sabath R, Ewing L, et al. Chest pain in otherwise healthy children and adolescents is frequently caused by exercise-induced asthma. Pediatrics 1992; 90(3):350–3.
17. Evangelista JA, Parsons M, Renneburg AK. Chest pain in children: diagnosis through history and physical examination. J Pediatr Health Care 2000;14:3–8.
18. Gilleland J, Blount RL, Campbell RM, et al. Brief Report: psychosocial factors and pediatric noncardiac chest pain. J Pediatr Psychol 2009;34:1170–4.
19. Laurell K, Larsson B, Eeg-Olofsson O. Headache in school children: association with pain, family history and psychosocial factor. Pain 2005;119:150–8.
20. Levy RL, Whitehead WE, Von Korff MR, et al. Intergenerational transmission of gastrointestinal illness behavior. Am J Gastroenterol 2000;95:451–6.
21. Craig TK, Cox AD, Klein K. Intergenerational transmission of somatization behaviour: a study of chronic somatizers and their children. Psychol Med 2002;32: 805–16.
22. Kadun GG, Shenker IR, Gootman N. Chest pain in adolescents. J Adolesc Health 1991;12(3):251–5.
23. Kato H, Sugimura T, Akagi T, et al. Long-term consequences of Kawasaki disease. A 10- to 21-year follow-up study of 594 patients. Circulation 1996;94: 1379–85.
24. Duvernoy CS, Bates ER, Fay WP, et al. Acute myocardial infarction in two adolescent males. Clin Cardiol 1998;21(9):687–90.
25. Perry RF, Garlisi AP, Hamrick CW, et al. Acute myocardial infarction in a 16-year-old boy with no predisposing risk factors. Pediatr Emerg Care 1997;13(6):413–6.
26. Kay ID, Flitter D, Wiggins J. Variant angina in an adolescent. Pediatr Cardiol 1994; 15(1):45–7.
27. Bisset GS 3rd, Schwartz DC, Meyer RA, et al. Clinical spectrum and long-term follow-up of isolated mitral valve prolapse in 119 children. Circulation 1980;62: 423–9.
28. Selbst SM, Ruddy RM, Clark BJ, et al. Chest pain in children: follow-up of patients previously reported. Clin Pediatr 1990;29(7):374–7.

A Teenage Fainter (Dizziness, Syncope, Postural Orthostatic Tachycardia Syndrome)

Thomas A. Pilcher, MD, MS, FHRS*, Elizabeth V. Saarel, MD, FHRS

KEYWORDS

- Syncope • Presyncope • Fainting • POTS • Vasovagal syncope
- Neurocardiogenic syncope • Dizziness

KEY POINTS

- Syncope (fainting) is a common complaint in the teenage population.
- Most fainting is benign; however, it is important for health care providers to differentiate benign fainting from life-threatening syncope.

SYNCOPE

Syncope is a sudden and brief loss of consciousness and postural tone secondary to hypoperfusion of the brain. Vasovagal syncope or neurocardiogenic syncope (fainting) results from a disturbance in the normal compensatory mechanisms of maintaining upright posture or from specific situations (**Box 1**) that cause hypotension and sometimes bradycardia. Syncope is common in teenagers, with some studies estimating that 15% experience at least 1 episode of syncope before adulthood. Other studies estimate a higher rate, with syncope in up to 47% of adolescent girls and 24% of adolescent boys.[1–3] For most patients who do faint, there is more than 1 episode (64% girls and 53% boys), but few seek medical attention.[1,4] Family history often reveals relatives with near fainting or fainting.[2] Most fainting is benign, but it is always important to distinguish simple fainting from more serious medical problems. A large prospective study of pediatric patients reported the causes and frequencies of pediatric syncope (**Box 2**).[5]

Details about primary neurologic causes are beyond the scope of this article but should be considered when evaluating a patient with syncope. This article focuses on distinguishing benign fainting from life-threatening syncope.

Funding Sources: None.
Conflict of Interest: None.
Division of Pediatric Cardiology, Primary Children's Medical Center, University of Utah, 100 North Mario Capecchi Drive, Salt Lake City, UT 84113, USA
* Corresponding author.
E-mail address: thomas.pilcher@imail.org

> **Box 1**
> **Common situations for syncope**
>
> Pain
>
> Fear
>
> Emotional distress
>
> Hair brushing
>
> Micturition
>
> Defecation
>
> Cyclical postural changes
>
> Prolonged stationary standing
>
> Immediately after rigorous exercise

VASOVAGAL SYNCOPE

In order to maneuver from a supine or sitting position and maintain upright posture, the body goes through a normal sequence of compensatory changes that overcome gravity-induced hydraulic changes on the blood volume. The following normal sequence takes place.

> **Box 2**
> **Relative frequency of syncope in 474 patients**
>
> | Cause | N (%) |
> | --- | --- |
> | Autonomic-mediated reflex syncope | 346 (73.0) |
> | Vasovagal syncope | 203 (42.8) |
> | Postural orthostatic tachycardia syndrome | 129 (27.2) |
> | Situational syncope | 8 (1.7) |
> | Orthostatic hypotension | 6 (1.3) |
> | Cardiac syncope | 14 (2.9) |
> | Congenital long QT syndrome | 4 (0.8) |
> | Sinus node dysfunction | 3 (0.7) |
> | Third-degree atrioventricular block | 2 (0.4) |
> | Supraventricular tachycardia | 1 (0.2) |
> | Hypertrophic cardiomyopathy | 1 (0.2) |
> | Dilated cardiomyopathy | 1 (0.2) |
> | Primary pulmonary hypertension | 2 (0.4) |
> | Neurologic syncope | 10 (2.1) |
> | Seizures attack | 9 (1.9) |
> | Migraine | 1 (0.2) |
> | Psychiatric syncope | 11 (2.3) |
> | Conversion reaction | 7 (1.4) |
> | Depressive disorder | 3 (0.7) |
> | School phobia | 1 (0.2) |
> | Metabolic syncope | 4 (0.8) |
> | Hypoglycemia | 2 (0.4) |
> | Severe anemia | 1 (0.2) |
> | Hyperventilation syndrome | 1 (0.2) |
> | Syncope of unknown origin | 89 (18.9) |
>
> *From* Zhang Q, Du J, Wang C, et al. The diagnostic protocol in children and adolescents with syncope: a multi-centre prospective study. Acta Paediatr 2009;98:882; with permission.

- Initial increase in heart rate: 10 to 15 beats per minute (bpm)
- Activation of renin-angiotensin-aldosterone system and vasopressin
- Baroreceptor-mediated increase in peripheral vascular resistance

If there is a disconnect or inability to coordinate any of these mechanisms, there can be failure to maintain adequate blood return to the heart, resulting in cerebral hypoperfusion and potential loss of consciousness.[2,4,6,7] Teenagers are prone to an autonomic instability in which there is an excessive decrease in blood pressure with sudden standing and almost all occasionally feel a brief light-headedness when standing from a squatting or supine position.[2]

During vasovagal fainting, most teenagers have prodromal symptoms before loss of consciousness (feeling lightheaded or dizzy, nausea, diaphoresis, muffled hearing, or visual changes). Most of them experience these symptoms in a warm environment or during predictable situations (see **Box 1**).[1,2,8]

SYNCOPE GAMES AND LARK

Some teenagers force themselves to pass out to obtain a high or to avoid an unwanted activity, such as a test at school. This state is achieved by hyperventilation followed by squeezing the chest or neck or performing a forceful Valsalva maneuver. The hyperventilation lowers P_{CO_2} levels, causing a compensatory cerebral vasoconstriction. The Valsalva maneuver decreases the venous return to the heart and in combination causes sufficient decrease in cerebral perfusion to lose consciousness.[1,2]

PSYCHOGENIC SYNCOPE

Psychogenic syncope was identified in 2.3% of pediatric patients in a large prospective study.[5] These patients either fain loss of consciousness or have a concurrent psychiatric disorder (conversion disorder, anxiety disorder, or depression). The loss of consciousness occurs without hypotension or identifiable change in transcranial Doppler or electroencephalography. Patients with conversion disorder are unaware of their actions.[8] Many of these patients are victims of abuse, and their symptoms may represent a cry for help, which should not be ignored.[8,9]

CARDIAC SYNCOPE

Cardiac syncope in teenagers is less common (2%–6%) than simple fainting but may represent episodes of aborted sudden death or periodic worsening of outflow tract obstruction.[4,10] A high index of suspicion should be held for primary cardiac causes of loss of consciousness. A thorough history and physical with an electrocardiogram (ECG) can usually be used to determine if cardiology referral is necessary.[10–13] Cardiac causes of syncope and some of the distinguishing findings are listed in **Box 3**.

DISTINGUISHING SIMPLE FAINTING FROM CARDIAC SYNCOPE

Historical factors that are most helpful in distinguishing vasovagal from cardiac syncope are sudden loss of consciousness during exercise or while supine.[10] **Table 1** shows a list of predictors of cardiac syncope in children and adolescents.

Palpitations before fainting may help differentiate vasovagal from cardiac syncope.[12,13] Specifically, palpitations are useful when differentiating children with long QT from those with vasovagal syncope.[14] However, palpitations failed to differentiate all forms of vasovagal from cardiac syncope in children and adolescents.[10]

Box 3
Cardiac causes of syncope

Cardiac Disease	Distinguishing Findings
Hypertrophic cardiomyopathy	Syncope during exercise
	Family history of sudden death
	Systolic murmur
	Left ventricular hypertrophy on ECG
Congenital heart disease	Abnormal cardiac examination
	Abnormal ECG
Myocarditis/other cardiomyopathy	History of heart failure symptoms
	Abnormal ECG
Wolf Parkinson White	Ventricular preexcitation on ECG
	History of episodes of palpitations
Supraventricular tachycardia	History of episodes of palpitations
Bradycardia	Second-degree or third-degree heart block on ECG
Long QT syndrome	Prolonged QTc on ECG (QTc $\geq$440 ms in teenage boys and QTc $\geq$460 ms in teenage girls)
	Syncope during exercise or startle
	Family history of sudden death
Other channelopathies	Abnormal ECG
	Family history of sudden death
	Syncope during exercise
Pulmonary hypertension	Abnormal ECG with RVH
	Loud P2 component or abnormal S2 splitting

Palpitations are the most reliable symptom in patients with arrhythmias, and special attention is needed to determine if cardiology referral is necessary.

A thorough family history is important to identify patients at risk for inherited rhythm-related disorders and cardiomyopathies. Patients with relatives who have died suddenly before the age of 30 to 40 years or with a family history of specific inherited rhythm disorders should be referred for cardiology evaluation.

An abnormal cardiac examination should also prompt further evaluation. An outflow tract murmur and cardiomegaly suggest congenital heart lesions, such as aortic stenosis or hypertrophic cardiomyopathy. Signs of heart failure such as jugular venous distension, crackles on lung examination, gallop, pathologic murmur, distended liver, or edema suggest other forms of cardiac disease, including dilated cardiomyopathy.

Many patients with inherited rhythm disorders have a normal physical examination, and an ECG should be obtained. Careful attention should be paid to specific ECG abnormalities, including

- QT, corrected QT interval (QTc), and T wave morphology (**Fig. 1**)
- Left or right ventricular hypertrophy or axis deviation
- Atrioventricular block (second or third degree) (**Fig. 2**)
- Wolff-Parkinson-White syndrome or preexcitation (δ wave) (**Fig. 3**)
- Ischemic changes (deep Q waves or ST segment changes)
- Brugada pattern (**Fig. 4**)[15]

Patients with a history consistent with benign syncope who have no concerning family history, a normal physical examination, and normal ECG should be treated for simple fainting. **Fig. 5** suggests an evaluation sequence to decide if cardiology referral is warranted.

Table 1 Predictors of cardiac syncope on univariate analysis in children and adolescents with syncope			
Clinical Feature	Cardiac Syncope (n = 31)	Vasovagal Syncope (n = 55)	P-Value
Age	8.5 ± 4.2	11.6 ± 2.6	.001
Sex (male/female)	15/16	21/34	.357
Course of disease (mo)	19.4 ± 22.4	22.3 ± 14.2	.566
Number of episodes	7.8 ± 17.6	5.0 ± 3.5	.376
Predisposing factors (%)	20/31 (64.5)	43/55 (78.2)	.169
Persistent standing (%)	1/31 (3.2)	21/55 (38.2)	.002
Warm and crowded place (%)	0	10/55 (18.2)	—
Fear–pain emotion (%)	0	10/55 (18.2)	—
Exercise (%)	19/31 (61.3)	8/55 (14.5)	.000
Position			
Standing (%)	22/31 (71.0)	53/55 (96.4)	.001
Supine (%)	8/31 (25.8)	2/55 (3.6)	.002
Various position (%)	6/31 (19.4)	2/55 (3.6)	.016
With prodromal symptoms (%)	16/31 (51.6)	48/55 (87.3)	.000
Dizziness (%)	1/31 (3.1)	33/55 (60.0)	.000
Headache (%)	2/31 (6.5)	13/55 (23.6)	.044
Chest discomfort (%)	3/31 (9.7)	17/55 (30.9)	.025
Palpitations (%)	6/31 (19.4)	9/55 (15.5)	.645
Sweating (%)	5/31 (16.1)	7/55 (12.7)	.662
Pale (%)	9/31 (29.0)	11/55 (20.0)	.314
Nausea, vomiting (%)	4/31 (12.9)	15/55 (27.3)	.123
Blurred vision (%)	4/31 (12.9)	19/55 (34.5)	.130
Fatigue (%)	1/31 (3.1)	5/55 (9.1)	.473
Duration of the loss of consciousness (min)	1.8 ± 3.4	4.8 ± 3.8	.000
≤1 min (%)	17/31 (54.8)	13/55 (23.6)	—
1–5 min (%)	13/31 (41.9)	14/55 (25.5)	—
>5 min (%)	1/31 (3.1)	28/55 (50.9)	—
Accompanying symptoms (%)	17/23 (54.8)	11/55 (20.0)	.001
Physical injury (%)	2/31 (6.5)	7/55 (12.7)	.905
Convulsion (%)	4/23 (12.9)	3/55 (5.5)	.251
Urine or fecal incontinence (%)	8/31 (25.8)	1/55 (1.8)	.001
Family history of sudden death or syncope (%)	2/31 (6.5)	1/55 (1.8)	.294
History of heart disease (%)	5/31 (16.1)	2/55 (3.6)	.042
Standard ECG abnormalities (%)	29/31 (93.5)	5/55 (9.1)	.000

From Zhang Q, Zhu L, Wang C, et al. Value of history taking children and adolescents with cardiac syncope. Cardiol Young 2013;23:58; with permission.

TILT TABLE TEST

Tilt table testing is often expected by referring physicians and is used more often by adult cardiologists than pediatric cardiologists. A recent survey of pediatric electro-physiologists found that 24% have stopped tilt testing all together and 76% performed

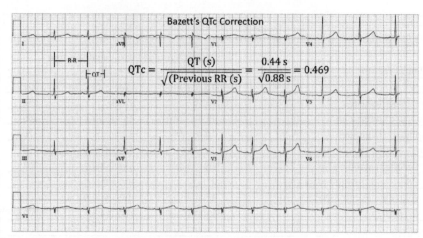

Fig. 1. ECG 1: Long QT with illustration of QTc correction.

fewer than 10 tests/y (median 3 tests/y). Most (68%) believed that the results of the tilt tests did not alter treatment.[16] Reasons for this practice were cited as low sensitivity and specificity of tilt testing as well as patient discomfort and cost. A study of control individuals showed that adolescent patients are more susceptible to orthostatic stress than adults. In this study,[17] 60% of normal control adolescents had syncope at a tilt angle of 80° and 30% at an angle of 60° to 70°. The reproducibility of tilt table testing in children is also questionable, with as many as 40% having a negative second tilt test; even among patients with long asystolic pauses (3 seconds), only 36% had a pause during a repeat tilt study.[18]

TREATMENT OF SIMPLE FAINTING

The natural history of teenagers with simple vasovagal fainting shows that most of them are symptom free within 24 months with or without treatment.[19] Education and nonpharmacologic interventions are the first-line treatment of vasovagal fainting

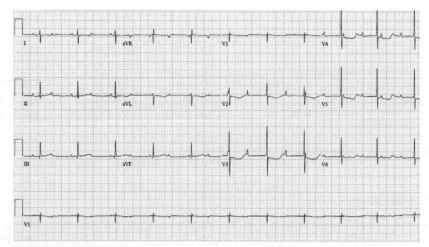

Fig. 2. ECG 2: Complete atrioventricular block with junctional escape rhythm.

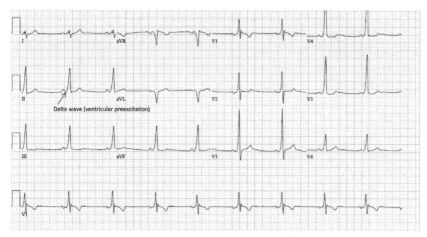

Fig. 3. ECG 3: Wolff-Parkinson-White syndrome or preexcitation (δ wave).

and should be started before pharmacologic therapy is prescribed, which should be reserved for extreme cases only. **Box 4** summarizes nonpharmacologic interventions.

Treatment begins with patient and family education about the mechanism of vasovagal fainting and giving insight into situations in which individuals are prone to faint. Patients should be taught to recognize the prodromal symptoms (feeling lightheaded or dizzy, nausea, diaphoresis, muffled hearing, and visual changes) that can alert them to an impending faint or near faint episode. If they feel these symptoms, they should sit down or lie down in an attempt to avoid complete loss of consciousness, which places them at a risk of serious injury from the fall.

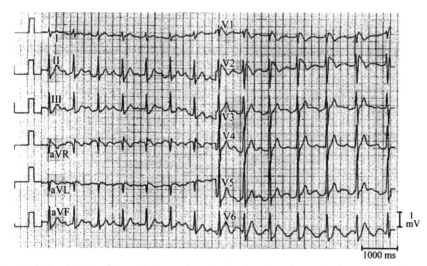

Fig. 4. 12-lead ECG of type 1 Brugada pattern showing the typical repolarization and depolarization abnormalities in V1 and V2. (*Adapted from* Antzelevitch C, Brugada P, Borggrefe M, et al. Brugada syndrome: report of the second consensus conference: endorsed by the heart rhythm society and the European heart rhythm association. Circulation 2005;111:661; with permission.)

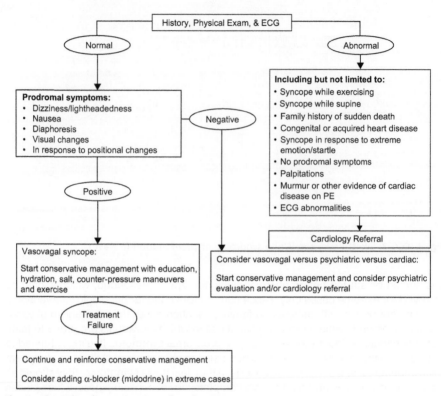

Fig. 5. Algorithm for evaluation of pediatric syncope.

Adolescents can benefit from the knowledge of counterpressure maneuvers, which can be performed to avoid an impending faint. These maneuvers include crossing the legs and tensing lower body and core muscles (legs, buttocks, and abdomen). Hand gripping and arm tensing can also be used. These maneuvers force blood centrally to the heart, increase cardiac output, and decrease the decrease in cerebral perfusion responsible for fainting.[20]

Along with education about trigger avoidance and symptom management, good hydration forms the cornerstone of treatment of adolescent patients with fainting or near fainting. Many teenagers do not drink fluids throughout the day and go until late in the afternoon before needing to urinate after the first postsleep morning void. These habits

---

Box 4
Conservative treatment of fainting

Education

Counterpressure maneuvers

Hydration with clear noncaffeinated beverages to the point of clear color frequent urination (≥4 voids per day not including the first postsleep void)

Add table salt to meals and in rare cases salt tablets

Aerobic exercise with lower extremity and core muscle strengthening

Wall stands with gradually increasing time

are often encouraged by strict rules about drinking fluids and using the bathroom at school. Often, a note for school with instructions for fluid intake are needed to institute proper hydration therapy. Patients should be instructed to drink clear noncaffeinated beverages, including water, throughout the day. Sports drinks containing salt and sugar can also be used and may be superior.[2] Patients should drink enough fluid that they urinate frequently throughout the day (minimum 2 times in the morning, not including the postsleep void and 2 times in the afternoon), and the urine color should be clear.[4] Some investigators suggest an intake goal of at least 2 to 3 L of fluid per day.[21]

Increasing dietary salt by adding table salt to the food or eating salty snacks can help increase the intravascular volume and reduce fainting and near fainting symptoms. In extreme cases, salt tablets with a daily intake of at least 2 g of sodium can be initiated.[21]

Aerobic exercise coupled with lower extremity and core muscle strengthening can improve symptoms in patients prone to fainting. Wall stands with progressive increase in time over 6 to 8 weeks can improve symptoms, possibly by retraining baroreceptor reflexes.[21,22] While the individual is standing, the upper back is positioned against a wall without arm and leg movement, beginning with 5-minute intervals twice daily and increasing gradually to 30-minute to 40-minute intervals over 6 to 8 weeks.

PHARMACOLOGIC TREATMENT

Despite institution of conservative measures, some patients continue to faint. Several medications have been used to treat vasovagal syncope, with varying results, and are listed later. However, the α agonist midodrine is the only medication with strong data supporting its use.

Medications frequently used to treat syncope[21]:

- α-adrenergic agonists (midodrine)
  - Encouraging results
- β-Blockers
  - Large randomized placebo-controlled trial showed that β-blockers are not effective, especially in patients younger than 42 years
  - No longer recommended in latest European guidelines
- Fludrocortisone
  - Shown to be ineffective in pediatric as well as large adult randomized placebo-controlled trials
- Selective serotonin reuptake inhibitors (SSRIs)
  - May be most useful in patients with anxiety and panic disorders

Midodrine

Midodrine is an α-adrenergic agonist and causes an increase in peripheral vascular resistance and decreases venous capacitance, which may decrease the amount of blood pooling with change in position. This effect can be achieved at doses that do not cause an increase in systemic blood pressure (2.5 mg twice daily).[23] A randomized controlled study of children[24] showed a significant reduction in syncope recurrence and few side effects. Midodrine does not cross the blood-brain barrier, eliminating some central nervous system side effects usually found with α agonists. However, some patients report nausea, gastrointestinal discomfort, headaches, and pilomotor reactions. Although midodrine has the most support as a pharmacologic agent for vasovagal fainting, a recent adult crossover placebo study showed no statistical difference in midodrine versus placebo in patients who failed nonpharmacologic treatment.[25] The patients in this study reported more side effects with placebo than midodrine, showing the complex body image and awareness issues in patients with syncope.

β-Blockers

Initial observational studies suggested that β-blockers reduced syncopal events. Hence, β-blockers were previously considered first-line pharmacologic therapy for vasovagal syncope. However, metoprolol was recently shown to be no better than placebo in a randomized, placebo-controlled trial (POST [Prevention of Syncope Trial]), and recent European guidelines for syncope treatment do not include β-blockers.[26,27]

Fludrocortisone

Fludrocortisone has also been used to treat vasovagal fainting, but a randomized placebo-controlled study in children showed that fludrocortisone was ineffective in preventing presyncope and syncope.[28] POST II (Prevention of Syncope Trial II) showed that recurrence of syncope was not reduced with fludrocortisone versus placebo.[29]

OTHER MEDICATIONS

Several other medications have been tested for vasovagal fainting but have limited data with mixed results. SSRIs have shown a significant improvement in quality of life but show mixed results in syncope recurrence.[30,31] SSRIs may be most useful in patients with concurrent psychiatric illness, such as anxiety or panic disorder.[21] Clonidine, pyridostigmine, erythropoietin, methylphenidate, desmopressin, and other agents have been tried but are not well tolerated or have little evidence supporting their use.[8]

PACING

Pacing is rarely indicated in teenagers who faint and often does not prevent syncope even in those with long asystolic pauses. In these patients, the vasodilatory effects are sufficient to cause a decrease in blood pressure and loss of consciousness despite a paced rhythm. However, in highly selected patients with no prodrome of symptoms and documented long asystolic pauses, pacing may prevent syncope or provide a brief episode of prodrome, which can be recognized before fainting, as shown in a recent adult study.[8,32] The benign nature of fainting along with the natural history of spontaneous resolution of fainting in teenagers should weigh heavily against pacemaker placement, especially if prodromal symptoms are present.

Key message

- Syncope in a teenager is most likely caused by vasovagal mechanism
- Disturbance in the normal sequence of changes that occur during change in position leads to cerebral hypoperfusion (fainting)
- Prodromal symptoms are usually present in simple fainting
- Cardiac syncope is less common; however, it may have serious implications
- Historical facts, physical examination, and a 12-lead ECG can be used to guide referral to cardiology
- Tilt table test is not useful in suspected vasovagal syncope and does not alter management
- Adequate hydration and parental/patient reassurance are the cornerstone of treatment
- Counterpressure maneuvers may be performed to abort an episode of fainting
- Midodrine is the only medication shown to have some benefit in this group of patients
- Pacing is rarely indicated for vasovagal syncope

POSTURAL ORTHOSTATIC TACHYCARDIA SYNDROME

Patients affected with postural orthostatic tachycardia syndrome (POTS) experience symptoms like light-headedness, weakness, near syncope, palpitations, and tachycardia, associated with standing upright. Most patients are young women, commonly presenting a few years after puberty or during rapid growth. Severely affected individuals experience chronic fatigue and can be debilitated to the point of inability to attend school, work, or recreational activities. The syndrome can develop slowly, but there is often a preceding trigger illness, such as Epstein-Barr virus, common cold, or other infections. Others begin after a prolonged recovery period from an operation or trauma.[33,34] Patients with POTS are chronically ill and rarely faint as opposed to patients with vasovagal fainting, who are well in general and faint sporadically.[35] **Box 5** lists common initial symptoms associated with POTS.

DIAGNOSIS

In teenagers, POTS is defined as chronic (>6 months) orthostatic intolerance and increase in heart rate of 40 bpm (compared with 30 bpm in adults) within 10 minutes of upright posture without hypotension (no more than a 20 mm Hg systolic or 10 mm Hg diastolic decrease in blood pressure).[36,37] Other disorders that may cause orthostatic intolerance should be excluded, including hypothyroidism, collagen vascular disorders, anemia, diabetes, systemic infections, inflammatory disorders, eating disorders, and paraneoplastic syndromes. Careful attention to the ECG during tachycardia should show sinus tachycardia, with a gradual acceleration of heart rate and not a sudden increase in heart rate, suggesting ectopic atrial tachycardia or other forms of supraventricular tachycardia.

Box 5
Common presenting symptoms from POTS

Tachycardia

Palpitations

Headaches

Weakness

Exercise intolerance

Nausea

Abdominal discomfort

Fatigue

Anxiety

Inappropriate sweating

Light-headedness/dizziness

Near syncope

Edema

Sleep disorder

Data from Johnson JN, Mack KJ, Kuntz NL, et al. Postural orthostatic tachycardia syndrome: a clinical review. Pediatr Neurol 2010;42:77–85.

Patients with POTS have a low total blood volume and a small left ventricle with low left ventricular end-diastolic volume.[34,35,37] A similar condition is seen in astronauts after extended periods in microgravity, and cardiac deconditioning plays an important role in this disorder.[38] The most effective treatment is centered on maintaining superhydration and a gradual reconditioning.

TREATMENT

Treatment of POTS begins with education. Patients should be given insight into their relative hypovolemia and deconditioning. Hydration and gradual exercise over 3 months have been shown to cure 53% of patients with POTS.[34] All patients reported improved quality of life after training in this study. The treatment used is as follows:

- Hydration (usually 2–3 L per day) with clear noncaffeinated beverages to the point of frequent urination with clear urine color (4 voids per day, not including the first postsleep void)
- Increased salt intake, with either table salt or salt tablets
- Elevation (10–15 cm [4–6 inches]) of the head of the bed
- Gradually increasing exercise program over 3 months
  - First month could be seated (rowing machine) or supine (recumbent bike) exercises, with swimming as an alternative
  - Starting with an easily obtainable goal and gradually increasing intensity and duration daily 6 days a week

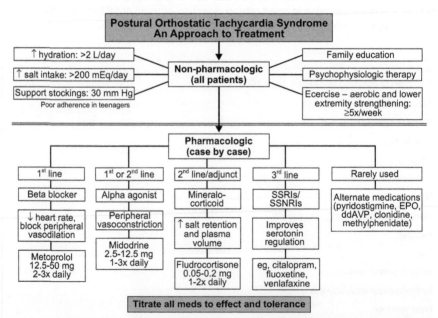

Fig. 6. Proposed treatment algorithm for postural orthostatic tachycardia syndrome (POTS), including pharmacologic and nonpharmacologic therapies. Of note, SSRI and selective serotonin norepinephrine reuptake inhibitor (SSNRI) agents have not been fully studied or approved for use in children and adolescents with POTS. ddAVP, desmopressin; EPO, erythropoietin. (*Modified from* Johnson JN, Mack KJ, Kuntz NL, et al. Postural orthostatic tachycardia syndrome: a clinical review. Pediatr Neurol 2010;42:82; with permission.)

○ During the second and third month, exercise should be changed to more traditional exercise bikes or treadmills, along with lower extremity and core muscle strengthening

MEDICATIONS FOR TREATING POTS

Similar medications as discussed for patients with syncope have been studied in patients with POTS. **Fig. 6** shows a suggestive algorithm for medication use in POTS.[33]

Initial studies showed some promising results for β-blockers.[39] However a more recent comparison between propranolol and exercise showed that β-blockers made patients worse, whereas exercise fostered significant improvement in most patients.[40] Randomized placebo-controlled studies are needed to evaluate the effectiveness of medications in POTS. Given the encouraging results of recent studies, conservative treatment with gradual exercise reconditioning should be used first. In teenagers who fail to respond to conservative measures, medications can be tried.

Key message

- Some adolescents with POTS can be severely debilitated
- Symptoms include light-headedness, weakness, near syncope, or palpitations with upright posture
- Symptoms for more than 6 months and an increase in heart rate of more than 40 bpm with upright posture without hypotension are diagnostic for POTS
- Education, hydration, and an exercise program form the mainstay of management and the role for medications is minimal

---

SUMMARY

Syncope is a common but usually benign problem in adolescence. History is the most important element of evaluation. Most patients do not seek medical attention for simple fainting. Those who do consult a physician often show a high level of anxiety. For most patients, symptoms are not life threatening and spontaneously resolve over time, so often conservative treatment with hydration and behavioral management is all that is required.

REFERENCES

1. Ganzeboom KS, Colman N, Reitsma JB, et al. Prevalence and triggers of syncope in medical students. Am J Cardiol 2003;91:1006–8.
2. Wieling W, Ganzeboom KS, Saul JP. Reflex syncope in children and adolescents. Heart 2004;90:1094–100.
3. Lewis DA, Dhalia A. Syncope in the pediatric patient. The cardiologist's perspective. Pediatr Clin North Am 1999;46:205–19.
4. Driscoll DJ, Jacobsen SJ, Porter CJ, et al. Syncope in children and adolescents. J Am Coll Cardiol 1997;29:1039–45.
5. Zhang Q, Du J, Wang C, et al. The diagnostic protocol in children and adolescents with syncope: a multi-centre prospective study. Acta Paediatr 2009;98:879–84.
6. Wieling W, VanLieshout JJ. Maintenance of postural normotension in humans. In: Low P, editor. Clinical autonomic disorders. Philadelphia: Lippincott-Raven; 1997. p. 73–82.

7. Thompson WO, Thompson PK, Dailey ME. The effect of upright posture on the composition and volume of the blood in man. J Clin Invest 1988;5: 573–609.
8. Grubb BP. Neurocardiogenic syncope and related disorders of orthostatic intolerance. Circulation 2005;111:2997–3006.
9. Kouakam C, Lacriox D, Klug D, et al. Prevalence and significance of psychiatric disorders in patients evaluated for recurrent neurocardiogenic syncope. Am J Cardiol 2002;89:530–5.
10. Zhang Q, Zhu L, Wang C, et al. Value of history taking in children and adolescents with cardiac syncope. Cardiol Young 2013;23:54–60.
11. Calkins H, Shyr Y, Frumin H, et al. The value of clinical history in differentiation of syncope due to ventricular tachycardia, atrioventricular block, and neurocardiogenic syncope. Am J Med 1995;98:365–73.
12. Rosso AD, Ungar A, Maggi R, et al. Clinical predictors of cardiac syncope at initial evaluation in patients referred urgently to a general hospital: the EGYS score. Heart 2008;94:1620–6.
13. Strickberger SA, Benson DW, Biaggioni, et al. American Heart Association Councils on Clinical Cardiology, Cardiovascular Nursing, Cardiovascular Disease in the Young, and Stroke; Quality of Care and Outcomes Research Interdisciplinary Working Group; American College of Cardiology Foundation; Heart Rhythm Society; American Autonomic Society. AHA/ACCF Scientific Statement on the evaluation of syncope. Circulation 2006;113:316–27.
14. Coleman N, Bakker A, Linzer M, et al. Value of history-taking in syncope patients: in whom to suspect long QT syndrome. Europace 2009;11:37–43.
15. Antzelevitch C, Brugada P, Borggrefe M, et al. Brugada syndrome: report of the second consensus conference: endorsed by the Heart Rhythm Society and the European Heart Rhythm Association. Circulation 2005;111:659–70.
16. Batra AS, Balaji S. Usefulness of tilt testing in children with syncope: a survey of pediatric electrophysiologists. Indian Pacing Electrophysiol J 2008;8:242–6.
17. Lewis DA, Zlotocha J, Henke L, et al. Specificity of head-up tilt testing in adolescents: effect of various degrees of tilt challenge in normal control subjects. J Am Coll Cardiol 1997;30:1057–60.
18. Foglia-Manzillo G, Romano M, Corrado G, et al. Reproducibility of asystole during head-up tilt testing in patients with neutrally mediated syncope. Europace 2002; 4:365–7.
19. Biffi M, Boriani G, Bronzetti G, et al. Neurocardiogenic syncope in selected pediatric patients–natural history during long-term follow up and effect of prophylactic pharmacological therapy. Cardiovasc Drugs Ther 2001;15:161–7.
20. Krediet CT, Van Dijk N, Linzer M, et al. Management of vasovagal syncope: controlling or aborting faints by the combination of legcrossing and muscle tensing. Circulation 2002;106:1684–9.
21. Guzman JC, Armaganijan LV, Morillo CA. Treatment of neutrally mediated reflex syncope. Cardiol Clin 2013;31:123–9.
22. Ector H, Reybrouck T, Heidbuchel H, et al. Tilt training: a new treatment for recurrent neurocardiogenic syncope or severe orthostatic intolerance. Pacing Clin Electrophysiol 1998;21:193–6.
23. Kaufmann H, Saadia D, Voustianiouk A. Midodrine in neutrally mediated syncope: a double blind randomized crossover study. Ann Neurol 2002;52: 342–5.
24. Qingyou Z, Junbao D, Chaoshu T. The efficacy of midodrine hydrochloride in the treatment of children with vasovagal syncope. J Pediatr 2006;149:777–80.

25. Romme J, Van Dijk N, Go-Schon IK, et al. Effectiveness of midodrine treatment in patients with recurrent vasovagal syncope not responding to non-pharmacological treatment (STAND-trial). Europace 2011;13:1639–47.
26. Sheldon R, Connolly S, Rose S, et al. Prevention of syncope trial (POST) a randomized, placebo-controlled study of metoprolol in the prevention of vasovagal syncope. Circulation 2006;113:1164–70.
27. Moya A, Sutton R, Ammirati F, et al. Guidelines for the diagnosis and management of syncope. Eur Heart J 2009;30:2631–71.
28. Salim MA, Di Sessa TG. Effectiveness of fludrocortisone and salt in preventing syncope recurrence in children: a double blind, placebo controlled, randomized trial. J Am Coll Cardiol 2005;45:484–8.
29. Sheldon R, Morillo CA, Krahn A, et al. A randomized clinical trial of fludrocortisone for the prevention of vasovagal syncope (POST II). Can J Cardiol 2011;27: S335–6.
30. Theodorakis GN, Leftheriotis D, Livanis EG, et al. Fluoxetine vs. propranolol in the treatment of vasovagal syncope: a prospective, randomized, placebo-controlled study. Europace 2006;8:193–8.
31. Di Girolamo E, Di Iorio C, Sabatini P, et al. Effects of paroxetine hydrochloride, a selective serotonin reuptake inhibitor, on refractory vasovagal syncope: a randomized, double-blind, placebo-controlled study. J Am Coll Cardiol 1999;33: 1227–30.
32. Brignole M, Menozzi C, Moya A, et al. Pacemaker therapy in patients with neutrally mediated syncope and documented asystole: Third International Study on Syncope of Uncertain Etiology (ISSUE-3): a randomized trial. Circulation 2012; 125:2566–71.
33. Johnson JN, Mack KJ, Kuntz NL, et al. Postural orthostatic tachycardia syndrome: a clinical review. Pediatr Neurol 2010;42:77–85.
34. Fu Q, VanGundy TB, Galbreath MM, et al. Cardiac origins of the postural orthostatic tachycardia syndrome. J Am Coll Cardiol 2010;55:2858–68.
35. Stewart JM. Postural tachycardia syndrome and reflex syncope: similarities and differences. J Pediatr 2009;154:481–5.
36. Raj SR, Levine BD. Postural tachycardia syndrome (POTS) diagnosis and treatment: basics and new developments. Cardiac rhythm management. 2013. Available at: CardioSource.org. Accessed July 19, 2013.
37. Singer W, Sletten DM, Opfer-Gehrking TL, et al. Postural tachycardia in children and adolescents: what is abnormal? J Pediatr 2012;160:746–52.
38. Levine BD, Pawelczyk JA, Ertl AC, et al. Human muscle sympathetic neural and haemodynamic responses to tilt following spaceflight. J Physiol 2002;538: 331–40.
39. Lai CC, Fischer PR, Brands CK, et al. Outcomes in adolescents with postural orthostatic tachycardia syndrome treated with midodrine and beta-blockers. Pacing Clin Electrophysiol 2009;32:234–8.
40. Fu Q, VanGundy TB, Shibata S, et al. Exercise training versus propranolol in the treatment of the postural orthostatic tachycardia syndrome. Hypertension 2011; 58:167–75.

The Asymptomatic Teenager with an Abnormal Electrocardiogram

Harinder R. Singh, MD, FHRS, CEPS, CCDS

KEYWORDS

- Abnormal electrocardiograms • Normal ECG variants • Asymptomatic • Children

KEY POINTS

- Electrocardiograms (ECGs) in children and young adults need to be interpreted by an individual trained in reading pediatric ECG, because the computerized interpretation of ECGs is fraught with errors.
- ECGs in children may show age-related evolutionary changes, normal variation, or abnormal findings representing cardiac disease.
- In this article, the ECG findings that may be encountered in an asymptomatic teen are discussed. Some findings may be benign and do not require further testing, whereas others may have a higher likelihood of being associated with heart disease or risk of sudden death. Personal history, family history, and the specific ECG findings dictate further management, which is discussed in detail.

INTRODUCTION

Electrocardiograms (ECGs) are performed in children and young adults as a part of evaluation for symptoms and signs related to the cardiovascular system, such as palpitations, chest pain, syncope, or cardiac murmurs; a screening test before sports participation or initiation of medications in conditions such as attention-deficit hyperkinetic disorders (ADHD). The ECG in the young shows evolutionary changes with age as well as benign variants seen in a few normal individuals. However, there are certain findings detected in asymptomatic teenagers with potential clinical significance that may require further investigations and management. These abnormal findings in asymptomatic individuals have a sensitivity of 51%, specificity of 61%, positive predictive accuracy of 7%, and negative predictive accuracy of 96% for identifying cardiovascular abnormalities.[1] In this article, the benign and potentially significant ECG findings in asymptomatic teenagers and their management are discussed.

Disclosures: None.
Division of Cardiology, The Carman and Ann Adams Department of Pediatrics, Children's Hospital of Michigan, Wayne State University School of Medicine, 3901 Beaubein, Detroit, MI 48201, USA
E-mail address: hsingh6@dmc.org

Pediatr Clin N Am 61 (2014) 45–61
http://dx.doi.org/10.1016/j.pcl.2013.09.015
0031-3955/14/$ – see front matter © 2014 Elsevier Inc. All rights reserved.

NORMAL VARIANTS

Findings like sinus arrhythmia, sinus bradycardia, sinus tachycardia, right ventricular conduction delay, or incomplete right bundle branch block without right ventricular hypertrophy (RVH) or right axis deviation, isolated intraventricular conduction delay, right axis deviation in patients 8 years of age or younger, early repolarization, normal variant of ST-T elevation, juvenile T wave pattern, QTc 0.45 seconds or greater reported by computer but normal by manual calculation, and borderline QTc 0.44 to 0.45 seconds without significant family history do not require any further testing or evaluation (**Box 1**). These findings are not associated with heart disease and are termed normal variants. Trained athletes (≤80%) may show sinus bradycardia, first-degree atrioventricular (AV) block, and or early repolarization, which result from physiologic adaptation of the cardiac autonomic nervous system to athletic conditioning.[2]

ABNORMAL ECG FINDINGS IN ASYMPTOMATIC TEENAGERS

Computerized ECG readouts must be treated with caution, because they are fraught with errors in interpretation and measurements. ECG findings that may be suggestive of heart disease are regarded as abnormal findings. Abnormal ECG findings that are confirmed by trained individuals for reading pediatric ECGs are discussed in the following section. These findings can be seen in asymptomatic individuals and may be related to the altered autonomic tone or structural remodeling secondary to intense physical training, or can be a true indicator of significant heart disease. Based on the type, intensity, and level of training, varying degrees of abnormal ECGs are seen in about 40% of athletes. The most common changes detected include early repolarization, chamber hypertrophy, repolarization abnormalities, and deep Q waves.[1] Some of the abnormal ECG findings have a low likelihood of being related to cardiac abnormality; however, there are other findings that would warrant further evaluation to rule out life-threatening cardiac conditions. Further evaluation in these asymptomatic teenagers with abnormal ECG findings is dependent on the indication for obtaining an ECG, personal and family history, physical examination, and the abnormality detected on the ECG (**Box 2**).

Chamber Enlargement or Hypertrophy

The principal ECG changes associated with hypertrophy or enlargement of cardiac chambers are associated with amplitude, duration of complexes, and vectors of

---

Box 1
Normal variants and findings on ECG with unlikely presence of heart disease

1. Sinus arrhythmia

2. Sinus bradycardia

3. First-degree atrioventricular block

4. Wenckebach phenomena

5. Incomplete right bundle branch block (without RVH or right axis deviation)

6. Early repolarization

7. Right axis deviation 8 years of age or younger

8. Juvenile pattern of repolarization

Data from Pelliccia A, Maron BJ, Culasso F, et al. Clinical significance of abnormal electrocardiographic patterns in trained athletes. Circulation 2000;102(3):278–84.

Box 2
ECG patterns associated with likelihood of heart disease

1. Voltage criteria for chamber enlargement or hypertrophy

2. Axis deviation

   • Right axis deviation (>8 years of age)

   • Left axis deviation

3. Abnormal rhythm

   • Escape rhythm

4. Ectopies

5. Bundle branch block pattern

   • Left bundle branch block

   • Right bundle branch block ± axis deviation

6. AV block

   • Second-degree type II AV block

   • Third-degree AV block

7. Wolff-Parkinson-White pattern

8. Abnormal repolarization

9. Abnormal QT interval

Data from Pelliccia A, Maron BJ, Culasso F, et al. Clinical significance of abnormal electrocardiographic patterns in trained athletes. Circulation 2000;102(3):278–84.

---

corresponding complexes and segments. There are age-specific criteria for left ventricular hypertrophy (LVH) and RVH based on the normal data established for infants and children.[3,4]

Detection of LVH in pediatrics, using ECG, has a sensitivity of only 25% to 30% when compared with echocardiogram.[5] The commonly used criteria in pediatrics includes the QRS amplitude greater than the upper limits of normal for age, the adaptation of adult criteria for LVH, presence of axis deviation, deep Q waves, and the presence of repolarization abnormalities. The most widely accepted adult criteria for LVH (**Box 3**) include the voltage criteria by Sokolow-Lyon,[6] the Cornell voltage criteria,[7] and the point score of Romhilt and Estes.[8] Even although the specificity of an individual criterion for LVH is high, the sensitivity is poor. QRS voltages are influenced not only by left ventricular size or mass but also by other factors like age, gender, race, body habitus, and sites of electrode placement. Their effect contributes to the limited accuracy of the ECG criteria. Use of ECG criteria for LVH with ST segment and T wave abnormalities increases the specificity and sensitivity to detect LVH (**Fig. 1**).[9]

The sensitivity of criteria for RVH is even lower. The criteria for RVH include voltage criteria with QRS amplitudes greater than upper limits of normal for age in the right precordial leads, right axis deviation, secondary ST-T–wave abnormalities specific for age, and presence of Q waves.

Biventricular hypertrophy is suggested by the presence of criteria for both LVH and RVH. Right axis deviation in presence of LVH and combined tall R waves and deep S waves in the midprecordial leads greater than 60 mm (Katz-Wachtel criteria, see **Fig. 1**) suggest biventricular hypertrophy.[10]

Box 3
Criteria for chamber hypertrophy

LVH:

1. QRS voltage greater than upper limits of normal for age

2. Sokolow-Lyon criteria: (SV1 or V2 + RV5 or V6) 35 mm or greater

3. Cornell criteria: (RaVL + SV3) 28 mm or greater for men and 20 mm or greater for women

4. Point score of Romhilt-Estes: (LVH, 5 points; probable LVH, 4 points)

    1. Amplitude (3 points)

        Any of the following:

        a. Largest R or S wave in the limb leads 20 mm or greater

        b. S wave in V1 or V2 30 mm or greater

        c. R wave in V5 or V6 30 mm or greater

    2. ST-T segment changes (typical pattern of left ventricular strain with the ST-T segment vector shifted in direction opposite to the mean QRS vector)

        Without digitalis (3 points)

        With digitalis (1 point)

    3. Left atrial involvement (3 points)

        Terminal negativity of the P wave in V is 1 mm or more deep with a duration of 0.04 seconds or more

    4. Left axis deviation −30° or more (2 points)

    5. QRS duration 0.09 seconds or more (1 point)

    6. Intrinsicoid deflection in V5, V6 0.05 seconds or more (1 point)

5. Associated QRS axis deviation, secondary ST-T changes and deep Q waves

RVH:

1. QRS voltage in the right precordial leads greater than upper limits of normal for age

2. Right axis deviation

3. Secondary ST-T changes, based on evolutionary changes

4. Presence of Q waves in the right precordial leads

Biventricular hypertrophy:

1. Presence of criteria for both LVH and RVH

2. Right axis deviation in presence of LVH

3. Combined tall R waves and deep S waves in the midprecordial leads greater than 60 mm (Katz-Wachtel criteria)

Left atrial abnormality:

1. P wave duration 120 milliseconds or greater

2. Widely notched P wave 40 milliseconds or greater

3. Left axis of the terminal P wave between −30° and −90°

Right atrial abnormality:

1. Increase in amplitude of the P wave

2. Rightward shift of the P wave vector

3. Prominent initial positivity of the P wave in V1 or V2 1.5 mm or greater

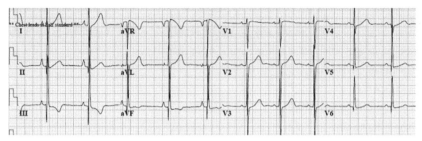

Fig. 1. LVH with mild ST changes. ECG of a 14-year-old girl, suggestive of LVH based on voltage greater than upper limit of normal for age, positive Sokolow-Lyon, Cornell, Romhilt-Estes criteria as well as presence of secondary ST segment changes. Also fulfills the Katz-Wachtel criterion for biventricular hypertrophy. The findings were confirmed with an echocardiogram.

Abnormal P waves are usually referred to as right or left atrial abnormality. The ECG criteria for atrial abnormality are highly specific but insensitive when compared with cardiac magnetic resonance imaging (MRI).[11] Left atrial abnormality is suggested by P wave duration 120 milliseconds or greater, widely notched P wave 40 milliseconds or greater, and left axis deviation of the terminal P wave between −30 and −90°.[12,13] Right atrial abnormality is manifested as an increase in amplitude of the P wave, a rightward shift of the P wave vector, and prominent initial positivity of the P wave in V1 or V2 of 1.5 mm or greater.

Because the sensitivity of ECG criteria for chamber hypertrophy in pediatrics is low, it is used only as a screening tool[14] and is correlated with other measurements for the assessment of hypertrophy or chamber enlargement. Because the sensitivity and specificity of individual criteria are low, further evaluation is usually based on presence of more than 1 criterion and clinical suspicion. Further evaluation is usually in the form of detailed personal and family history, physical examination, and echocardiogram.

Axis Deviation

The QRS axis is defined as the average direction in which the excitatory process spreads throughout the ventricular myocardium.[15] A similar vector can be obtained for the P and the T waves. The normal QRS axis is age dependent. The QRS axis is rightward at birth and progressively shifts leftward to reach the normal adult range of 0° to 90° by 8 years of age. Thereafter, the shift remains stable, with further shifts dependent on conduction tissue abnormality seen in the older age. An abnormal QRS axis is not a specific finding. However, it should prompt a detailed history, physical examination, detailed evaluation of the ECG, and possibly an echocardiogram. About 15% of individuals among all age groups have rightward QRS frontal plane axis (>90°). About 8.7% of normal children have QRS axis leftward of 30°, and 1.8% have QRS axis leftward of 0°.[16]

Persistence of rightward axis or right axis deviation in teenagers (**Box 4**)[17] may need further evaluation. Left axis deviation in teenagers can occasionally be seen as a normal variant but needs further evaluation in the form of an echocardiogram to rule out other possible causes (**Box 5**).[18]

Abnormal Rhythm

Low right atrial rhythm, wandering atrial pacemaker, and sinus arrhythmia are benign rhythm variants that do not require any further workup or evaluation. Sinus

> **Box 4**
> **Causes of rightward axis or right axis deviation (>8 years of age) in asymptomatic teenagers**
>
> - Normal variant, inherited as autosomal-dominant trait
> - Tall asthenic individuals
> - Dextrocardia
> - Right ventricular hypertrophy
> - Pulmonary causes
> - Wolff-Parkinson-White syndrome
> - Atrial septal defects
>
> *Data from* Stephen JM, Dhindsa H, Browne B, et al. Interpretation and clinical significance of the QRS axis of the electrocardiogram. J Emerg Med 1990;8(6):757–63.

bradyarrhythmia, junctional rhythm, and first-degree AV block or Wenckebach phenomena are commonly seen in trained teenagers related to a heightened vagal tone and need no further evaluation.[19]

Sinus tachycardia is sinus rhythm at a rate faster than normal for patient's age. It is usually related to increased sympathetic tone or as a compensatory response to increase the cardiac output. In an asymptomatic teenager, the context may be important. It may be secondarily related to hypovolemia, anxiety, toxins, medications, anemia, hyperthyroidism, or catecholamine-secreting tumors. Of greater concern is that persistent sinus tachycardia may be related to decreased cardiac function. Rarely, sinus node reentry tachycardia and inappropriate sinus tachycardia may mimic sinus tachycardia. It requires detailed evaluation, including personal history, physical examination, rhythm monitoring, and blood and urine tests, to rule out secondary causes. A persistent sinus tachycardia should prompt an echocardiogram to evaluate cardiac function.[20]

> **Box 5**
> **Causes of left axis deviation in asymptomatic teenagers**
>
> - Normal variant
> - LBBB or LAHB
> - Left ventricular hypertrophy
> - Wolff-Parkinson-White syndrome
> - Congenital heart defects
>   Endocardial cushion defect
>   Tricuspid atresia
>   Congenitally corrected transposition of the great arteries
>   Single ventricle
>   Double-outlet right ventricle with infracristal ventricular septal defect
> - Mechanical factors: obesity, chest wall deformities, ascites, pregnancy
>
> *Data from* Stephen JM, Dhindsa H, Browne B, et al. Interpretation and clinical significance of the QRS axis of the electrocardiogram. J Emerg Med 1990;8(6):757–63.

Sinus bradycardia is sinus rhythm at a rate slower than normal for patient's age. It is commonly seen in athletic, well-conditioned individuals. It may also be seen with extracardiac causes like hypoxia, poisoning, electrolyte disorders, infection, sleep apnea, drugs, hypoglycemia, hypothyroidism, hypothermia, and increased intracranial pressure. Unless associated with symptoms or poor perfusion, it does not warrant further investigations or treatment.[21]

Junctional escape rhythm is a slow narrow-complex rhythm without preceding atrial activity, originating from the AV node. It may suggest high vagal tone or sinus node dysfunction. Rhythm monitoring and exercise stress test are indicated only in the presence of symptoms or evidence of poor perfusion.[22]

Ventricular escape rhythm is a slow wide-complex rhythm originating from the ventricles. It usually indicates significant sinus bradycardia or AV block. Unless the cause is a known reversible cause, it usually warrants cardiology evaluation and possible intervention.

Ectopic Beats

Ectopic beats may originate from the atrium, junction, or ventricles. Isolated premature ventricular complexes (PVCs) may be identified on a routine resting ECG in 0.2% to 2.2% of normal children (**Fig. 2**).[23] PVCs are common, occurring in 20% to 30% of younger children and up to 40% of teenage boys on Holter monitoring.[24] They may be related to an idiopathic cause, electrolyte abnormalities, stimulant intake, drugs, or cardiomyopathy, as well as channelopathies like long QT syndrome (LQTS). The frequency of PVC is usually no more than 1 to 5 per hour, but occasional individuals may have more frequent ectopic activity or prolonged periods of ventricular bigeminy (every other beat is a PVC). Couplets (2 PVCs in a row) and multifocal extrasystoles (PVC of different morphology) are occasionally seen in a few individuals. Ventricular ectopies that are isolated, uniform in morphology, and accompanied by structurally normal heart and are suppressed on exercise are almost certainly benign.[23] In some cases, PVCs may need to be evaluated with an echocardiogram to rule out significant structural or functional causes. A Holter monitor should be obtained to assess the frequency load, morphology, and presence of sustained or nonsustained ventricular tachycardia. If the PVC is incidental (not perceived by the patient), uniform in morphology, isolated, and suppressed during light activity on the Holter, then generally no further workup is required. Patients with PVCs that fall out of these parameters may be referred to a cardiologist for evaluation. An exercise

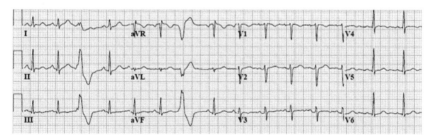

Fig. 2. PVC is an early ventricular beat originating from below the bifurcation of the bundle of His, characterized by a premature wide QRS complex that is morphologically different compared with the baseline QRS complexes with a compensatory pause (ie, R-R interval produced by atrial initiated QRS complexes on either side of the PVC is equal to twice the normal R-R interval).

stress test may be useful to assess suppression with exercise (an indicator of benign PVC). If cardiac muscle disease is suspected, a cardiac MRI with late gadolinium enhancement may be performed.

Isolated premature atrial complexes (PACs) are common at all ages (**Fig. 3**). The prevalence of premature atrial contraction in junior high school, high school, and university students is 0.13%, 0.17%, and 0.16%, respectively, with no differences noted for gender.[25] Holter monitoring in young adults with normal hearts has shown that approximately 10% to 73% have PACs, but only 2% have more than 100 PACs in a 24-hour period and less than 1% have frequent PACs.[26,27]

Premature junctional complexes (PJCs) are less frequent than PACs and PVCs. PJCs are noted in 0.2%, with an equal distribution in all age groups.[28] Asymptomatic patients with either PACs or PJCs do not require any investigations or treatment.

Bundle Branch Block Pattern

Bundle branch block pattern can be seen as a normal variant in a few individuals.

The criteria for diagnosis of left bundle branch block (LBBB) is QRS duration 140 milliseconds or greater (men) or 130 milliseconds or greater (women) or more than 2 standard deviations (SD) of normal for age, QS or rS pattern in leads V1 and V2 and mid-QRS notching or slurring in 2 or more of leads V1, V2, V5, V6, I, and aVL.[29] LBBB is seen in 0.1% of normal athletes.[30] The presence of LBBB mandates evaluation to rule out potential causes (**Box 6**). A detailed cardiology evaluation including echocardiogram, Holter monitoring, and exercise stress test should be performed.[31]

The criteria for diagnosis of right bundle branch block pattern (RBBB) is QRS duration 120 milliseconds or greater, rsr prime or rsR prime or rSR prime or M shaped with R prime usually greater than initial R wave in V1, V2, and wide S wave in I, V5, V6 (S wave duration >R wave).[32] RBBB is reported in 0.11% of normal children. The potential causes are listed in **Box 7**.[33] Isolated RBBB pattern mandates evaluation, including family history, echocardiogram, stress test, and Holter monitoring.

Incomplete RBBB (IRBBB) pattern is similar to complete RBBB except the QRS duration is 120 milliseconds or less. It is prevalent in 0.32% to 0.7% of normal children.[34,35] It is related to either a conduction delay in the right bundle branch that may be a normal variant or caused by a congenital lesion like atrial septal defects or pulmonary stenosis, degeneration, ischemic or inflammatory damage, or RVH caused by lung disease. In an otherwise healthy teenager with an unremarkable family

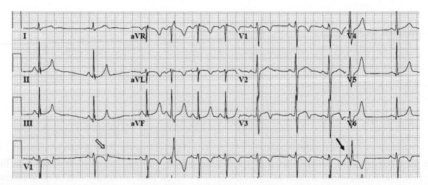

Fig. 3. PAC is an early beat arising from an atrial focus other than the sinoatrial node, with 3 possible outcomes: (1) blocked PAC as a result of AV nodal refractoriness (*pale arrow*), (2) aberrantly conducted PAC (*solid arrow*), and (3) normally conducted PAC.

Box 6
Causes of LBBB in asymptomatic teenagers

- Normal variant
- Cardiomyopathy (overt or latent)
- Systemic hypertension
- Ischemic heart disease
- Sclerotic (Lev) or degenerative (Lenegre) disease of the cardiac skeleton
- Type B Wolff-Parkinson-White pattern

---

history and normal cardiac examination, no further testing is indicated for IRBBB. Echocardiography is indicated in the presence of heart murmur with fixed split-second heart sound (suspect atrial septal defect). In patients with a family history of cardiac conduction defects, periodic follow-up may be warranted.

The presence of changes in the QRS axis along with RBBB may indicate an associated left fascicular hemiblock and warrant more extensive investigations. Left axis deviation in the presence of RBBB usually indicates bifascicular block involving the RBBB and the left anterior hemiblock (LAHB) (**Fig. 4**). This is the most common type of bifascicular block. Right axis deviation with RBBB indicates bifascicular block involving the RBBB and left posterior hemiblock (**Fig. 5**). Even although bifascicular blocks are mostly related to coronary artery disease in the adult population, the few causes that may be applicable to previously asymptomatic younger individuals include cardiomyopathy, aortic valve disease, and degenerative fibrotic disease of the cardiac skeleton.[36] These patients may require an echocardiogram and periodic follow-up to assess progression of cardiac conduction delays.

AV Block

The prevalence of AV block in the young is between 0.2% and 0.6 %. First-degree AV block is a prolongation of the PR interval greater than 2 SD for the age. It is seen in

---

Box 7
Causes of RBBB in asymptomatic teenagers

- Normal variant
- Congenital heart diseases (atrial septal defect)
- Ischemic heart disease
- Systemic hypertension
- History of open heart surgery
- Sclerotic (Lev) or degenerative (Lenegre) disease of the cardiac skeleton
- Systemic diseases: diabetes mellitus
- Chronic airways disease: bronchial asthma
- Type A Wolff-Parkinson-White pattern

Data from Agarwal AK, Venugopalan P. Right bundle branch block: varying electrocardiographic patterns. Aetiological correlation, mechanisms and electrophysiology. Int J Cardiol 1999;71(1):33–9.

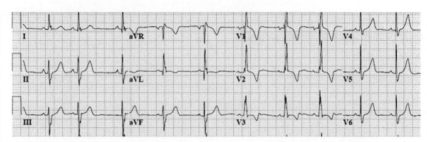

Fig. 4. Bifascicular block (RBBB with left axis deviation suggestive of LAHB).

about 0.8%,[37] frequently related to the high parasympathetic tone in the athletic individuals. The disappearance of the pattern with exercise or hyperventilation confirms the benign prognosis. Other causes of first-degree AV block include normal variance, medications, rheumatic fever, myocarditis, collagen vascular disease, tumors, trauma, hypothermia, hypothyroidism, and electrolyte disturbances.[38] The patients with first-degree AV block are usually asymptomatic, except for patients with PR interval greater than 300 milliseconds, who may manifest symptoms related to AV dyssynchrony, resulting in decreased cardiac output and cannon A waves, termed 'pseudopacemaker syndrome'. First-degree AV block usually does not warrant any further testing or follow-up, unless it is associated with bundle branch block.

Second-degree Mobitz type I AV block (Wenckebach phenomena) is progressive prolongation of the PR interval followed by a nonconducted P wave. It is seen in patients with high vagal tone, drugs, myocarditis, ischemia, and after cardiac surgery.[39] It does not usually produce any symptoms. However, rare individuals may experience symptoms similar to pseudopacemaker syndrome. It does not usually require any additional testing but may be followed intermittently. In patients with known abnormal cardiac structure or function, type I second-degree AV block may indicate a more guarded prognosis.

Second-degree Mobitz type II AV block is seen with a fixed PR interval before a nonconducted P wave. It may be caused by age-related fibrous degeneration of the conduction system, myocardial infarction with ischemia of the AV node, myocarditis, infection, or in patients who are taking drugs that block the AV node. It is always permanent and may progress to higher grades of AV block. Therefore, asymptomatic patients with Mobitz type II AV block require cardiology consultation and evaluation for pacemaker implantation at the time of detection.[40]

Third-degree AV block is the total failure of the atrial impulses to conduct to the ventricles. It is seen in about 0.002% of normal asymptomatic children.[35] It is suspected

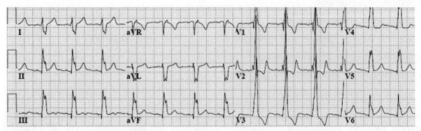

Fig. 5. Bifascicular block (RBBB with right axis deviation suggestive of left posterior hemiblock).

by finding a slow heart rate. The cause is usually related to asymptomatic congenital complete AV block related to maternal lupus, sclerotic (Lev disease) or degenerative (Lenegre disease) disease of the cardiac skeleton, congenital heart defects like the congenitally corrected transposition of the great arteries, myocarditis, or cardiomyopathy, or may be postsurgical or iatrogenic. Patients with third-degree AV block need cardiology evaluation and follow-up. Thorough investigations to find the cause of the AV block can guide the need and timing of intervention.

Wolff-Parkinson-White Pattern

A Wolff-Parkinson-White (WPW) pattern on the ECG is seen in about 1 to 3 per 1000 individuals (**Fig. 6**).[41] Of these individuals, 65% of the adolescents with WPW pattern are asymptomatic.[42,43] It is detected in 0.13% of asymptomatic schoolchildren. A common misconception is that all WPW leads to tachyarrhythmia such as supraventricular tachycardia (SVT). However, this finding, even in absence of SVT, is not entirely benign. In patients with structurally normal hearts, the incidence of sudden death ranges between 1.1 per 1000 patient-years and 1.5 per 1000 patient-years.[43,44] Because of the risk of sudden death even for the asymptomatic individuals with WPW pattern on ECG, it is recommended that they undergo initial risk stratification with an exercise stress test and Holter monitoring. Sudden disappearance of preexcitation or the WPW pattern during an exercise stress test is an indicator of a low-risk accessory connection. Persistence of preexcitation at peak exercise, difficulty in interpreting the exercise stress test, or inability to perform the exercise stress test mandates an invasive electrophysiology study.[45]

Abnormal Repolarization (ST Wave and T Wave Changes)

Abnormal repolarization has been reported to occur in 2% to 4% of young trained athletes.[1,46] This condition is defined as inverted T waves ($\geq$2 mm deep) in at least 3 leads (exclusive of standard lead III), and predominantly in the anterior and lateral precordial leads V2 to V6. In a cohort of athletes with repolarization abnormalities, about 6% of the patients were subsequently diagnosed to have cardiomyopathies, implying that abnormal repolarization may be an initial expression of underlying cardiomyopathy.[47] Inverted T waves may represent the first and only sign of an inherited heart muscle disease, in the absence of any other features and before structural changes in the heart can be detected. Alternative causes of T wave inversion include drugs (eg, digoxin/cocaine/amphetamines), acute pulmonary embolism, myocardial ischemia, myopericarditis, electrolyte disturbance/hypokalemia, and LQTS (particularly type 2). Current evidence suggests that anterior (V1–V4) T wave inversion seems benign in adolescents and black athletes, whereas lateral (V5–V6) T wave inversion should always

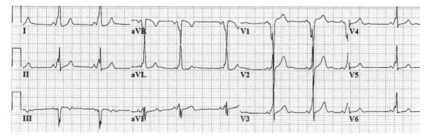

Fig. 6. WPW pattern with a short PR interval, δ wave, and wide QRS complex.

be viewed with suspicion. Asymptomatic individuals with T wave inversion (≥2 contiguous anterior, inferior, or lateral leads but not aVR, and III) should undergo thorough personal symptom and family history inquiries, physical examination, echocardiography, late gadolinium-enhanced cardiac MRI, exercise stress testing, and Holter monitoring (including 1 exercise training session). If feasible, first-degree relatives should undergo 12-lead ECG and echocardiography (>10 years).[48]

A benign variant of ST elevation (STTNV) is reported in 0.88% of normal adult ECGs, with 96% in the black population.[49] STTNV is distinctively different from early repolarization. In STTNV, the T waves are inverted in the midprecordial (V3–V4) and the lateral precordial (V5–V6) leads (**Fig. 7**), whereas they are upright and tall in early repolarization (**Fig. 8**).[50] STTNV can be easily mistaken for acute myocardial infarction or pericarditis.[51]

Brugada syndrome is characterized by early, high takeoff (≥2 mm), and downsloping ST segment increase (J wave) of either the coved (negative T wave) or saddle-back (positive T wave) type in V1 to V2/V3 and the increased vulnerability to ventricular fibrillation and sudden cardiac death, in the absence of clinical evidence of structural heart disease.[52] Dynamic ECG changes over time are common and may lead to a transient, complete normalization of the ECG. A febrile state, electrolyte disturbances, maneuvers/circumstances associated with an increased vagal tone, or provocation tests have been reported to produce ST segment elevation and trigger a polymorphic ventricular tachycardia or ventricular fibrillation in patients with Brugada syndrome.[53] Individuals with a suspected Brugada ECG should undergo further clinical cardiology workup, including a pharmacologic test with sodium channel blocking, risk stratification, and familial evaluation.

Deep Q Waves

An abnormal Q wave is greater than 0.04 seconds in width and greater than 25% of the height of the R wave in most ECG leads. Presence of a Q wave up to 0.05 seconds wide in lead III is a normal variant. The presence of Q wave in the right precordial leads (V1, V2, and V3) is considered abnormal.[54] Deep Q waves are detected in 1.26% of asymptomatic children.[55] The noninfarction causes of deep Q waves include normal variation as seen in athletes, misplacement of chest electrodes, chamber hypertrophy, LBBB or LAHB, WPW pattern, and pulmonary causes.[56] Teenagers with pathologic deep Q waves may be evaluated with detailed history, physical examination, and an echocardiogram.

Abnormal QT Interval

The QT interval represents the sum of depolarization and repolarization duration of a cardiac cycle.[57] LQTS may present dramatically, with sudden cardiac death in 10% of

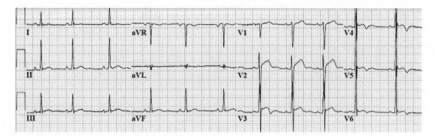

Fig. 7. Normal variant of ST segment elevation with T wave inversion.

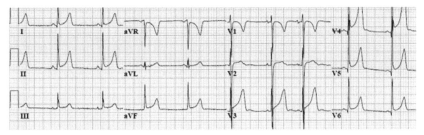

Fig. 8. Early repolarization.

children or with syncope or seizures in 30% to 40% as the first symptom.[58] The prevalence of QT interval prolongation in asymptomatic elite athletes is 0.4%, or 1 in 286 patients.[59] An abnormal QT interval is detected in 0.024% of asymptomatic young children. Corrected QT interval (QTc) beyond the so-called normal range is seen in 10% to 20% of otherwise healthy postpubertal individuals.[60] The abnormality in QT intervals can be related to heart rate, gender, abnormal QRS complexes, medications or drugs, electrolyte disturbance in the form of hypocalcemia, hypokalemia, hypomagnesemia, hypothyroidism, and patients with LQTS. The normal cutoff for QTc in females is 460 milliseconds or less and for males is 450 milliseconds or less. The computer-generated reporting of the measurement of QTc interval is frequently inaccurate. When there is a suspicion of abnormal QTc, the ECG should be evaluated by an experienced cardiologist, and QTc should be calculated manually. Because patients with LQTS have an increased risk of sudden death, it is important to investigate these patients with thorough personal and family history, ECG, Holter monitoring, echocardiogram, exercise stress test, and genetic testing before establishing a diagnosis, and serial follow-up is crucial.

Key message

- Preparticipation sports physical examination and use of medications for attention-deficit hyperkinetic disorders are common reasons for performing ECG in an asymptomatic teen

- Routine use of ECG is not recommended by the American Academy of Pediatrics and American Heart Association because of concerns for false-negative and false-positive results and availability of resources

- Computer interpretation of an ECG for the pediatric population, including adolescents, is fraught with errors and can lead to unwarranted referral and anxiety for parents and patient

- It is important that all pediatric ECGs are reviewed by health care providers trained in interpreting pediatric ECGs

- Primary-care providers should familiarize themselves with the benign variation on an ECG, age-related evolutionary changes, and changes related to physical conditioning

- Primary providers should be trained to recognize findings on an ECG that may suggest a cardiac disease so that appropriate referral to a subspecialist can be made

- Detailed personal and family history along with a comprehensive examination may aid interpretation of an ECG and further management

- There may be risk of sudden death even in asymptomatic patients with WPW pattern on an ECG, hence appropriate referral is warranted for risk stratification

- Inaccurate prolongation of the corrected QT interval is frequently encountered in computer-generated reports; QTc should be calculated manually in these situations and appropriate referral should be made

SUMMARY

It is important to distinguish between the evolutionary changes, benign variants, and abnormal findings on an ECG. Abnormal findings can be related to significant heart disease. Trusting a computer-generated interpretation in pediatrics can lead to unwarranted referral and parental anxiety. All ECGs in this age group should be read by individuals knowledgeable in pediatric ECG interpretation. The further workup in patients with abnormal ECG findings is based on personal and family history, physical examination, and the kind of abnormality detected, because certain findings have a higher likelihood of heart disease and risk of sudden cardiac death.

REFERENCES

1. Pelliccia A, Maron BJ, Culasso F, et al. Clinical significance of abnormal electrocardiographic patterns in trained athletes. Circulation 2000;102(3): 278–84.
2. Corrado D, Pelliccia A, Heidbuchel H, et al. Recommendations for interpretation of 12-lead electrocardiogram in the athlete. Eur Heart J 2010;31(2):243–59.
3. Davignon A, Rautaharju PM, Boisselle E, et al. Normal ECG standards for infants and children. Pediatr Cardiol 1980;1(2):123–31.
4. Rijnbeek PR, Witsenburg M, Schrama E, et al. New normal limits for the paediatric electrocardiogram. Eur Heart J 2001;22(8):702–11.
5. Rijnbeek PR, van Herpen G, Kapusta L, et al. Electrocardiographic criteria for left ventricular hypertrophy in children. Pediatr Cardiol 2008;29(5):923–8.
6. Sokolow M, Lyon TP. The ventricular complex in left ventricular hypertrophy as obtained by unipolar precordial and limb leads. Am Heart J 1949;37(2): 161–86.
7. Casale PN, Devereux RB, Alonso DR, et al. Improved sex-specific criteria of left ventricular hypertrophy for clinical and computer interpretation of electrocardiograms: validation with autopsy findings. Circulation 1987;75(3):565–72.
8. Romhilt DW, Estes EH Jr. A point-score system for the ECG diagnosis of left ventricular hypertrophy. Am Heart J 1968;75(6):752–8.
9. Shah N, Chintala K, Aggarwal S. Electrocardiographic strain pattern in children with left ventricular hypertrophy: a marker of ventricular dysfunction. Pediatr Cardiol 2010;31(6):800–6.
10. Jain A, Chandna H, Silber EN, et al. Electrocardiographic patterns of patients with echocardiographically determined biventricular hypertrophy. J Electrocardiol 1999;32(3):269–73.
11. Tsao CW, Josephson ME, Hauser TH, et al. Accuracy of electrocardiographic criteria for atrial enlargement: validation with cardiovascular magnetic resonance. J Cardiovasc Magn Reson 2008;10:7.
12. Alpert MA, Munuswamy K. Electrocardiographic diagnosis of left atrial enlargement. Arch Intern Med 1989;149(5):1161–5.
13. Josephson ME, Kastor JA, Morganroth J. Electrocardiographic left atrial enlargement. Electrophysiologic, echocardiographic and hemodynamic correlates. Am J Cardiol 1977;39(7):967–71.
14. Hancock EW, Deal BJ, Mirvis DM, et al. AHA/ACCF/HRS recommendations for the standardization and interpretation of the electrocardiogram: part V: electrocardiogram changes associated with cardiac chamber hypertrophy: a scientific statement from the American Heart Association Electrocardiography and Arrhythmias Committee, Council on Clinical Cardiology; the American College of Cardiology Foundation; and the Heart Rhythm Society. Endorsed by the

International Society for Computerized Electrocardiology. J Am Coll Cardiol 2009;53(11):992–1002.

15. Ziegler RF. Electrocardiographic studies in normal infants and children. Springfield (IL): Charles C Thomas; 1951.

16. Wershing JM, Walker CH. Influence of age, sex, and body habitus on the mean QRS electrical axis in childhood and adolescence. Br Heart J 1963; 25:601–9.

17. Stephen JM, Dhindsa H, Browne B, et al. Interpretation and clinical significance of the QRS axis of the electrocardiogram. J Emerg Med 1990;8(6):757–63.

18. Perloff JK, Roberts NK, Cabeen WR Jr. Left axis deviation: a reassessment. Circulation 1979;60(1):12–21.

19. Choo JK, Abernethy WB 3rd, Hutter AM Jr. Electrocardiographic observations in professional football players. Am J Cardiol 2002;90(2):198–200.

20. Neumar RW, Otto CW, Link MS, et al. Part 8: adult advanced cardiovascular life support: 2010 American Heart Association guidelines for cardiopulmonary resuscitation and emergency cardiovascular care. Circulation 2010;122(18 Suppl 3):S729–67.

21. Mangrum JM, DiMarco JP. The evaluation and management of bradycardia. N Engl J Med 2000;342(10):703–9.

22. Knoebel SB, Fisch C. Accelerated junctional escape. A clinical and electrocardiographic study. Circulation 1974;50(1):151–8.

23. Jacobsen JR, Garson A Jr, Gillette PC, et al. Premature ventricular contractions in normal children. J Pediatr 1978;92(1):36–8.

24. Nagashima M, Matsushima M, Ogawa A, et al. Cardiac arrhythmias in healthy children revealed by 24-hour ambulatory ECG monitoring. Pediatr Cardiol 1987;8(2):103–8.

25. Tsuda J, Niimura I, Matsuo M. Statistics of arrhythmias in school age. Health guidance of heart disease in childhood [in Japanese]. Jpn Med J 1982;3035: 43–8.

26. Sobotka PA, Mayer JH, Bauernfeind RA, et al. Arrhythmias documented by 24-hour continuous ambulatory electrocardiographic monitoring in young women without apparent heart disease. Am Heart J 1981;101(6):753–9.

27. Brodsky M, Wu D, Denes P, et al. Arrhythmias documented by 24 hour continuous electrocardiographic monitoring in 50 male medical students without apparent heart disease. Am J Cardiol 1977;39(3):390–5.

28. Hiss RG, Lamb LE. Electrocardiographic findings in 122,043 individuals. Circulation 1962;25:947–61.

29. Strauss DG, Selvester RH, Wagner GS. Defining left bundle branch block in the era of cardiac resynchronization therapy. Am J Cardiol 2011;107(6):927–34.

30. Pelliccia A, Culasso F, Di Paolo FM, et al. Prevalence of abnormal electrocardiograms in a large, unselected population undergoing pre-participation cardiovascular screening. Eur Heart J 2007;28(16):2006–10.

31. Francia P, Balla C, Paneni F, et al. Left bundle-branch block–pathophysiology, prognosis, and clinical management. Clin Cardiol 2007;30(3):110–5.

32. Goldman MJ. Principles of clinical electrocardiography. 12th edition. Los Altos (CA): Lange Medical; 1986.

33. Agarwal AK, Venugopalan P. Right bundle branch block: varying electrocardiographic patterns. Aetiological correlation, mechanisms and electrophysiology. Int J Cardiol 1999;71(1):33–9.

34. Chiu SN, Wang JK, Wu MH, et al. Cardiac conduction disturbance detected in a pediatric population. J Pediatr 2008;152(1):85–9.

35. Niwa K, Warita N, Sunami Y, et al. Prevalence of arrhythmias and conduction disturbances in large population-based samples of children. Cardiol Young 2004;14(1):68–74.
36. Surawicz B, Knilans TK. Chou's electrocardiography in clinical practice: adult and pediatric. 5th edition. Philadelphia: WB Saunders; 2001.
37. Kobza R, Cuculi F, Abacherli R, et al. Twelve-lead electrocardiography in the young: physiologic and pathologic abnormalities. Heart Rhythm 2012;9(12): 2018–22.
38. Sornsin S. First degree atrioventricular block. J Emerg Med 1987;5(1):29–34.
39. Zeppilli P, Fenici R, Sassara M, et al. Wenckebach second-degree A-V block in top-ranking athletes: an old problem revisited. Am Heart J 1980;100(3):281–94.
40. Wogan JM, Lowenstein SR, Gordon GS. Second-degree atrioventricular block: Mobitz type II. J Emerg Med 1993;11(1):47–54.
41. Guize L, Soria R, Chaouat JC, et al. Prevalence and course of Wolf-Parkinson-White syndrome in a population of 138,048 subjects. Ann Med Interne (Paris) 1985;136(6):474–8.
42. Goudevenos JA, Katsouras CS, Graekas G, et al. Ventricular pre-excitation in the general population: a study on the mode of presentation and clinical course. Heart 2000;83(1):29–34.
43. Munger TM, Packer DL, Hammill SC, et al. A population study of the natural history of Wolff-Parkinson-White syndrome in Olmsted County, Minnesota, 1953-1989. Circulation 1993;87(3):866–73.
44. Cain N, Irving C, Webber S, et al. Natural history of Wolff-Parkinson-White syndrome diagnosed in childhood. Am J Cardiol 2013;112(7):961–5.
45. Pediatric and Congenital Electrophysiology Society (PACES), Heart Rhythm Society (HRS), American College of Cardiology Foundation (ACCF), et al. PACES/HRS expert consensus statement on the management of the asymptomatic young patient with a Wolff-Parkinson-White (WPW, ventricular preexcitation) electrocardiographic pattern: developed in partnership between the Pediatric and Congenital Electrophysiology Society (PACES) and the Heart Rhythm Society (HRS). Endorsed by the governing bodies of PACES, HRS, the American College of Cardiology Foundation (ACCF), the American Heart Association (AHA), the American Academy of Pediatrics (AAP), and the Canadian Heart Rhythm Society (CHRS). Heart Rhythm 2012;9(6):1006–24.
46. Sharma S, Whyte G, Elliott P, et al. Electrocardiographic changes in 1000 highly trained junior elite athletes. Br J Sports Med 1999;33(5):319–24.
47. Pelliccia A, Di Paolo FM, Quattrini FM, et al. Outcomes in athletes with marked ECG repolarization abnormalities. N Engl J Med 2008;358(2):152–61.
48. Wilson MG, Sharma S, Carre F, et al. Significance of deep T-wave inversions in asymptomatic athletes with normal cardiovascular examinations: practical solutions for managing the diagnostic conundrum. Br J Sports Med 2012; 46(Suppl 1):i51–8.
49. Roukoz H, Wang K. ST elevation and inverted T wave as another normal variant mimicking acute myocardial infarction: the prevalence, age, gender, and racial distribution. Ann Noninvasive Electrocardiol 2011;16(1):64–9.
50. Goldman MJ. RS-T segment elevation in mid- and left precordial leads as a normal variant. Am Heart J 1953;46(6):817–20.
51. Wang K, Asinger RW, Marriott HJ. ST-segment elevation in conditions other than acute myocardial infarction. N Engl J Med 2003;349(22):2128–35.
52. Antzelevitch C, Brugada P, Borggrefe M, et al. Brugada syndrome: report of the second consensus conference. Heart Rhythm 2005;2(4):429–40.

53. Junttila MJ, Gonzalez M, Lizotte E, et al. Induced Brugada-type electrocardiogram, a sign for imminent malignant arrhythmias. Circulation 2008;117(14): 1890–3.
54. Conover MB. Understanding electrocardiography. 8th edition. St Louis (MO): Mosby; 2003.
55. Bross U, Bruggemann G, Schmaltz AA. Deep Q waves in the ECG of children– an electro-, vector- and echocardiographic study. Monatsschr Kinderheilkd 1985;133(7):476–82.
56. Goldberger AL. Pathogenesis and diagnosis of Q waves on the electrocardiogram. In: Rose BD, editor. Waltham (MA): 2006.
57. Kautzener J. QT interval measurements. Card Electrophysiol Rev 2002;6(3): 273–7.
58. Garson A Jr, Dick M 2nd, Fournier A, et al. The long QT syndrome in children. An international study of 287 patients. Circulation 1993;87(6):1866–72.
59. Basavarajaiah S, Wilson M, Whyte G, et al. Prevalence and significance of an isolated long QT interval in elite athletes. Eur Heart J 2007;28(23):2944–9.
60. Johnson JN, Ackerman MJ. QTc: how long is too long? Br J Sports Med 2009; 43(9):657–62.

The Teenager with Palpitations

Farshad Sedaghat-Yazdi, MD*, Peter R. Koenig, MD

KEYWORDS

- Palpitations • Teenager • Pediatric • Supraventricular tachycardia
- Sinus tachycardia

KEY POINTS

- The history and physical examination, along with an ECG, should provide a general diagnostic category of the palpitations.
- Every portion of the history is important: the history of present illness; review of systems; and medical, family, social, as well as medication history; including information of drugs of abuse. Issues specific to teenagers should be addressed.
- Further testing (if needed), should be able to provide a specific diagnosis.
- Patients with a cardiac cause of palpitations and/or nonsinus tachycardia should be referred to a pediatric cardiologist for further evaluation.

INTRODUCTION

Palpitations are a common complaint in teenagers,[1–3] and are defined as a feeling or awareness of an irregular, rapid, or strong beating of the heart.[4] They can result from cardiac awareness (increased conscious perception of the heart beating) or from a fast or irregular cardiac rhythm. The term palpitation is typically used by older children or adolescents, instead of than toddlers or young children. The causes of palpitations are typically benign, though they can cause anxiety and concern to the family and individual. It is important to differentiate cardiac from noncardiac causes of palpitations, given the potential risk of sudden death or injury in those patients with an underlying cardiac cause. The history and physical examination is the physician's most useful tool, followed by specific diagnostic testing to distinguish cardiac causes from noncardiac causes of palpitations. A standard 12-lead ECG is an excellent additional screening tool. Further laboratory testing may be needed, based on whether or not there are concerns for noncardiac causes such as dehydration, anemia, or hyperthyroidism. In most cases, an immediate diagnosis cannot be made and additional testing might be necessary, such as ambulatory ECG monitoring, exercise stress testing, or

Department of Cardiology, The Willis J. Potts Heart Center, Ann & Robert H. Lurie Children's Hospital of Chicago, Feinberg School of Medicine, Northwestern University, 225 East Chicago Avenue, Box 21, Chicago, IL 60611-2605, USA
* Corresponding author.
E-mail address: fsedaghatyazdi@luriechildrens.org

Pediatr Clin N Am 61 (2014) 63–79
http://dx.doi.org/10.1016/j.pcl.2013.09.010
0031-3955/14/$ – see front matter © 2014 Elsevier Inc. All rights reserved.

echocardiography. Most causes for palpitations in the teenager can be diagnosed with minimal testing. Patients with an abnormal ECG (eg, long QT, Wolff-Parkinson White syndrome, heart block, ST-segment and T-wave abnormalities), abnormal cardiac examination, concerning family history, or palpitations associated with activity or syncope should be referred to a pediatric cardiologist. This article discusses the evaluation, testing, and management of teenagers with palpitations. It also provides a general guideline for referral for subspecialty evaluation.

EPIDEMIOLOGY

The incidence of palpitations in the teenage population varies greatly depending on the study. Adult studies have shown that the incidence of palpitations in the primary care setting is estimated to be approximately 16%.[5,6] Of patients presenting with palpitations, a cardiac cause accounted for 43% of cases; whereas 31% were due to as a psychiatric disorder, 6% to drugs, and 4% to other causes.[6] An arrhythmia, typically supraventricular tachycardia (SVT), has been reported to correlate with palpitations in 10% to 15% of young patients.[7] Despite frequent occurrences in some patients, a particular cause for the palpitations may not be found.

Key message

- Palpitations are a common complaint during adolescence in a primary care setting.
- Most commonly, palpitations are benign; however, they can cause tremendous anxiety for parents and patients.
- It is important to differentiate increased cardiac awareness from other cardiac or noncardiac causes of palpitations.
- A history and physical with ECG in selected cases may be a sufficient initial work up.
- Palpitation in patients with an abnormal ECG, abnormal cardiac examination, concerning family history, or in association with activity or syncope should be referred for a subspecialty evaluation.

DIFFERENTIAL DIAGNOSIS

The differential diagnosis of palpitations is extensive, though they can be grouped into similar broad categories (**Box 1**). This list is not comprehensive but is a general list of the wide range of the different causes of palpitations.

DIAGNOSTIC APPROACH TO A TEENAGER WITH PALPITATIONS

Evaluation of a teenager with a complaint of palpitations begins with a history, physical examination, and an ECG. Any further testing should be obtained based on findings and suspicion. **Fig. 1** is an algorithm approach to the teenager presenting with palpitations. The general thought is to differentiate palpitations into enhanced cardiac awareness, an irregular rhythm, or a tachycardia. If a tachycardia is confirmed, it should be differentiated into either sinus or nonsinus tachycardia. The detailed history is comprised of several parts, each of which may provide clues as to the cause of the palpitations.

History

History of present illness
There is a wide variety of terms used to describe the sensation of palpitations, including fluttering, racing, skip beats, or pounding. Important aspects of the

Box 1
Differential diagnosis of palpitations

1. Cardiac awareness
2. Sinus tachycardia
   a. Cardiac causes (nonarrhythmia)
      - Cardiomyopathy, myocarditis, pericardial effusion
      - Congenital heart disease
        Large left-to-right shunts
        Valve lesions with a reduced stroke volume
   b. Extracardiac causes
      - Anemia
      - Fever
      - Hyperthyroidism
      - Hypoglycemia
      - Hypovolemia or dehydration
      - Neurocardiogenic syncope
      - Pheochromocytoma
   c. Psychiatric causes
      - Anxiety
      - Panic attacks
   d. Drugs, medications, and substance abuse
      - Alcohol
      - Caffeine or energy drinks
      - Drugs of abuse (cocaine, phenylcyclohexyl piperidine [PCP], marijuana, tobacco)
      - Over-the-counter medications (cold medicines)
      - Prescription medications (stimulants, beta agonists)
   e. Inappropriate sinus tachycardia
3. Arrhythmia and nonsinus tachycardia
   - Premature atrial and ventricular contractions
   - Atrial flutter and fibrillation
   - Supraventricular tachycardia (including Wolff-Parkinson-White)
   - Ectopic atrial tachycardia
   - Junctional tachycardia
   - Ventricular tachycardia

subjective details from the patient include the onset of the palpitations, frequency, and duration of symptoms, occurrence with exertion, and associated symptoms such as chest pain, dizziness, or syncope. Each of these aspects of history may provide suggestions for the next step in evaluation. For example, symptoms with exercise should raise a red flag. These may be best evaluated by an exercise stress test that reproduces the symptoms in a controlled environment. Palpitations with a

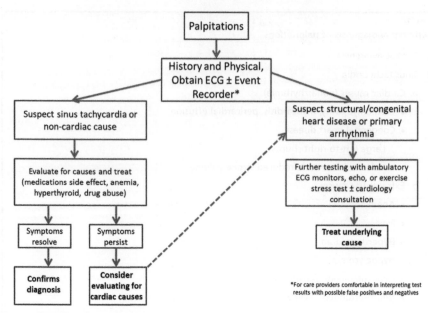

Fig. 1. Algorithm for evaluating a teenager with palpitations.

sudden onset and complete resolution after several minutes are suggestive of an arrhythmia, such as paroxysmal SVT or ventricular tachycardia (VT).[8] Symptoms that last for a second or a single heartbeat are suggestive of isolated ectopic beats. Symptoms that are present all of the time and have vague descriptions are unlikely to be cardiac in origin. If palpitations precede any syncopal episodes, the physician should obtain specific details and inquire about associated symptoms. Symptoms of blurry or tunnel vision, nausea, pallor, and dizziness with positional changes are suggestive of a vasovagal cause. Palpitations are a frequent complaint with neurocardiogenic syncope (see article elsewhere in this issue for detailed discussion of syncope) and are most likely secondary to an appropriate increase in the patient's heart rate in an attempt to increase the cardiac output.[9] If this is a suspected diagnosis, a detailed diet history should be obtained, including specific amounts of daily fluid intake and types of beverages consumed. Unfortunately, many teenage patients are poor historians and may not be able to give an accurate description of their symptoms.

A simple starting point for many patients may be to advise them or their parents to count the pulse during an episode of palpitations and record the rate, duration, and subjective assessment of the onset and termination of the sensation (gradual or sudden) in a diary or journal. There may be some resistance to this strategy, but most parents can be encouraged by teaching them a simple technique of counting the pulse. Clinically useful information can emerge from this attempt. Writing down the results of their efforts is crucial.

Review of systems
A thorough review of systems should be performed. Focused questions regarding each system should be included in every history. This can be especially helpful in teenagers who have a difficult time describing their symptoms. Each item in the review of systems may lead to further questions in a directed manner that may help guide the

differential diagnosis. **Table 1** lists positive findings and associated causes of palpitations in teenagers.[10]

Past medical history and review of medications

The past medical history is another valuable clue to assess possible causes of palpitations. Many medical problems may predispose patients to feelings of palpitations, such as hypoglycemia in a patient with diabetes after receiving an inappropriate amount of insulin or an asthmatic receiving albuterol treatments (which will increase the heart rate). A detailed review of the medications, both prescribed and over-the-counter should be performed because increased heart rates and arrhythmias can be common side effects of many medications. Patients with chronic medical problems and a history of prolonged hospitalization could be at higher risk for other medical problems, which may explain the cause of their palpitations (eg, infection or anemia). Any patient with a history of congenital or acquired heart disease, arrhythmias, or cardiac surgery presenting with palpitations warrants more urgent evaluation and further discussion with the patient's cardiologist.

Family and social history

The family history should include any history of congenital heart disease and surgery, sudden or unexplained death, arrhythmias, and pacemaker or defibrillator placement (especially at a young age). In addition, it should include a detailed history of other noncardiac problems such as endocrine (thyroid disorder), rheumatologic (systemic lupus erythematosus), hematologic (anemia, bleeding disorder, sickle cell disorder),

Table 1
Review of systems and potential causes of palpitations

System	Differential Diagnosis
General—weight change, fever, night sweats	Thyroid disorder, anorexia, infection
Head, ears, eyes, nose, and throat—frequent sore throat	Rheumatic fever
Respiratory—wheezing, cough, shortness of breath	Pneumonia, asthma, heart failure
Cardiovascular—chest pain, syncope, dyspnea on exertion, edema	Acquired or congenital heart disease
Gastrointestinal—persistent vomiting, diarrhea, abdominal distention, blood in stool	Dehydration, electrolyte imbalance, heart failure, anemia
Genitourinary—dysuria, nocturia and polyuria	Infectious (sexually transmitted disease or urinary tract infection or pyelonephritis)
Muscular or skeletal—joint pain or swelling	Rheumatic fever, infection
Skin—rash, dry or oily skin	Infection, thyroid disorder
Neurologic—headaches, syncope, abnormal movement	Seizure disorder, intracranial process with autonomic dysfunction
Hematologic—history of easy bruising and bleeding	Anemia or pancytopenia
Endocrine—thyroid enlargement, heat or cold intolerance, polyuria	Thyroid disorder, diabetes (possibility of overdose from insulin therapy causing hypoglycemia)
Menses—onset, prolonged duration or heavy periods	Anemia
Psychiatric—anxiety, depression	Anxiety, panic disorder

neurologic (seizure disorder), and psychiatric disorders. The social history in the teenager should address any associated emotional and social problems, such as change of school systems, bullying, parental arguments, smoking, and illegal drug use (see later discussion).

Physical Examination

A comprehensive physical examination should be performed in every patient. Vital signs should include the heart rate in the supine, sitting, and standing positions, and they should be referenced with age-appropriate normal ranges (**Table 2**). Elevated heart rates may be secondary to normal physiologic responses such as anxiety or dehydration. Blood pressure should also be obtained in the supine and standing positions. The heart rate and blood pressure may help diagnose orthostatic hypotension or postural orthostatic tachycardia syndrome (see article elsewhere in this issue for further discussion of the latter).

All portions of the physical examination are important and should not be overlooked. **Table 3** lists abnormal physical examination findings, which may help narrow the differential diagnosis of possible causes of the palpitations. Specifically, the cardiac examination should evaluate for heart rate and rhythm, pathologic murmurs, clicks, rubs, peripheral and central pulses, and perfusion. If there are any concerns with the cardiac examination, further testing or referral to a pediatric cardiologist may be necessary.

ECG

A standard 12-lead ECG should be an initial test for evaluating a patient with palpitations. The ECG defines the rhythm at rest and may be diagnostic if the patient is having symptoms at the time of the ECG. Findings that should not be missed are abnormal atrioventricular (AV) nodal conduction, a prolonged QT interval (which may suggest polymorphic VT), delta wave or short PR interval (which may suggest preexcitation), or ST-segment and T-wave abnormalities (which may suggest coronary artery abnormalities, myocarditis, or cardiomyopathy).

Echocardiogram

An ECG is used to evaluate cardiac anatomy, origin of the coronary arteries, valve abnormalities, heart size and thickness, shunts, function, and effusion. An echocardiogram is typically not obtained for isolated palpitations in a patient with a normal ECG.[11] Abnormalities on history, physical examination, or ECG suggesting structural or mechanical heart disease should be evaluated with an echocardiogram.

Laboratory Testing

A complete blood count should be ordered in patients with suspicion for anemia or an infectious cause. A free T4 and a thyroid-stimulating hormone test should be ordered if there is suspicion of hyperthyroidism. This is more likely in the setting of a persistent,

Table 2 Normal heart rates for age	
Age	Heart Rate (beats per minute)
12–16 y	60–110 (85)
≥16 y	60–100 (80)

Data from Gajewski KK. Cardiology. In: Robertson J, Shilkofski N, editors. The John Hopkins Hospital: the Harriet Lane handbook: a manual for pediatric house officers. 17th edition. Philadelphia: Elsevier Mosby; 2005. p. 159–209.

Table 3	
Pertinent physical examination findings and possible causes of palpitations	
Physical Examination Finding	**Differential Diagnosis**
General—weight, mood and appearance of patient	Obese (deconditioned), anorexia, anxiety
Eyes—exophthalmos	Hyperthyroidism
Ears, nose, throat, or mouth—goiter, tonsillar erythema	Thyroid disorder, rheumatic disease
Respiratory—wheezing, rales, crackles	Asthma (and side effects from asthma medication), infection (pneumonia), pulmonary edema from heart failure
Cardiovascular—heart rate or rhythm, pathologic murmur, abnormal pulses, poor perfusion	Structural heart defect, arrhythmias, heart failure
Abdomen—liver size, ascites	Heart failure, renal disease and changes in volume status
Muscular—joint pain or swelling, edema	Rheumatic disease, heart failure
Neurologic—abnormal neurology examination	Possible intracranial process

mostly continuous, sinus tachycardia. Electrolytes should be evaluated in patients with persistent vomiting or diarrhea, concern for anorexia, or chronic medication use, which could affect electrolyte levels. A urine-specific gravity can be ordered to evaluate the hydration status of a patient. Currently, there is no consensus regarding the best diagnostic test for pheochromocytoma. The two major tests available are a 24-hour urinary fractionated catecholamine and metanephrine level and a plasma fractionated metanephrine level. Further discussion of specific laboratory testing is beyond the scope of this article and consultation should take place with an expert if there is a high suspicion of pheochromocytoma.[12,13]

Ambulatory ECG Monitors (Holter Versus Event Monitor)

A normal resting ECG does not exclude cardiac arrhythmias, especially if the patient is not experiencing symptoms at the time of this very brief test. If the suspicion for an arrhythmia is high and the office ECG is normal, further investigation should include ambulatory ECG monitoring. Determining which type of monitor to order is based on the frequency and duration of symptoms. **Table 4** summarizes the indications and advantages of the various ambulatory ECG monitors.

A Holter monitor is a continuous ambulatory monitor that is placed for 24 to 48 hours and it continuously records the rhythm for that period. If a patient is complaining of daily symptoms, a Holter monitor is the ideal monitor. These recorders are widely available and easy to set up. A patient can manually record the time and type of symptoms on a diary, or electronically press an event entry to match the symptoms with the ECG tracing. There are several limitations with the Holter monitor: its relatively short duration of time to evaluate an arrhythmia and noncompliant teenagers who may not record their symptoms. Studies have shown that Holter recordings have a low diagnostic yield[14] and, therefore, might be more useful in other clinical situations (such as determining average heart rate, heart rate variability, or clinically silent arrhythmias in high-risk groups). Despite the limitations, Holter monitoring gives the best global, extended picture of heart rate over time. A "negative" Holter, even without the symptom occurring during the recording period, still offers insight into the rate and rhythm related behavior of the heart during sleep and wake cycles.

Table 4
Ambulatory monitoring in teenagers with palpitations: indications, advantages, and disadvantages

Type of Device	Indications	Advantages	Disadvantages
Holter	• Daily symptoms	• Widely available • Easy setup	• Short monitoring duration • Requires patient to record symptoms • Lower diagnostic yield
Looping Event Recorder	• Infrequent and short duration of palpitations	• Useful in correlating symptoms to rhythm • Records onset of arrhythmia (if present)	• Requires patient compliance (must wear monitor continuously or very frequently) • Requires frequent lead replacement
Nonlooping Event Recorder	• Infrequent and longer duration of palpitations	• Small and lightweight device • No lead placement (device applied directly to chest or body part)	• Requires patient compliance • Does not record onset of arrhythmia (if present)
Autotriggered Event Recorder	• Infrequent episodes when patient cannot activate monitor (syncope or if arrhythmia is clinically silent and patient is asymptomatic)	• Can program specific heart rate and rhythm triggers to activate monitor • Records onset of arrhythmia	• Requires patient compliance • Many triggers may be secondary to artifact
Implantable Loop Recorder	• Infrequent episodes of palpitations associated with syncope • Negative results from other forms of monitoring and persistent symptoms	• Long monitoring period (months to year) • Can program to capture events on predetermined settings • Patient may activate if symptomatic	• Surgical procedure to place and remove device • Risk of infection

If palpitations do not occur on a daily basis, an event monitor is a more cost-effective and practical method to evaluate for an arrhythmia.[15,16] Event monitors are typically ordered for 30 days but can be extended for longer periods if needed. These monitors record ECG activity only when activated by the patient. Data can be transmitted over a telephone line, which can then be interpreted by a cardiologist. There are typically two kinds of event monitors, looping and nonlooping event monitors.

A looping event monitor is worn by patients whose symptoms are infrequent and short lived. The monitor needs to be worn most of the time, if not continuously, with the goal of trying to capture as many episodes as possible. Looping recorders have a continuous memory loop, which, on patient activation, stores several minutes of rhythm data before and after activation, which can then be transmitted for interpretation. An important benefit of this type of recording is that if an arrhythmia is detected, the preactivation rhythm, initiation, and perhaps termination of the arrhythmia may be recorded. The limitation with this type of monitor is that it requires compliance from the patient to wear the monitor daily for most of the time, which may be difficult for a teenager.

A nonlooping event monitor is ideal for patients who have infrequent episodes that last for a longer duration (usually several minutes). The patient must have enough time to obtain the monitor and place it appropriately on his/her bare chest (or other body part) to record the electrical activity. The advantage of this monitor is that they are lightweight and do not require wearing chest electrodes. The major limitations are compliance among teenagers (they may forget to keep the monitor with them, or not use it) and the inability to record the initiation of the arrhythmia.

There are other, more complex, types of monitors available. One such monitor is similar to a telemetry system used in the hospital, except that it is worn by the patient outside of the hospital. The device continuously monitors the patient's rhythm and automatically detects arrhythmias or elevated heart rates with subsequent transmission for immediate evaluation. An implantable loop recorder placed subcutaneously is yet another option in patients in whom the suspicion of an arrhythmia is very high but an arrhythmia has not been captured with the forms of testing already discussed.[17] Further discussion of these types of monitors is beyond the scope of this article.

According to the American College of Cardiology/American Heart Association guidelines, ambulatory ECG monitoring is a class I indication in patients with palpitations who have a history of surgery for congenital heart disease and significant residual hemodynamic abnormalities. It is also a class IIa indication in patients with palpitations "in the absence of a reasonable explanation and where there is no overt clinical evidence of heart disease."[7]

Exercise Stress Testing

Patients who experience palpitations with exercise should cause concern, especially if there is associated chest pain or syncope. In addition to possible cardiology consultation and an echocardiogram (to rule out a major coronary artery anomaly or cardiomyopathy), these patients should be evaluated with an exercise stress test to monitor for reproducible symptoms and evaluate the rhythm during exercise with an attempt to correlate symptoms with the underlying rhythm. It is also useful to evaluate for ischemia secondary to coronary artery disease or cardiomyopathy and for catecholamine-sensitive arrhythmias (see later discussion). The latter diagnosis is of importance because undiagnosed cases could potentially place the patient at an increased risk of mortality, especially with exercise.

Electrophysiology Study

An electrophysiology study (EPS) is typically performed in patients after the first tier of diagnostics are completed. The two common types of EPSs are transesophageal pacing (TEP) and intracardiac EPSs. TEP uses an esophageal electrode pair, placed through the nose or mouth, to induce arrhythmias, assess for accessory pathways, and study the properties of the AV node or accessory pathway. This technique is most frequently used in infants with arrhythmias and for risk-stratification in older children with Wolff-Parkinson-White (WPW) syndrome.[18,19] An intracardiac EPS involves placement of catheters directly into the heart via percutaneous approach. It is able to perform the same diagnostic functions as TEP; however, it may additionally localize an arrhythmogenic focus or pathway. In some cases, the arrhythmia focus can be altered or eradicated during the same procedure. Although the risks of an EPS are relatively modest, EPSs are typically reserved for patients with structural heart disease and concern of an arrhythmia or for patients with a structurally normal heart and a documented arrhythmia or abnormal conduction (especially SVT and WPW syndrome).

Key message

- All aspects of history of present illness are important in evaluating palpitations.
- A simple starting point for many patients may be counting and recording a pulse during the symptoms.
- A detailed examination may guide further testing or referral to a subspecialist.
- ECG is diagnostic if performed during the symptoms.
- Based on the frequency of symptoms, a continuous ambulatory (Holter monitor) or an event monitor can be performed to capture the ECG during symptoms.
- Selective use of echocardiogram, exercise stress test, and/or EPS may be helpful.

SPECIFIC CAUSES AND MANAGEMENT
Sinus Tachycardia

Appropriate sinus tachycardia: physiologic and nonphysiologic causes

Sinus tachycardia is an increase in the heart rate while maintaining a normal conduction sequence between the atria and ventricle. On an ECG, it is seen as a normal P-wave morphology followed by a normal QRS morphology and a heart rate greater than expected for the patient's age. Because the heart rate multiplied by the stroke volume of the heart equals the cardiac output, increasing the heart rate will increase cardiac output. The sinus rate is determined by the sinus node (pacemaker of the heart), which is in turn influenced by several factors. The brain (which senses cardiac output, namely oxygen and glucose delivery) and the autonomic nervous system play an important part in maintaining cardiac output by controlling and increasing the heart rate through mechanisms that increase endogenous catecholamines and/or increase sympathetic tone, which then feed back on the sinus node. The heart rate may be increased due to a perceived (eg, stress, anxiety, fear) or physiologic (eg, exercise) need to increase cardiac output. It may also be increased due to pathologic causes (eg, with severe anemia or desaturation to increase oxygen delivery, or with hypoglycemia to maintain glucose delivery). Sinus tachycardia may also occur to maintain cardiac output, when stroke volume has decreased to maintain the metabolic needs of the body. Thus, with a low volume (preload) as seen with dehydration or other causes of low intravascular volume, or with decreased cardiac function (contractility) as seen with myocarditis or a cardiomyopathy, the heart rate will increase appropriately to maintain cardiac output. Because sinus tachycardia causes increased cardiac output, the patient may perceive this as an "increased forcefulness" in the heartbeat and may describe it as palpitations.

The history and physical examination, as well as limited testing, should provide the cause of sinus tachycardia based on the generalizations previously listed. Many teenagers may have a noncardiac cause for their palpitations. The most common cause of an elevated heart rate is sinus tachycardia and most of the time it is secondary to a normal physiologic (no underlying pathologic organ condition) response. With the obesity epidemic, deconditioned teenagers might be more likely to complain of palpitations due to a greater need to augment cardiac output with activity. However, there is also a wide variety of pathologic causes for sinus tachycardia, such as fever, hypoglycemia, anemia, or hyperthyroidism. In patients with a low suspicion of cardiac disease or arrhythmia, observation with a minimal amount of laboratory testing should be the first-line of testing, instead of more advanced cardiac testing.

Congenital and acquired heart disease

Most often, significant congenital heart disease is diagnosed during infancy, especially if there are associated symptoms of cyanosis, murmurs, poor weight gain, or exercise intolerance. Acquired heart diseases may be diagnosed at any age by abnormal cardiac signs or symptoms or due to the associated cardiac disease (eg, Kawasaki disease or rheumatic fever). Any cardiac pathologic condition resulting in a reduced stroke volume (eg, diastolic dysfunction due to pericardial constriction, severe valve regurgitation, reduced systolic dysfunction from a cardiomyopathy, or systemic steal from a large left-to-right shunt) may result in a compensatory sinus tachycardia to maintain cardiac output. The differential diagnosis within these categories is vast. However, all of these diagnoses are effectively detected with the detailed history, physical examination, ECG, and echocardiography.

Medications and substance abuse

As previously mentioned, the patient's list of medications should be reviewed. This should not only include prescription medications, but also over-the-counter medications and any herbal supplements.

Stimulant medications prescribed for attention deficit hyperactivity disorder (ADHD) present a diagnostic conundrum when patients complain of palpitations. The resting heart rate is frequently increased under the influence of these medications. As the resting heart rate increases, small perturbations in rate may produce the subjective sensation of palpitations. As previously mentioned, counting the pulse may help in evaluating this situation. However, the work-up may include ambulatory heart rate monitors.

Drugs of abuse should be discussed and reviewed in every teenager with palpitations. A 2001 survey in youths revealed that 10% of participants used cocaine or methamphetamine.[20] Cocaine is a well-known cause of cardiac ischemia and arrhythmias in adults, which are typically secondary to coronary artery spasms and increased cardiac oxygen demands. Inhalant use has remained prevalent among youths because it is easily available and inexpensive (eg, glue, paint, gasoline). Inhalants sensitize the myocardium to endogenous catecholamines and can predispose the heart to dangerous arrhythmias.[9] It is appropriate to obtain a drug screen in a teenager with unexplainable palpitations if there is suspicion of drug use. Finally, daily caffeine use should be reviewed, including soda, tea, and coffee intake.

Energy drink consumption has increased over the recent years, especially in the teenage and young adult populations. These drinks are specifically targeted with advertising slogans claiming to help increase energy, performance, concentration, and endurance. The main active ingredient in energy drinks is caffeine. A recent study showed that the most common adverse symptom reported with consumption of energy drinks was palpitations.[21] Even small amounts of caffeine can induce tachycardia. Although it is rare, serious toxicity may lead to significant cardiac arrhythmias. The caffeine content in these energy drinks may be higher than that listed on the ingredient list because some ingredients in the drink may contain additional caffeine, which are not labeled on the packaging. In addition, there is a high correlation of coingestion of alcohol and other drugs with energy drinks, which may further precipitate the symptom of palpitations. Teenagers presenting with palpitations should be questioned directly about the use of energy drinks or other substance abuse. More education and awareness is necessary in the community about the dangerous and unpleasant side effects of energy drinks.

Anxiety

Anxiety is a common noncardiac cause of palpitations.[6,22] The prevalence of panic disorders in youth is approximately 2% with the most common symptom in those patients being palpitations (91%), followed by trembling or shaking (86%), dizziness (76%), fainting (71%), and chest pain (64%).[23] These patients also have a difficult time describing the palpitations and have many positive symptoms in their review of systems. One useful description from the history is to determine whether the sense of anxiety started before or after the palpitations. However, it is still important to evaluate carefully patients with known anxiety or psychiatric problems because they may have significant cardiac arrhythmias. In one study of adult subjects with SVT, 67% were diagnosed with panic, stress, or anxiety disorder and 50% had an unrecognized arrhythmia on the initial evaluation. The median time from presentation to diagnosis of SVT was 3.3 years.[24]

Eating disorders

Teenagers, especially females, suffering from anorexia nervosa or bulimia nervosa may commonly present with complaints of palpitations, in addition to dizziness and syncope.[9] This is typically a result of dehydration. Palpitations may also occur because of the use of appetite suppressants or due to arrhythmias secondary to electrolyte imbalances (either from vomiting or chronic use of diuretics). If the diagnosis of anorexia or bulimia is suspected, a collaborative team approach might be necessary to correct the weight carefully with refeeding and to improve the symptoms of palpitations.

Inappropriate sinus tachycardia

Inappropriate sinus tachycardia (IST) is a "syndrome characterized by unexpectedly fast sinus rates at rest, with minimal physical activity, or both," in which associated symptoms (palpitations, weakness, fatigue) may be present.[25] Many patients may not have any associated symptoms and they are referred for elevated heart rates during well examinations and sports physicals. To rule out sinus tachycardia simply from anxiety, it might be appropriate to place a 24-hour Holter monitor to evaluate heart rates in a nonmedical environment. IST is a diagnosis of exclusion and it is crucial to exclude psychological and physiologic triggers that may cause appropriate sinus tachycardia. When evaluating the ECG, the P-wave morphology can be used to determine if the rhythm is sinus and not atrial tachycardia. However, it is not always easy to differentiate between sinus and ectopic atrial tachycardia. An echocardiogram should be obtained to assure that the cardiac function is normal and that there is no pericardial effusion. IST is more common in the female population; however, the exact incidence is not known.[25] The mechanism for IST is complex and not completely understood. Thus, treatment is challenging. Long-term outcomes seem to be benign, so treatment is typically not necessary in asymptomatic patients. Exercise and physical training are helpful and recommended. For patients with persistent symptoms, a trial of beta blockade might be attempted. Lowering the heart rate does not always eliminate symptoms, though, and may even worsen symptoms. Ablation therapy is controversial and beyond the scope of this discussion.

Nonsinus Tachycardia and Other Causes of Palpitations

In a teen presenting with palpitations, it is crucial to exclude life-threatening arrhythmias when the ventricular rate is so fast or unorganized that it reduces cardiac output. Teenagers with a history of repaired congenital or acquired heart disease are at an increased risk of serious arrhythmias. For example, patients with repaired tetralogy of Fallot are at an increased risk of both atrial and ventricular arrhythmias.[26]

Atrial and ventricular premature beats

Atrial premature contractions are common and typically benign. They are commonly seen in patients with and without cardiac disease. Isolated, monomorphic premature ventricular contractions are a common, benign variant. Treatment is typically not warranted for isolated ectopy unless the patient is symptomatic, has underlying heart disease or cardiac dysfunction, a history of syncope, a concerning family history, or if the palpitations are disruptive to the patient's lifestyle. Patients with more complex, frequent, consecutive, or multiform ectopy might require further evaluation and therapy.

SVT

SVT, literally meaning a tachycardia originating above the ventricles, is a common and important cause of palpitations. SVT may include several arrhythmias (sinus tachycardia, ectopic or multifocal atrial tachycardia, atrial flutter, atrial fibrillation, junctional tachycardia, or reentry tachycardia involving the AV node). An important and common cause of SVT in teens is re-entry tachycardia involving the AV node. Two forms of tachycardia involve the AV node. One is AV nodal reciprocating tachycardia (AVNRT) and the other is accessory pathway-mediated tachycardia. In AVNRT, the AV node has two pathways and the tachycardia can circle between the two, causing the atrium and the ventricle to contract rapidly every time the arrhythmia goes around the circle. In accessory pathway-mediated tachycardia, the pathway is separate from the AV node. During tachycardia, conduction goes down the AV node and back up the abnormal pathway. Thus, in both forms of re-entry tachycardia (AVNRT and accessory pathway-mediated tachycardia) a fast, circuitous electrical pathway exists, resulting in stimulation of both the atria and ventricles, as long as this reentry conduction is maintained.

AVNRT rarely appears in infants and it is typically seen in the older child and adolescent.[27-29] Although accessory pathway-mediated tachycardia is commonly seen earlier in life, the first presentation may also occur in teenagers and it should be considered in the evaluation of palpitations. SVT due to these common mechanisms may present as frequent, recurrent paroxysmal episodes of palpitations. In most cases, patients with these arrhythmia mechanisms will have a structurally normal heart.

Accessory pathways can conduct electricity in only one direction (usually from the ventricle back toward the atrium) or in both directions across the AV groove. When conduction occurs downward from the atrium to the ventricle over an accessory pathway, instead of waiting for the AV node to conduct, the ventricle is excited, or preexcited, ahead of schedule via the accessory pathway. This preexcitation manifests as a short PR interval, delta wave, and wide QRS morphology on the resting ECG (**Fig. 2**). The observation of preexcitation on a resting ECG, especially in a patient with accessory pathway-mediated tachycardia, is WPW syndrome. The incidence of WPW in the general population is 3 out of 1000.[5] In addition to being at risk for SVT, these patients have a slightly increased risk of atrial fibrillation, even as a teenager. The accessory conduction pathway is different from pathways in other types of SVT because the accessory conduction pathway allows for anterograde conduction from the atrium to the ventricle, bypassing the AV node (other common pathways allow for only retrograde conduction). Thus, if a patient were to develop atrial fibrillation and the accessory conduction were to allow for fast conduction of the atrial beats, the patient would be at high risk for extremely fast ventricular rates (ventricular fibrillation). There is a very small, but well documented, risk of sudden death in patients with WPW due to ventricular fibrillation by this mechanism. Therefore, patients with WPW, even in absence of tachycardia, warrant evaluation by a pediatric cardiologist for risk stratification.

Because both accessory pathway-mediated tachycardia and AVNRT involve the AV node, most therapies (including vagal maneuvers, pharmacologic therapy, and ablation), are intended to slow or stop conduction through either the abnormal pathway

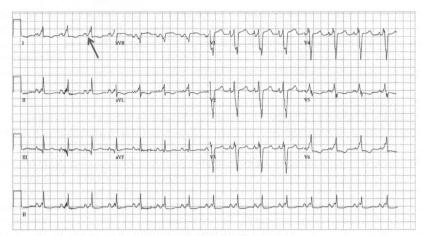

Fig. 2. ECG of a patient with WPW. Note delta wave (*arrow*).

or the AV node and thus terminate the tachycardia.[30] Further evaluation and treatment of SVT is beyond the scope of this article.

VT

Ventricular tachycardia (VT) is rapid, repetitive activation of the heart that is initiated from a location in the ventricle. The morphology, rate, and correlated symptoms are important in determining severity and treatment of the arrhythmia. VT at faster rates with a polymorphic nature (different ventricular complex morphologies on ECG) is more concerning than monomorphic VT at slower rates. Patients found to have VT are typically referred to a pediatric cardiologist, especially if there is a history of syncope.

The causes of VT in the teenager with a structurally normal heart can vary from benign to dangerous pathologic state. A benign cause of VT in the teenage population is right ventricular outflow tract tachycardia. This does not seem to be related to underlying heart disease and has a good prognosis. The cause of this form of VT is unclear but is thought to be secondary to foci of cells in the right ventricular outflow tract with pacemaker properties.[31] This type of VT is usually well tolerated. It is responsive to medical therapy and amenable to catheter ablation in symptomatic patients. A more serious form of VT is catecholaminergic polymorphic VT, which is an abnormally fast and irregular tachycardia that is typically triggered by physical activity or emotional stress. The inheritance pattern can be autosomal dominant or recessive with familial occurrence noted in about 30% of cases.[32] The gene mutations involve receptors that regulate intracellular calcium levels. Most cases present in the first or second decade of life with syncope or palpitations during exercise and emotional stress.[32] Patients for whom there is a high suspicion of this diagnosis may undergo an exercise stress test to monitor for arrhythmias in a controlled environment. The resting ECG is typically normal but, with exercise, bidirectional or polymorphic VT may be induced. There can be increased mortality in untreated cases. Management therapy is beyond the scope of this article but can vary from antiarrhythmic mediations to implantable cardioverter-defibrillator placement.

Long QT Syndrome

Patients with congenital long QT syndrome (LQTS) may have a prolonged QT interval on ECG. LQTS is an ion channelopathy, which can prolong ventricular repolarization and predispose patients to dangerous ventricular arrhythmias, especially torsade de pointes.[27] The rapid ventricular rhythm may result in syncope with short-lived episodes and sudden death if sustained. Palpitations may result from a transient and self-limited run of ventricular arrhythmia. Symptomatic patients (history of syncope) with LQTS who are untreated have a relatively high mortality rate.[27] LQTS should be considered in teenagers with palpitations and syncope when there is a strong family history of sudden death, seizures, unexpected drowning, or single-person car accidents and an abnormal QT interval on ECG. Because LQTS is an inherited disorder, it is important to screen close family members of a patient diagnosed with LQTS. Further discussion regarding the different forms of LQTS and treatment is beyond the scope of this article.

Key message

- Sinus tachycardia is the most common cause of palpitations.
- Sinus tachycardia can be due to physiologic need to increase heart rates or due to a pathologic cause.
- Energy drink consumption is commonly seen in teens can result in palpitations.
- Inappropriate sinus tachycardia is a diagnosis of exclusion.
- Repaired congenital or acquired heart disease patients are at increased risk for arrhythmias.
- Premature contractions, atrial or ventricular, are commonly benign.
- SVT and VT may present as palpitations; therefore, it is important to differentiate them from the other benign causes.

SUMMARY

This article shows an approach to palpitations in the teenager, most of which are diagnosed and categorized based on the history, physical examination, and ECG or other type of recording monitor. Most teenagers with palpitations have either sinus tachycardia, premature beats, or no specific arrhythmogenic cause for their palpitations. The treatment should be within the realm of the general pediatrician without the need for cardiac consultation in most cases. For patients with an underlying cardiac disease, or suspected disease, referral to a pediatric cardiologist is indicated.

REFERENCES

1. Rajagopalan K, Potts JE, Sanatani S. Minimally invasive approach to the child with palpitations. Expert Rev Cardiovasc Ther 2006;4(5):681–93.
2. Batra AS, Hohn AR. Consultation with the specialist: palpitations, syncope, and sudden cardiac death in children: who's at risk? Pediatr Rev 2003;24(8):269–75.
3. Freed MD. Advances in the diagnosis and therapy of syncope and palpitations in children. Curr Opin Pediatr 1994;6(4):368–72.
4. Zimmernam F. Palpitations. In: Koenig P, Hiajzi ZM, Zimmerman F, editors. Essential pediatric cardiology. New York: McGraw-Hill; 2004. p. 23–7.
5. Lawless CE, Briner W. Palpitations in athletes. Sports Med 2008;38(8):687–702.
6. Weber BE, Kapoor WN. Evaluation and outcomes of patients with palpitations. Am J Med 1996;100(2):138–48.
7. Crawford MH, Bernstein SJ, Deedwania PC, et al. ACC/AHA Guidelines for Ambulatory Electrocardiography. A report of the American College of Cardiology/American Heart Association Task Force on Practice Guidelines (Committee

to Revise the Guidelines for Ambulatory Electrocardiography). Developed in collaboration with the North American Society for Pacing and Electrophysiology. J Am Coll Cardiol 1999;34(3):912–48.

8. Mirvis DM. Palpitations. In: Walker HK, Hall WD, Hurst JW, editors. Clinical methods: the history, physical, and laboratory examinations. 3rd edition. Boston: Butterworth Publishers; 1990. p. 76–7.

9. DiVasta AD, Alexander ME. Fainting freshmen and sinking sophomores: cardio-vascular issues of the adolescent. Curr Opin Pediatr 2004;16(4):350–6.

10. Seidel HM, Ball JW, Dains JE, et al. The history and interviewing process. In: Seidel HM, editor. Mosby's guide to physical examination. 5th edition. St Louis (MO): Mosby; 2003. p. 1–37.

11. Daniels CJ, Franklin WH. Common cardiac diseases in adolescents. Pediatr Clin North Am 1997;44(6):1591–601.

12. Sawka AM, Prebtani AP, Thabane L, et al. A systematic review of the literature examining the diagnostic efficacy of measurement of fractionated plasma free metanephrines in the biochemical diagnosis of pheochromocytoma. BMC Endocr Disord 2004;4(1):2.

13. Lenders JW, Pacak K, Walther MM, et al. Biochemical diagnosis of pheochromo-cytoma: which test is best? JAMA 2002;287(11):1427–34.

14. Ayabakan C, Ozer S, Celiker A, et al. Analysis of 2017 Holter records in pediatric patients. Turk J Pediatr 2000;42(4):286–93.

15. Kinlay S, Leitch JW, Neil A, et al. Cardiac event recorders yield more diagnoses and are more cost-effective than 48-hour Holter monitoring in patients with palpi-tations. A controlled clinical trial. Ann Intern Med 1996;124(1 Pt 1):16–20.

16. Abbott AV. Diagnostic approach to palpitations. Am Fam Physician 2005;71(4): 743–50.

17. Rossano J, Bloemers B, Sreeram N, et al. Efficacy of implantable loop recorders in establishing symptom-rhythm correlation in young patients with syncope and palpitations. Pediatrics 2003;112(3 Pt 1):e228–33.

18. Ko JK, Ryu SJ, Ban JE, et al. Use of transesophageal atrial pacing for documen-tation of arrhythmias suspected in infants and children. Jpn Heart J 2004;45(1): 63–72.

19. Fenici R, Ruggieri MP, di Lillo M, et al. Reproducibility of transesophageal pacing in patients with Wolff-Parkinson-White syndrome. Pacing Clin Electrophysiol 1996;19(11 Pt 2):1951–7.

20. Grunbaum JA, Kann L, Kinchen SA, et al. Youth risk behavior surveillance—United States, 2001. MMWR Surveill Summ 2002;51(4):1–62.

21. Gunja N, Brown JA. Energy drinks: health risks and toxicity. Med J Aust 2012; 196(1):46–9.

22. Wexler RK, Pleister A, Raman S. Outpatient approach to palpitations. Am Fam Physician 2011;84(1):63–9.

23. Diler RS, Birmaher B, Brent DA, et al. Phenomenology of panic disorder in youth. Depress Anxiety 2004;20(1):39–43.

24. Lessmeier TJ, Gamperling D, Johnson-Liddon V, et al. Unrecognized paroxysmal supraventricular tachycardia. Potential for misdiagnosis as panic disorder. Arch Intern Med 1997;157(5):537–43.

25. Olshansky B, Sullivan RM. Inappropriate sinus tachycardia. J Am Coll Cardiol 2013;61(8):793–801.

26. Gatzoulis MA, Balaji S, Webber SA, et al. Risk factors for arrhythmia and sudden cardiac death late after repair of tetralogy of Fallot: a multicentre study. Lancet 2000;356(9234):975–81.

27. Doniger SJ, Sharieff GQ. Pediatric dysrhythmias. Pediatr Clin North Am 2006; 53(1):85–105, vi.
28. Sacchetti A, Moyer V, Baricella R, et al. Primary cardiac arrhythmias in children. Pediatr Emerg Care 1999;15(2):95–8.
29. Ko JK, Deal BJ, Strasburger JF, et al. Supraventricular tachycardia mechanisms and their age distribution in pediatric patients. Am J Cardiol 1992;69(12): 1028–32.
30. Wen ZC, Chen SA, Tai CT, et al. Electrophysiological mechanisms and determinants of vagal maneuvers for termination of paroxysmal supraventricular tachycardia. Circulation 1998;98(24):2716–23.
31. Kannankeril PJ, Fish FA. Disorders of cardiac rhythm and conduction. In: Allen AD, Driscoll DJ, Shaddy RE, et al, editors. Moss and Adams' heart disease in infants, children, and adolescents including the fetus and young adult. Philadelphia: Lippincott Williams & Wilkins; 2008. p. 293–341.
32. Francis J, Sankar V, Nair VK, et al. Catecholaminergic polymorphic ventricular tachycardia. Heart Rhythm 2005;2(5):550–4.

Management of a Hyperactive Teen and Cardiac Safety

Heather Sowinski, DO, Peter P. Karpawich, MSc, MD, FHRS*

KEYWORDS

- Attention deficit hyperactivity disorder • ADHD • Arrhythmias
- Sudden cardiac death • Electrocardiogram • QT interval • Hypertension
- Tachycardia

KEY POINTS

- Stimulants improve behavior yet can be associated with cardiovascular effects of increased heart rate and blood pressure changes.
- The risk of sudden death is not increased over that of the general population.
- Routine ECG monitoring is not indicated.
- Patient compliance with medication regimens is often suboptimal.

INTRODUCTION

Although possibly described as early as the 17th century, distraction of attention was recognized and reported as an adverse behavioral condition by Dr Alexander Crichton in 1789 in his medical treatise on mental illness, "An Inquiry into the Nature and Origin of Mental Derangements." In his series of 3 books, he describes patients who are easily distracted by even the slightest extraneous stimuli. This inability to focus on any one task, which he describes as a morbid alteration of attention among such patients, causes them to become hyperexcited and exhibit what was described as having the fidgets.[1] In 1846, as 1 of 10 short stories of various childhood behaviors included in his children's book, *Struwwelpeter* (Slovenly Peter), Dr Heinrich Hoffmann introduced the fictitious character of "Zappel-Philipp" (Fidgety Philip).[2] Fidgety Philip, although perhaps not directly implying any mental disorder, does illustrate several of the now-accepted criteria for attention deficit hyperactivity disorder (ADHD): inattention, hyperactivity, and impulsivity. In addition, he describes his character's behavioral effects on parents and family.

However, a more definitive description of the disorder was published by Dr George Still (of the innocent Still's murmur fame). A pediatrician, Dr Still became involved in

No Author disclosures.
Section of Pediatric Cardiology, The Carmen and Ann Adams Department of Pediatrics, The Children's Hospital of Michigan, School of Medicine, Wayne State University, 3901 Beaubien Boulevard, Detroit, MI 48201, USA
* Corresponding author.
E-mail address: pkarpawi@dmc.org

Pediatr Clin N Am 61 (2014) 81–90
http://dx.doi.org/10.1016/j.pcl.2013.09.021   pediatric.theclinics.com

childhood disease research and in his treatise, "On Some Abnormal Psychical Conditions in Children," published in 1902, he described children with a morbid defect of moral control but without evidence of physical disease or impairment of intellect, to distinguish these children from those with associated physical conditions such as meningitis, brain tumor, head injury, or mental illness.[3] His work was followed by numerous authors over the ensuing decades, with descriptions of childhood hyperactivity, inattentiveness, compulsive behavior, ease of excitability, and inability to concentrate.[4] Accordingly, the condition itself has been associated with controversy as to its actual existence as a neurodevelopmental disorder and has undergone several name changes, culminating in the current ADHD designation in 1987.

In 1994, the condition was subdivided according to clinical presentation:

- ADHD inattentive
- ADHD hyperactive-compulsive
- ADHD combined.

Between 5% and 20% of school-aged children are currently diagnosed with ADHD; boys more frequently than girls. Although previously thought to be only a childhood disorder, over 50% of individuals diagnosed in childhood continue to exhibit symptoms as adults. Causal theories have varied over the years. Although a precise single cause of ADHD remains controversial, at present, environmental, genetic, as well as neuropsychological factors have been included. A genetic inheritance factor has been indicated in 75% of affected children.[5]

Possible cause includes

1. Environmental factors
   - Preterm and very low birth weight infants
   - Fetal alcohol and tobacco exposure
   - Fetal or childhood infections
   - Lead exposure
   - Food additives
   - Polychlorinated biphenyls exposure
   - History of physical or emotional abuse
   - Congenital heart repair before 1 year of age
2. Genetics
   - Genes associated with dopamine transportation
   - LPHN3 gene, which facilitates responsiveness to stimulant medications
3. Neuropsychological
   - Inability to regulate and manage daily tasks (executive functioning)

Because executive functioning evolves with age and brain maturation, this last concept helps to explain why symptoms of ADHD may not become fully manifest until adolescence or young adulthood.

DIAGNOSIS

Depending on which criteria are used (DSM-IV or ICD-10), children may or may not be correctly identified as actually having ADHD. It is beyond the scope of this writing to elaborate on actual testing techniques but suffice to say that all are based on an assessment of individual behavior and cognitive development, especially in regards to age-matched peers, taking in account parental and educator assessments. ADHD is based on behavior and is not a neurologic disease. As such, it differs from other psychotic/mental disorders, such as schizophrenia, anxiety, or personality disorders. It is classified as a disruptive behavior disorder with oppositional defiance associated with adverse conduct and social interaction. As indicated above, currently ADHD is classified according to symptoms (inattention, hyperactive-impulsive, or combination). Most children are diagnosed as having the combination type.

MANAGEMENT

Once the appropriate diagnosis of ADHD is made, effective management is required to permit the child to function appropriately. This managements typically includes psychotherapy, medications, or both.[6,7] Among psychological interventions, behavioral, cognitive, and interpersonal therapies have been advocated. Other modalities include school-based interventions, social skill training, parental management, and neurofeedback. Medications included amphetamine and methylphenidate stimulants, atomoxetine, α-adrenergic agonists as well as antidepressants and antihypertensives. A study done by the National Institute of Mental Health-funded multisite trial showed that parent and teacher ratings had greater improvement with pharmacotherapy when compared with behavioral therapy alone. The response to both methylphenidate and amphetamine has been shown to be greater than 70% as compared with 12% for placebo controls. There have been multiple studies that have confirmed the importance of treating ADHD from not only a patient standpoint but also the effect a patient with ADHD has on a family and society. As might be expected, management issues differ between the young child and adolescent, as discussed below. Because psychological counseling would not be expected to have any adverse cardiac effects, this review focuses primarily on pharmacologic interventions.

PHARMACOLOGIC TREATMENT

Effective pharmacologic treatment of ADHD was found by chance.[8] While attempting to treat headaches associated with pneumoencephalograms, performed to examine structural brain abnormalities in the 1930s, Dr Charles Bradley noticed that use of Benzedrine to stimulate the choroid plexus resulted in behavioral improvement in some children. In addition, previously hyperactive and inattentive children were found to exhibit improved school performance as well as a decrease in motor activity. This seemingly paradoxic effect of stimulant medications laid the foundation for current therapeutic modalities of ADHD intervention.

As the term implies, "stimulant" medications can be associated with secondary cardiovascular effects such as sinus tachycardia and hypertension. These effects have caused considerable debate recently as to the cost/risk/benefits as well as need for or against close cardiac monitoring of patients prescribed pharmacologic agents, such as methylphenidate, amphetamine, or atomoxetine. Concerns of adverse cardiovascular events associated with use of such stimulant medications, including sudden cardiac death, have lead to conflicting scientific publications.

Key message

- Five to 20% of children are currently diagnosed with ADHD
- Symptoms of ADHD can be seen during adolescence and adulthood
- A precise cause for ADHD is not known
- ADHD is diagnosed after detailed assessment of the behavior of the individual
- Management includes medications and psychotherapy
- Cardiovascular adverse effects have become a significant concern in society

CONTROVERSIAL ISSUES

Major issues in any study involving patients are demographics, especially patient selection, age, and numbers. Multiple case reports and some small population-based studies published since the 1980s, although reporting some adverse cardiovascular patient events, have generally failed to show any definitive correlation between use of stimulant medications and adverse events in children and adolescents. On the other hand, the elderly and those patients with other health issues contributing to cardiac morbidity may demonstrate a correlation.[9]

Patients with other health issues, particularly those on prescribed medications, tend to be more sensitive to the potential problems than those without comparable issues. Therefore, although children and adolescents on stimulant medications may present more frequently to emergency rooms with complaints of palpitations or sensed tachycardia, ostensibly related to direct adrenergic agonist effects of the drugs, there has been no evidence of any actual adverse cardiovascular events. In one population study of 89,031 patients that used stimulant medications to treat ADHD, there was no increased risk of a severe cardiovascular event (myocardial infarction, stroke, respiratory arrest, or sudden death) compared with matched controls. In another large population-based study of 124,932 person-years of observation over 10 years, 5 children of a reported 73 deaths died of cardiac causes. None of these children were prescribed stimulant medications. Of note, this latter study did include patients with congenital circulatory diseases. The authors recognized that the incidence of fatal and serious events due to circulatory causes in the study age group is extremely low.[10–12]

Screening ECG are not always accurate, especially in the current era of computerized ECG interpretations.[13] For this reason, practitioners should be aware that false negative and false positive reports are commonplace. As a result, general ECG screening even for athletes remains controversial in this country.[14] In a study, correlated with the 2008 American Heart Association (AHA) publication of the usefulness of screening ECGs in association with ADHD of 372 patients with screening ECGs, 24 (6.4%) were interpreted as being abnormal, resulting in some medication administration delay. Of these 24 patients, 18 were referred to a cardiologist. The cardiac evaluation including consultation, echocardiogram, and stress testing, all with their respective financial charges, resulted in no patient being found to have any cardiac disease.[15]

PERTINENT "GUIDELINE" PUBLICATION ISSUES

- 2005 Safety concerns of methylphenidate, including cardiovascular risks, issued by the Pediatric Advisory Committee of the United States Food and Drug Administration (FDA)[16]
  - 2005 Adderall removed from the Canadian market
    - Decision revoked 6 months later
- 2008 AHA statement that ECG screening prior to initiation of stimulant therapy was reasonable[17]
- 2008 American Academy of Pediatrics rebuttal of the AHA publication indicating that routine ECG screening was not effective[18]
- 2011 American Academy of Pediatrics Subcommittee on ADHD, Steering Committee on Quality Improvement and Management, Practice Guidelines published[19]

Controversies raised by the publications noted above have created much uncertainty among primary caregivers as to how to monitor patients best for whom stimulant medications are being considered. Routine cardiac testing (ECG or echocardiography) has not been shown to offer any enlightenment to the clinician or safety to this issue. Although medications useful to treat children and teens with ADHD are associated with some side effects, to date, there is no evidence that the risk of serious cardiovascular events (sudden cardiac death, myocardial infarct, stroke) is any greater than that found in the general population. Reports of methylphenidate overdose have failed to substantiate any ECG changes or adverse arrhythmias.[20] Unfortunately, the "Black Box" warning placed on stimulant medication use for ADHD in children by the FDA in 2006 (in deference to recommendations by their own Pediatric Advisory Committee that such was not warranted) appears, at the time of this writing, to still be in effect. The Black Box warning also provides "warning" but no direction for action to either primary caregivers or specialists and therefore has little practical impact on care. It is hoped this will be removed soon, especially considering the 2011 FDA publication indicating that ADHD medications are not associated with an increased risk of cardiovascular events in children.[21] At present there are at least 13 different pharmacologic agents approved for use in ADHD therapy.

Key message

- There is no evidence of increase in serious cardiovascular events in patients on stimulant medications when compared with the general population
- Benefits of screening ECG or cardiac ultrasound has not been shown
- Unnecessary testing may be associated with patient/family anxiety and delay of therapy

---

CURRENT MEDICATION ISSUES

Medications used to treat ADHD can be divided into 2 main categories, stimulants and nonstimulants. **Table 1** provides a list of the drug categories, drug names, mechanism of action, cardiac effects, ECG changes, and commonly seen noncardiogenic side effects. The main stimulant medications are methylphenidate and amphetamine. They act by increasing circulating catecholamine at the synapse in the central nervous system. The nonstimulant medications include Atomoxetine, Clonidine, Guanfacine, and Bupropion. The most commonly used and often first-line medication is a stimulant. All of the medications come in various dosages and are typically titrated to achieve maximum symptom improvement with the least side effects.

Methylphenidates are sympathomimetics that act by inhibiting both dopamine and norepinephrine reuptake. There are several new long-acting preparations that allow the medication to be released over an extended time period. The older medications such as Ritalin are found in shorter acting forms and work for 6 to 8 hours. The longer acting preparations work for approximately 8 to 12 hours and include Metadate, Focalin, and Concerta. There is also a transdermal patch preparation, Daytrana, that offers an alternative to oral medication.

The cardiac effects of methylphenidate use are small and there has been no documentation of ECG changes after starting the medication. Although the patient's blood pressure and heart rate can increase, they still remain in the normal range for age.

- Average increase in systolic blood pressure by 3–4 mm Hg
- Average increase in diastolic blood pressure by 1–2 mm Hg
- Average increase in heart rate of 3–4 beats per minute.

Table 1
Common pharmacotherapy used to treat ADHD

Medication	Drugs	Action	Cardiac Effects	ECG Effect	Side Effects
Methylphenidate	Concerta, Focalin, Metadate, Ritalin, Daytrana	Inhibition of dopamine and norepinephrine reuptake	Increased HR and BP, ventricular arrhythmias, decreased cardiac function in overdose	None	Decreased appetite, sleep problems, stomachaches, headaches
Amphetamine	Adderall, Dexedrine	Release of norepinephrine from stores, block dopamine uptake, central nervous system stimulant	Increased HR and BP	None	Decreased appetite, sleep problems, stomachaches, headaches
Atomoxetine	Strattera	Selectively blocks norepinephrine uptake	Increased HR, increased systolic and diastolic BP	None	Decreased appetite, somnolence, nausea, stomachaches
Clonidine	Catapress	α_2-Adrenergic agonist	Decreased peripheral vascular resistance, decreased BP and HR	None	Mild sedation, rebound hypertension with abrupt cessation
Guanfacine	Tenex, Intuiv	α_2-Adrenergic agonist	Decreased peripheral vascular resistance, decreased BP and HR	None	Mild sedation, rebound hypertension with abrupt cessation
Bupropion	Wellbutrin, Zyban	Decreased norepinephrine- and serotonin-releasing neurons	Increased BP in adults, cardiac toxicity in overdose	None	Agitation, insomnia, dry mouth, nausea, vomiting, headache

Abbreviations: BP, blood pressure; HR, heart rate.

Amphetamines are also adrenergic agonists that act both centrally and peripherally. Centrally, they act to stimulate release of norepinephrine from stores and increase dopamine by blocking its reuptake, resulting in an improvement in patient's focus. Peripherally, it has sympathomimetic effects by stimulating both β- and α-receptors. It is the peripheral action that leads to increased heart rate and blood pressure. Their action is similar to methylphenidates and the efficacy and adverse effects are similar as well. There are short-acting and long-acting preparations that have comparable duration of effect to the short- and long-acting methylphenidates, respectively. Even though the medications have similar profiles, an individual patient may respond differently to each medication category. Thus, it may be beneficial to switch a patient from methylphenidate to an amphetamine if they are not responding favorably and vice versa. The Multimodal Treatment of Attention-Deficit Hyperactivity Disorder study showed that 38% of patients respond to either medication, 35% respond to amphetamines only, and 26% respond to methylphenidate only.[22]

The cardiac side effects of amphetamines are similar to that of methylphenidates and, again, no ECG changes are seen after starting the medication.

- Average systolic blood pressure increased by 3–4 mm Hg
- Average heart rate increased by 1–2 beats per minute.

The average increase in blood pressure of healthy children with ADHD who take stimulant medication is less than 5 mm Hg and heart rate is less than 10 beats per minute. It is estimated that 5% to 15% of patients will experience cardiac side effects. The noncardiogenic side effects are usually mild and can abate over time or resolve with stopping the medication or switching to a different class of medication. The most common side effects include decreased appetite and stomachache. Any observed slowing of growth is typically corrected after stopping the medication with no effect on final adult height. There is some question that if there is a slowing of growth in patients, it is part of the disease process as opposed to a side effect of the medication as slowed growth in patients with ADHD can be observed even without stimulant medications. The sleep disturbances seen in patients taking stimulant medication usually consist of insomnia or difficulty falling asleep. It appears to be worse in patients taking amphetamines as opposed to methylphenidate.

Atomoxetine, a nonstimulant medication and thus having a lower risk of abuse potential, acts specifically by blocking norepinephrine uptake. This medication has been shown to be effective compared with placebo and also to have similar efficacy compared with stimulant medications. Quality of life of patients on Atomoxetine is comparable to those on stimulant medications. The noncardiac side-effect profile is similar to a stimulant medication with the most common being decreased appetite, nausea, and abdominal pain. However, Atomoxetine can cause somnolence as opposed to insomnia.

The cardiac side effects of Atomoxetine are comparable to other medications:

- Slight increase in blood pressure
- Slight increase in heart rate
- No significant ECG changes

There are 2 direct α-agonist medications used to treat ADHD, Clonidine and Guanfacine. Both treat ADHD symptoms by directly stimulating the α-adrenergic receptors in the frontal cortex. These medications cause mild sedation and are often added to a medication regimen if there is significant insomnia or to treat other psychological issues such as oppositional or aggressive behavior. Rebound hypertension can occur with abrupt cessation of these medications, but is not seen if the medication is gradually weaned.

The cardiac side effects of α agonist medications are somewhat different from the other medications:

- Decrease in peripheral vascular resistance
- Decrease in blood pressure
- Decrease in heart rate
- No significant ECG changes

ADOLESCENTS WITH ADHD AND CHALLENGES

Patients with ADHD are typically diagnosed before the age of 12 years and most will continue to have symptoms into their adolescent years. It becomes more of a diagnostic challenge as the normal adolescent need for autonomy and growing peer influences become evident. Teenagers commonly run the risk of increasing comorbidities, such as substance abuse, conduct disorders, anxiety, and depression. Oppositional defiant disorders may become more evident. It is not uncommon for any teenager to counteract parental efforts to obtain appropriate treatment for them. Teenage pregnancy and potential fetal effects of any prescribed medications may become an issue.

It is beyond the scope of this review to discuss all the issues pertaining to all aspects of ADHD therapy in the teen. An excellent overview can be found elsewhere.[23] However, from a cardiac safety concern viewpoint, there are little reported issues specific to the teenager that are different when compared with the child. Again, a careful family history for any cardiac issues as well as comprehensive physical examination to rule out cardiac disease is mandatory. A screening ECG, as discussed above, is not necessarily required. In a recent study from Canada, children who underwent congenital heart repair before 1 year of age exhibited an increase in ADHD symptoms compared to age-match controls. Therefore, continued observation is recommended throughout childhood and adolescence.[24] Among current prescribed ADHD medications, dopamine agonists are available as sustained release preparations that can assist with compliance issues of the teenager. Side effects of norepinephrine uptake inhibitors, such as loss of appetite, insomnia, rash, and edema, need to be discussed. Concomitant use of antidepressant medications, such as tricyclics, may be associated with increased sensed tachycardia. Orthostatic complaints, already quite common in teenagers, may be exacerbated. However, previous tricyclic-related reports of fetal limb defects have not been confirmed by more recent studies. Antihypertensive medications can be associated with sensed tachycardia as well as orthostatic

---

Key message

- Detailed inquiries into significant cardiac family history are necessary to determine any pre-existing cardiovascular susceptibilities to a drug
- Choice of the medication needs to be individualized based on other issues
- Increased risk of substance abuse, conduct disorders, anxiety, depression, oppositional defiant disorders during adolescence
- Noncompliance is high in this age group
- Teenage pregnancy and potential adverse fetal effects of a prescribed medication can add complexity
- Side effects of the prescribed medication should be discussed in detail with the teenager and may improve compliance

complaints. Side effects of the prescribed medication should be discussed in detail with the teenager to aid with better compliance.

SUMMARY

ADHD is not a new diagnosis. However, clinical recognition has increased over the years. There are multiple causes. Although typically a childhood condition, symptoms can continue into adolescence and adulthood, requiring lifelong therapy. Therapeutic intervention includes a combined approach: psychotherapy and medications. Although psychotherapy would not be expected to be associated with any adverse cardiac problems, the various stimulant pharmacologic agents can have some cardiac and cardiovascular effects (tachycardia, hypertension, or hypotension). However, to date, there have been no definitive studies demonstrating that young patients receiving such drugs for ADHD control are at any greater risk than the general population for serious adverse cardiac or cardiovascular events, which is in contradiction to studies among the elderly or those with preexisting medical conditions, placing them at high risk for cardiovascular problems. Unfortunately, to date, there are no studies among teenagers specifically with repaired congenital heart defects, who are on these medications.

As with any medical condition requiring pharmacologic intervention, a detailed family history is mandatory before initiation of the drug. In this instance, inquiries into family history of sudden cardiac death, genetically inherited cardiovascular conditions, such as channelopathies or long QT syndrome, are necessary to determine any pre-existing cardiovascular susceptibilities to a drug. At present, genetic testing is available for most of these inherited conditions to help determine inheritance patterns. Routine ECG (or echocardiographic) screening, on the other hand, has not been shown to add any benefit and may actually be associated with unnecessary patient/family anxiety and delay of therapy.

Because the potential for abuse as well as noncompliance is high among teenagers, there are now extended release preparations of both stimulant and nonstimulant medications to help defray these age-related problems. Discussion of all potential medication side effects is recommended when dealing with an adolescent.

ACKNOWLEDGMENTS

The authors wish to thank Arthur L. Robin, PhD for his assistance in the preparation of this article.

REFERENCES

1. Lange KW, Reichi S, Lange KM, et al. The history of attention deficit hyperactivity disorder. Atten Defic Hyperact Disord 2010;2:241–55.
2. Thome J, Jacobs K. Attention deficit hyperactivity disorder (ADHD) in a 19th century children's book. Eur Psychiatry 2004;19:303–96.
3. Still GF. Some abnormal psychical conditions in children: the Goulstonian lectures. Lancet 1902;1:1008–12.
4. Barkley RA. The relevance of the Still lectures to attention-deficit/hyperactivity disorder: a commentary. J Atten Disord 2006;10:137–40.
5. Franke B, Farone SV, Asherson P, et al. International Multicentre persistent ADHD CollaboraTion. Mol Psychiatry 2012;17(10):960–87.
6. Goldman LS, Genel M, Bezman RJ, et al. Diagnosis and treatment of attention-deficit/hyperactivity disorder in children and adolescents. JAMA 1998;279:1100–7.

7. Barkley RA. Adolescents with attention-deficit/hyperactivity disorder: an overview of empirically based treatments. J Psychiatr Pract 2004;10(1):39–56.

8. Bradley C. The behavior of children receiving benzedrine. Am J Psychiatry 1937; 94:577–85.

9. Cooper WO, Habel LA, Sox CM, et al. ADHD drugs and serious cardiovascular effects in children and young adults. N Engl J Med 2011;365:1896–904.

10. Westover AN, Halm EA. Do prescription stimulants increase the risk of adverse cardiovascular events?: a systemic review. BMC Cardiovasc Disord 2012;12: 41–50.

11. Winterstein AG, Gerhard T, Shuster J, et al. Cardiac safety of central nervous system stimulants in children and adolescents with attention-deficit/hyperactivity disorder. Pediatrics 2007;120:e1494–501.

12. Olfson M, Huang C, Gerhard T, et al. Stimulants and cardiovascular events in the young with attention-deficit/hyperactivity disorder. J Am Acad Child Adolesc Psychiatry 2012;51(2):147–56.

13. Shah N, Chintal K, Aggarwal S. Electrocardiographic strain pattern in children with left ventricular hypertrophy: a marker of ventricular dysfunction. Pediatr Cardiol 2010;31:800–6.

14. Roberts WO, Stovitz SD. Incidence of sudden cardiac death in Minnesota High School Athletes 1993-2012 screened with a standardized preparticipation evaluation. J Am Coll Cardiol 2013. http://dx.doi.org/10.1016/j.jacc.2013.05.080.

15. Thomas PE, Waldemar CF, Decker JA, et al. Impact of the American Heart Association Scientific Statement of screening electrocardiograms and stimulant medications. Arch Pediatr Adolesc Med 2011;165(2):166–70.

16. FDA Statement. Available at: http://www.fda.gov/ohrms/dockets/ac/05/briefing/ 2005-4152b1_00_05a_Statement%20for%20June%2030.pdf.

17. Vetter VL, Elia J, Erickson C, et al. Cardiovascular monitoring of children and adolescents with heart disease receiving medications for attention deficit/hyperactivity disorder. Circulation 2008;117:2407–23.

18. Perrin JM, Friedman RA, Knilans TK, Black Box Working Group, Section on Cardiology and Cardaic Surgery. Cardiovascular monitoring and stimulant drugs for attention-deficit/hyperactivity disorder. Pediatrics 2008;122:451–3.

19. Subcommittee on Attention-Deficit/Hyperactivity Disorder, Steering Committee on Quality Improvement and Management, Wolraich M, et al. ADHD: clinical practice guideline for the diagnosis, evaluation, and treatment of attention-deficit/ hyperactivity disorder in children and adolescents. Pediatrics 2011;128:1007–22.

20. Hill SL, El-Khayat RH, Sandilands EA, et al. Electrocardiographic effects of methylphenidate overdose. Clin Toxicol (Phila) 2010;48(4):342–6.

21. FDA Statement. Available at: http://www.fda.gov/downloads/Drugs/DrugSafety/ UCM277931.pdf.

22. Jensen PS, Hinshaw SP, Swanson JM, et al. Findings from the NIMH Multimodal Treatment Study of ADHD (MTA): implications and applications for primary care providers. J Dev Behav Pediatr 2001;22(1):60–73.

23. Robin AL. Family intervention for home-based problems of adolescents with attention-deficit/hyperactivity disorder. Adolesc Med State Art Rev 2008;19(2): 268–77.

24. Drew CY, Porter AA, Conway JL, et al. Early repair of congenital heart disease associated with increased rate of attention deficit hyperactivity disorder symptoms. Canadian Journal of Cardiology 2013. [Epub ahead of print].

Sports Participation During Teenage Years

James M. Galas, MD

KEYWORDS

- Athletes • Athletic heart • Preparticipation screening • Sports cardiology
- Sudden cardiac arrest

KEY POINTS

- American Academy of Pediatrics and American Heart Association recommendations for preparticipation screening include the use of patient history, family history, and physical examination, with additional testing if there is clinical suspicion of heart disease.
- Chest pain or syncope with exercise should raise concern for underlying cardiac disorder; further cardiac evaluation is appropriate.
- The athlete's heart is a constellation of adaptive changes in response to intense athletic training. Differentiation from pathologic cardiac enlargement or hypertrophy can be challenging.

INTRODUCTION

More than 7.5 million young people are estimated to participate in competitive high school athletics annually in the United States,[1] with additional youth participate in recreational sports. Though infrequent, sudden cardiac arrest (SCA) in young athletes is devastating to families, schools, and communities when it occurs. With this in mind, local, county, and statewide initiatives for preparticipation sports screening have grown in recent years. Although formal nationwide screening programs exist elsewhere, controversy remains within the United States as to what type of screening is most appropriate for young US athletes. As a result, providing sports clearance is often to the responsibility of individual pediatric practitioners. Given this setting, this article provides:

- A summary of current screening philosophies and preparticipation sports guidelines put forth by the American Association of Pediatrics (AAP) and the American Heart Association (AHA)

Disclosures: None.
Division of Pediatric Cardiology, The Carman and Ann Adams Department of Pediatrics, Wayne State University School of Medicine, 3901 Beaubien Boulevard, Detroit, MI 48201-2119, USA
E-mail address: jgalas@dmc.org

Pediatr Clin N Am 61 (2014) 91–109
http://dx.doi.org/10.1016/j.pcl.2013.09.020

- Pertinent screening history and physical examination with red flags of which to be aware
- Understanding of the athlete's heart
- A brief review of the most common disorders associated with risk of SCA

PREPARTICIPATION SCREENING

Although it is generally agreed that some form of preparticipation screening should take place before allowing involvement in competitive athletics, controversy remains as to what, if any, testing should be conducted on a screening basis. Advocacy for routine electrocardiogram (ECG) screening of athletes has been well reported in the literature.[2–4] Corrado and colleagues,[5] based in Italy, are perhaps the most prominent of these advocates. Following the initiation of a mandatory national screening program consisting of personal and family history, pointed physical examination, and screening ECG, they showed an 89% decrease in the annual incidence of sudden cardiac deaths.[5,6] The principle behind this ECG-based program has been that hypertrophic cardiomyopathy (HCM) and arrhythmogenic right ventricular cardiomyopathy, two leading entities responsible for sudden cardiac death, may be detectable via ECG in asymptomatic individuals.[5]

Furthermore, the use of echocardiographic screening has been proposed by some cardiologists.[7] Proponents cite the ability to obtain technically adequate imaging that can augment history, physical examination, and screening ECG, but also acknowledge that a significant learning curve exists in order to do so.[7] This screening usually takes place outside the medical office using portable echocardiogram devices and obtaining images via a specific screening protocol, which differs from the routine adult or pediatric examination in both comprehensiveness and time in which it is completed.[7,8]

Despite the merits of the screening programs mentioned earlier, the feasibility of applying universal athletic screening to the population of young athletes in the United States has come into question.[5,6] Halkin and colleagues[9] argued that implementation of a similar program in the United States is not as economically feasible as implementation of secondary prevention strategies such as lay person cardiopulmonary resuscitation (CPR) and external automatic defibrillator (AED) training. Maron and colleagues[6] refuted the idea that the United States' screening process was inferior to the Italian process in a study that compared the rate of sudden cardiac death in Minnesota versus Veneto, Italy. Despite the absence of routine ECG screening in Minnesota, there was no statistically significant difference in sudden death rates between the two geographic locations over a similar time span.

The use of history and physical alone in screening US high school athletes has been detailed in recent publications. Roberts and Stovitz[10] reported an incidence of 0.24 sudden cardiac deaths per 100,000 athlete years in a population of high school athletes and proposed that ECG screening may not add any significant benefit to screening. At the same time, they cautioned that their results may not be applicable to other populations that differ demographically in terms of age, race, or gender.[10–12]

Furthermore, concern has been raised that false-positive screening may lead to additional testing, unnecessary restrictions or therapies, and unwarranted patient and family anxiety.[13] A recent meta-analysis from Tuft's University School of Medicine reviewed the literature between 1950 and 2010 to determine the efficacy of ECG and/or echocardiogram testing to diagnose HCM, long QT syndrome (LQTS), and Wolff-Parkinson-White syndrome in asymptomatic individuals.[14] They concluded that, although ECG and/or echocardiogram screening had an excellent ability to reassure that patients had no disease (nearly 100% negative predictive value), it was at the expense of too many false-positive reports.[14]

ACKNOWLEDGING REASONS FOR DIFFERENCES IN OUTCOME/PHILOSOPHY

In trying to reconcile these polarized opinions by respected leaders in medicine, it is important to understand the fundamental differences in experience and the populations served by these various groups. The success or failure of a screening program may depend more on the infrastructure of the health care system, diversity of the population (ie, age, ethnicity, gender, level and type of activity), and prevalence of disease in that area than on the screening examination or tests. With this in mind, it is important to interpret the data from the literature in the context of the parameters discussed earlier in order to better gauge its applicability to a population.

CURRENT RECOMMENDATIONS FOR PREPARTICIPATION SCREENING IN THE UNITED STATES

With these concerns in mind, the American Academy of Pediatrics and AHA have chosen to take a more conservative approach to their screening recommendations than their European counterparts. The 2007 AHA scientific statement on preparticipation screening in competitive athletes does not recommend the routine use of ECG or echocardiography in the context of mass, universal screening and concludes that mandated 12-lead ECG screening is, "probably impractical and would require considerable resources that do not currently exist."[13]

In its 2012 policy statement on pediatric SCA, the AAP echoes this sentiment and endorses the use of standardized preparticipation evaluation forms to obtain a specific patient and family history and physical examination to solicit warning signs of those who may be at risk for SCA, as well as to identify individuals and families who may benefit from referral to a pediatric cardiologist.[15] Several such preparticipation forms have been published.[16] The policy statement goes on to state that, "Not all SCA can be foreseen, even in the best of circumstances. No screening protocol has yet proven to be effective in this role or validated as highly effective."[15] The article states that primary prevention of SCA should be specific to an individual's cardiac disorder and should consist of a combination of medical therapy, device implantation, activity restriction, and avoidance of particular medications.[15] Because this form of primary prevention requires a specific diagnosis, and the initial presentation of these occult cardiac diseases is often SCA or aborted SCA, secondary preventative measures are advocated. These measures include early symptom recognition, ability to provide effective CPR, and access to an AED.[15] Through implementation of secondary prevention programs, the ability to successfully resuscitate both individuals previously diagnosed and those undiagnosed with cardiac disorders at the time of an SCA has been shown.[17]

Key message

- Considerable controversies exist as to the best type of screening in athletic adolescents
- Routine use of ECG or echocardiography is currently not recommended by the AAP and AHA because of concerns for false-negative and false-positive results and availability of resources
- In the absence of a perfect screening tool, secondary preventative measures including early symptom recognition, ability to provide effective CPR, and access to an AED are advocated

APPROACH TO CARDIAC HISTORY AND PHYSICAL EXAMINATION IN THE ATHLETE

Although limitations of the preparticipation evaluation have been described, there is merit in obtaining a thorough cardiac history and physical examination.[18] Positive findings can trigger further evaluation that may lead to a diagnosis of heart disease in the athlete or even an athlete's family member. The AHA has published a 12-element recommendation for cardiovascular screening in competitive athletes, which is reflected in the 2010 Preparticipation Physical Evaluation Monograph published by the American Academy of Family Physicians and the American Academy of Pediatrics (**Box 1**).[13,19]

History

The goal of the cardiac history should be to elicit an account of symptoms with exercise, including chest pain, shortness of breath, palpitations, near syncope, syncope, or easy fatigue.[20] Taking a careful history can help differentiate cardiac from noncardiac causes of these symptoms.

Chest pain

Chest pain is most likely to be of musculoskeletal origin in young athletes; however, chest pain that occurs with exercise should lead to further evaluation.[21] Location, radiation, intensity, character, duration, provocative and palliative factors, and associated symptoms need to be identified in order to describe the pain. The presence of associated symptoms, such as diaphoresis, pallor, palpitations, dizziness, or radiation of the pain to the jaw or left arm, can suggest cardiac chest pain. Chest pain that causes athletes to stop their activities is also worrisome. A history of recent viral illness

---

Box 1
Preparticipation screening elements. Based on the AHA recommendations

Patient history

Chest pain with exercise

Syncope or presyncope without clear noncardiac cause

Shortness of breath or fatigue out of proportion to activity

History of heart murmur on examination

History of systolic hypertension

Family history

Relative with unexpected death before 50 years of age

Close relative with cardiac disease or disability before 50 years of age

Relative with cardiomyopathy, LQTS, channelopathy, connective tissue disorder, or arrhythmia for which they receive treatment

Physical examination findings

Heart murmur

Increased blood pressure

Marfanoid body habitus

Weak femoral pulses

Data from Maron BJ, Thompson PD, Ackerman MJ, et al. Recommendations and considerations Related to preparticipation screening for cardiovascular abnormalities in competitive athletes: 2007 update. Circulation 2007;115:1643–55.

in a patient with cardiac symptoms may be caused by myocarditis or pericarditis. In addition, a previous history of Kawasaki disease should be elicited, which could place the athlete at risk for coronary artery disease.

Dyspnea on exertion

Dyspnea on exertion can be a nebulous symptom, but certain characteristics should raise concern for cardiac involvement. When shortness of breath occurs at a notably lower threshold than previously in a given individual, in the absence of a period of deconditioning or known respiratory illness, further cardiac evaluation is warranted. It is often also helpful to gauge the degree of shortness of breath against peers who were performing the same activity at that time. Symptoms that impair the athlete's performance are generally more concerning than those that they can work through. Referral to a pulmonary specialist may be warranted when cardiac causes are unlikely.

Palpitations

A palpitation is defined as a sensation of rapid or irregular beating of the heart and may represent different events to different young athletes.[22] Sensations of a pounding heart during exercise, in the absence of other associated symptoms, often represent a normal physiologic response to exercise. In this case, the increase and subsequent decrease in heart rate are gradual and correspond with the warm-up and cool-down period of the activity. A careful history of the nature of the onset and cessation of sensed tachycardia can provide clues to its cause. Supraventricular tachycardia characteristically has an abrupt onset and termination, often with a perceived prominent beat or thump ending the cycle. In all instances, knowledge of the heart rate at the time of sensed tachycardia is helpful in establishing its mechanism. Teaching athletes, parents, and coaches to take a pulse can help elicit valuable information should the symptoms recur. In general, heart rates of more than 180 beats per minute in teenagers should raise concern for arrhythmia.[23] Palpitations associated with near syncope, syncope, chest pain, diaphoresis, or pallor, are concerning for a cardiac disorder.

Syncope

Syncope and near syncope are common occurrences in teens. Classic vasovagal syncope consists of a prodrome of feeling unwell, followed by visual changes, culminating in a loss of consciousness. Intense fear, heat, pain, sight of blood, dehydration, prolonged standing, micturition, and even hair combing are all well-known triggers for benign syncope.[24] Syncope with exercise is less common and far more concerning.[25] Sudden loss of consciousness occurring in the middle of exercise, with no recollection of the events immediately surrounding the syncopal event is a harbinger of severe cardiac disease. This type of passing out is different from postexercise syncope, which is often accompanied by the prodrome of vasovagal syncope after the activity is completed.

Easy fatigue

Tiring with exercise can be a normal phenomenon in athletes undergoing intense training. It is most likely to occur following a period of deconditioning, when athletes are unable to perform to the level of exertion to which they were previously accustomed. It is noteworthy that significant physical deconditioning can occur within 3 weeks of cessation of training.[26] Easy fatigue is most concerning when it is of recent onset in an otherwise well-conditioned athlete or when the fatigue is disproportionate to that experienced by the athlete's peers of similar athletic ability. Associated symptoms of chest pain, diaphoresis, pallor, palpitations, dizziness, or syncope are all concerning. Recent viral prodrome may be innocuous or could raise concern for myocarditis. A history of worsening fatigue is more worrisome than improving fatigue.

Medications, supplements, and other substances

Investigating what teenage athletes are putting into their bodies can identify individuals with risky behavior. Although the use of prescription stimulant medications (under the guidance of a medical professional) has been shown to be safe, abuse of stimulants can be hazardous.[27,28] The athlete should be questioned and counseled about the use of energy drinks, so-called performance-enhancing drugs, recreational drugs, and dietary supplements.[20] Abuse of cocaine, amphetamines, ecstasy, LSD (lysergic acid diethylamide), psilocybin (mushrooms), narcotics, cannabis, and volatile substances have all been shown to have adverse, and sometimes deadly, effects on the cardiovascular system.[29] The use of synthetic marijuana has been shown to cause myocardial damage.[30] Knowledge of consumption habits can aid in the explanation of the symptom and may lead to prevention of a catastrophic event.

Family History

A history of cardiac problems in the family, particularly in first-degree relatives, portends an increased risk of quiescent cardiac disease in the young athlete.[31] History of congenital heart disease, sudden infant death syndrome, sudden cardiac death, cardiomyopathy, arrhythmias, pacemakers, familial hypercholesterolemia, connective tissue disorders (such as Marfan syndrome and the vascular form of Ehlers-Danlos syndrome), seizure disorder, congenital deafness, drownings, or other unexplained deaths in young people are noteworthy and deserve further investigation.[13] It is particularly appropriate to inquire specifically about relatives with hypertrophic or dilated cardiomyopathies, LQTS, cardiac ion channelopathies, Brugada syndrome, and Marfan syndrome.[13] A detailed review of the implications of positive family history is presented by Miller and colleagues, elsewhere in this issue.

Physical Examination

Great care should be taken in performing a physical examination, because findings may be subtle in certain heart diseases. The use of history and extracardiac physical findings to guide a more in-depth cardiac analysis can be helpful. The physical examination, as it pertains to the discovery of cardiac disease, is discussed later.

Vital signs

Heart rate, respiratory rate, and blood pressure should be routinely obtained, with the addition of pulse oximetry if there is any question of cyanosis. Tachypnea and tachycardia make up two-thirds of the clinical triad consistent with congestive heart failure (the third being organomegaly). Patients may often have essential hypertension, but coarctation of the aorta must be excluded. Palpating for weak or absent femoral pulses and obtaining upper and lower extremity blood pressures to look for a gradient is helpful to evaluate for coarctation. Height and weight are useful to estimate body mass index, and can identify those at risk for developing hypertension.

General appearance

Tall, lanky body habitus with abnormally long arm span should arouse suspicion for Marfan syndrome. Obese individuals may be at risk for development of metabolic syndrome.

Chest wall
The presence of pectus excavatum or carinatum can be a manifestation of Marfan syndrome.[32] The presence of reproducible chest tenderness on palpation favors a diagnosis of costochondritis or musculoskeletal chest pain, making cardiac chest pain unlikely.

Lung examination
Crackles in the lungs can have a variety of causes, but rales can be a manifestation of pulmonary congestion secondary to heart failure. Tachypnea can be a manifestation of pulmonary edema caused by left-sided heart failure or pulmonary overcirculation.

Cardiac examination
The chest wall should be palpated for displacement of the cardiac apex and the presence of any lifts, heaves, or thrills. Auscultation of rate and rhythm can differentiate between sinus arrhythmia (variation in heart rate with respiratory phase) and ectopic beats. Physiologic splitting of the second heart sound (S2), which varies with respiration, should be differentiated from a widely fixed split S2, which may represent a left-to-right shunt at the atrial level (atrial septal defect or partial anomalous pulmonary venous connection) or some form of intraventricular conduction delay (such as right bundle branch block). The presence of a third heart sound (S3) may be normal, whereas a fourth heart sound (S4) represents diastolic dysfunction, which can be present in cardiomyopathies or pathologic ventricular hypertrophy. The presence of systolic clicks may represent a bicuspid semilunar valve when associated with the ejection phase of the cardiac cycle or mitral valve prolapse when occurring during midsystole. Particular attention should be paid to the timing, intensity, and character of cardiac murmurs. In general, low-frequency, low-intensity, systolic murmurs are likely to be benign in the asymptomatic individual, although findings of atrial level shunts and mild pulmonary stenosis may be subtle. Murmurs that are loud, harsh, high frequency, radiate to the back, louder when standing, diastolic, or associated with symptoms warrant evaluation by a pediatric cardiologist.[20] An in depth review of teenage heart murmurs is given elsewhere in this issue.

Abdominal examination
Palpation for hepatosplenomegaly, as an indicator of right-sided heart failure, should be performed. Abdominal distension from ascites is unlikely to be present in an asymptomatic individual.

Extremities
Examination for cyanosis, clubbing, and edema is routine, but unlikely in the asymptomatic athlete.

Limitations of Testing

From a cardiologist's perspective, it is often most desirable to consult on a patient in person, and put together history, physical examination, and cardiac test results to form a complete picture of the patient before diagnosing or attempting to exclude cardiac disorders. Realizing that many geographic, economic, organizational, and temporal barriers may prevent this ideal situation, it is important to understand the strengths, weaknesses, and limitations of different forms of cardiac testing, particularly when they are performed in isolation. Resourceful use of testing, with a healthy respect for these limitations, can help practitioners diagnose occult disorders and minimize false reassurance or unwarranted alarm.

Some clinical pearls, helpful in understanding the limitations of cardiac testing, are as follows:

- Electrical diseases, such as supraventricular tachycardia and LQTS, often occur in a structurally normal heart with normal findings on echocardiogram.[33]
- Cardiomyopathies can develop at various stages of life. A normal echocardiogram does not preclude future development of disease.[34]
- Abnormal coronary artery origins and intramural coronary arteries can be difficult to appreciate on echocardiogram. High clinical suspicion for coronary artery disease should lead to additional imaging with different modalities.
- Risk of sudden cardiac death is never zero. Some disorders responsible for sudden cardiac death are diagnosed only on autopsy with a previously normal cardiac work-up.[35]

Key message

- The AHA recommends 12 elements for screening young athletes, including 8 items for personal and family history and 4 items for physical examination
- Symptoms with exercise including chest pain, shortness of breath, palpitations, near syncope, syncope, or easy fatigability should be taken seriously and referred to a cardiologist
- Further testing can be based on the findings of a comprehensive history and physical examination

---

RESTRICTION OF ATHLETIC PARTICIPATION

Restriction from participation in athletic activities centers on identification of cardiac disease, degree of severity of the disease, and classification of the desired athletic activity. The Bethesda Guidelines address specific cardiac disorders lesion by lesion and provide a blueprint for the parameters of disease that need to be followed.[36] Although a pediatric cardiologist should be involved in evaluating young people with known cardiac disease for sports eligibility, it is helpful for general practitioners to have an understanding of current guidelines and recommendations.

In these guidelines, different athletic activities have been classified by their components of static and dynamic demand. Based on these recommendations, a patient with certain cardiovascular disease may be cleared for participation in one form of activity, but restricted from another. For example, a patient with aortic regurgitation may be able to tolerate high levels of dynamic activity, such as long distance running, whereas caution should be exercised in engaging in activities with a high static demand, such as weight lifting. The Bethesda Guidelines are based primarily on expert consensus opinion and provide a framework for identifying the youth with heart disease who can be risk stratified for participation in athletics.

With a premium being placed on athletic achievement, both for its own sake and with the goal of funding higher education through athletic scholarship, it may be advisable to take into account the natural history of a patient's disease process and attempt to match it to the patient's selection of sports. Doing so early in an athletic career can often avoid the disappointment of having to give up or switch sports once a patient's disease process has progressed to a certain severity. Patients with congenital heart disease often face difficult decisions about when to proceed with additional surgeries during adolescence.

Key message

- The Bethesda Guidelines address specific cardiac disorders and provide a framework in which youth with heart disease can be risk stratified for participation in athletics
- It is helpful for general practitioners to have an understanding of current guidelines and recommendations

---

THE ATHLETE'S HEART

When a well-conditioned athlete undergoes cardiac testing, it is common to discover abnormalities in the ECG tracings or in the left ventricular dimensions on echocardiogram.[37–39] These findings can cause alarm and confusion in the evaluation of a young athlete. It is important to understand the physiologic changes that take place with intense cardiac conditioning and be able to decipher physiologically adaptive changes to exercise from pathologic changes associated with evolving heart disease.

The cardiac response to prolonged, high-intensity training is one of increased ventricular chamber size and wall thickness. Acknowledgments that physiologic changes take place in the heart in response to exercise date back to the nineteenth century.[40] Since that time, physical examination findings suggesting cardiac enlargement in athletes have been further substantiated by chest radiograph, ECG, echocardiogram, and cardiac magnetic resonance imaging findings. These changes in heart morphology are referred to as cardiac remodeling. The type of cardiac remodeling, whether chamber dilatation, hypertrophy, or both, is related to the specific type of conditioning performed. Endurance sports such as cycling, swimming, and canoeing have the greatest impact on left ventricular chamber size and wall thickness.[39] It is important to interpret findings of left ventricular enlargement in the context of the patient's athletic history.

ECG Findings in the Athlete's Heart

ECG findings that may be flagged as abnormal on a computer-generated preliminary report may represent normal physiologic adaptation to exercise. Physiologic dilatation of the left ventricle governs stroke volume (SV). Increased stroke volume allows cardiac output (CO) to be maintained at a lower heart rate (HR) ($CO = HR \times SV$). As a result, sinus bradycardia, with a resting heart rate less than 60 beats per minute, is a common finding in athletes.[41] In highly trained endurance athletes, heart rates may decrease to as low as 30 beats per minute, particularly while asleep. This finding is acceptable, as long as the athlete is asymptomatic and able to adequately increase the heart rate on demand.[37] Sinus bradycardia often coincides with an increase in vagal tone, which can result in the additional, and usually benign, findings of sinus arrhythmia, prolongation of the PR interval (first-degree atrioventricular block), and Mobitz type I or Wenckebach second-degree heart block.[42]

Variations in the QRS morphology and amplitude can also occur in young athletes. The presence of an incomplete right bundle branch block (QRS duration less than 120 milliseconds) or isolated voltage criteria for left ventricular hypertrophy (LVH) may reflect adaptive changes to exercise rather than abnormal hypertrophy.[41] These QRS variations are more concerning when accompanied by abnormalities in the P waves, QRS axis, or repolarization abnormalities than when found in isolation.[37]

A phenomenon of early repolarization, which is characterized as ST elevation most often seen in the precordial leads, is a common finding in well-conditioned athletes.[38] This finding is vagally mediated and should disappear with increased heart rate and exercise.[43] Care should be taken to differentiate benign early repolarization from ST segment changes seen in ischemic heart disease, Brugada syndrome, or LQTS.[37]

There are several abnormal ECG findings that are uncommon in athletes, and should be viewed as red flags, worthy of further evaluation. These include T-wave inversion (other than juvenile pattern seen in lead V1), ST segment depression, pathologic Q waves, left atrial enlargement, right or left bundle branch block, short PR interval with delta wave (preexcitation), QT interval abnormalities, and ST segment changes other than benign early repolariztion.[13]

ECG variations should be interpreted by those with experience in reading pediatric ECGs. Referral to a pediatric cardiologist for further evaluation is often appropriate aside from findings of sinus arrhythmia and sinus bradycardia. Knowledge of the ECG variants commonly seen in athletes can aid in understanding ECG results and allow proper counseling of patients during the cardiac evaluation process (a detailed discussion on ECG findings can be found elsewhere in this issue).

Echocardiographic Findings in the Athlete's Heart

The heart's physiologic response to high-intensity training is a combination of chamber dilatation and wall hypertrophy. These findings can be readily shown on echocardiogram, and must be interpreted in the context of age, body size, gender, and type of sports activity in which the athlete is engaged.[44,45] Left ventricular end diastolic dimension (LVEDD), left ventricular mass, septal and posterior wall thickness, left atrial dimensions, and right atrial and ventricular dimensions may all be increased in well-conditioned athletes.[46] Overall, the athletic heart may often have an LVEDD greater than 55 mm, but seldom greater than 60 mm in diameter.[47,48] Increases in left ventricular wall thickness may be 20% greater than nonathletic controls, but seldom measure more than 12 mm in diameter in men and 11 mm in women.[46,47,49] There is usually symmetry in the hypertrophy between the septal and posterior left ventricular wall in the athlete's heart, and systolic and diastolic function are preserved or enhanced.[44,46,50–52]

Physical Examination Findings in the Athlete's Heart

The cardiac portion of the physical examination of a well-trained athlete may reveal a number of variations from the norm. The athlete may have a heart rate less than 60 beats per minute and noticeable variation of heart rate with respiration (sinus arrhythmia), both owing to increased baseline vagal tone.[41] A physiologic third heart sound (S3) may be present, indicating physiologic vibration of the ventricular walls during passive filling in diastole. Benign systolic murmurs may be heard as well. The low-frequency, vibratory midsystolic murmur best heard between the left lower sternal border and the apex is consistent with a Still murmur, and is loudest when supine. The low-frequency, early to midsystolic murmur best heard at the left upper sternal border with a blowing quality is consistent with a benign pulmonary ejection murmur. These murmurs are not associated with any abnormal clicks, fixed splitting of S2, or thrills, and do not have a diastolic component.

Differentiating the Athlete's Heart from Hypertrophic Cardiomyopathy

Concern arises in differentiating a mild form of HCM from a heart that has hypertrophied because of adaptation to exercise. With adult-sized athletes, a ventricular septum dimension of 13 mm is often thicker than most ventricular septa seen in athletes, as described earlier.[46,47,49] However, because some athletes have been shown to develop a ventricular septal width greater than 13 mm in the absence of any disorder, a so-called gray zone can develop. Because hypertrophy in the athlete results from a physiologic adaptive process, the well-trained athlete with these findings generally should be able to show excellent maximal aerobic capacity with absence of any rhythm or T-wave abnormalities on exercise stress test.[48] Red flags for a diagnosis of HCM include lack of expected physiologic dilatation of the left ventricle, abnormal diastolic function, and family history of HCM.[48] Genetic testing may be useful in certain situations. However, the genetic mutations responsible for some forms of HCM have not been identified, making it difficult to rule out HCM in this fashion (a detailed discussion of HCM can be found elsewhere in this issue).[34]

Care should also be taken to exclude other disorders that can produce LVH in athletes, such as systemic hypertension and coarctation of the aorta. A thorough history and physical examination, including upper and lower extremity blood pressure measurements can be helpful in steering further evaluation of LVH.

When doubt remains as to whether LVH is physiologic or pathologic, a 3-month trial of deconditioning is often advised. In the athletic heart, a 2-mm to 5-mm reduction in septal thickness is expected.[53] Although this practice seems to be scientifically sound, in practice it may be difficult for a high school or college athlete to abstain from training for a period of 3 to 6 months. Many top athletes in this age group participate in multiple sports. In addition, intense off-season training programs may be necessary in order to compete for or retain an athletic scholarship. As a result, the recommendation of a deconditioning period may be met with reluctance. Therefore, the approach to differentiating a diagnosis of athletic heart from one of HCM should be coordinated with the athlete, the family, the primary physician, and specialists.

Key message

- It may be difficult to differentiate physiologic changes that occur in an athletic adolescent from pathologic findings associated with heart disease
- Scrutiny of ECG and echocardiographic findings may lead to differentiation between benign adaptation and pathologic changes. If doubt remains, a 3-month trial of deconditioning may be helpful

---

UNDERSTANDING DISORDERS RESPONSIBLE FOR SCA

A principal reason to provide cardiac clearance for sports participation is to identify those athletes who may be at increased risk for SCA. The incidence of SCA in young athletes in the United States is not known, largely because of a lack of mandated reporting or formal SCA registry. The US Centers for Disease Control and Prevention has estimated that 2000 sudden cardiac-related deaths occur annually in athletes less than 25 years of age.[54] Studies performed by Van Camp and colleages[55] and Maron and colleagues[56] estimated the incidence of SCA in high school athletes to be 1 in 100,000 to 1 in 200,000. Harmon and colleagues[11] arrived at a higher incidence of 1 in 43,000 sudden cardiac deaths among National Collegiate Athletic Association athletes when examining data from 2004 to 2008. Studies have shown that the incidence of sudden cardiac death is highest among highly competitive athletes, particularly male athletes of African descent.[57]

Attempts to provide cardiac clearance for sports participation should center on identifying athletes with risk factors for SCA, and possibly excluding the presence of those disorders responsible for SCA. Maron and colleagues[12] compiled the largest analysis of these causes to date by examining 1866 deaths in young competitive athletes. The leading causes of cardiovascular death included HCM, coronary anomalies, myocarditis, and arrhythmias (**Fig. 1**).[12] Other notable disorders associated with sudden cardiac death included connective tissue disorders and aortic stenosis.[12] Cardiac trauma, including commotio cordis as a cause of sudden death, is discussed elsewhere in this issue. The remainder of this article focuses on clinical identification of 4 cardiac diseases most commonly associated with increased risk of SCA. **Table 1** provides a summary of findings seen in these cardiac diseases.

Hypertrophic Cardiomyopathy

HCM consists of not only an abnormal thickening of the myocardium but also an abnormal arrangement of the myocardial fibers on a histologic level.[58] The patient with HCM is predisposed to both left ventricular outflow tract obstruction and cardiac arrhythmia. Inheritance of HCM follows an autosomal dominant pattern. A detailed family history is essential for screening. History in symptomatic individuals may reveal easy fatigability, dyspnea on exertion, chest pain, or palpitations. Syncope or near syncope is an ominous sign.[59] Physical examination shows a systolic ejection murmur over the left ventricular outflow tract when obstruction exists; however, a diagnosis of HCM is possible without having significant obstruction at a given point in time. If present, this murmur may be brought out by performing the Valsalva maneuver. The murmur becomes less prominent when squatting. A high-frequency, systolic regurgitant murmur at the cardiac apex of mitral regurgitation may be present as well, owing to systolic anterior motion of the mitral valve. The most common ECG findings include LVH and abnormalities in repolarization (T-wave morphology) (**Fig. 2**).[60] Echocardiographic findings may include LVH (often asymmetric and most prominent in the ventricular septum), systolic anterior motion of the mitral valve with mitral regurgitation, and varying degrees of pressure gradient across the left ventricular outflow tract.[61] The degree of left ventricular outflow tract obstruction can progress throughout childhood and adolescence. Patients with HCM are at risk for ventricular arrhythmia, with ventricular fibrillation being the most common cause of death.[62] Management involves avoidance of a hyperdynamic physiologic state and prevention of arrhythmia (with or without implantation of an automatic internal defibrillator device). First-degree relatives should be evaluated by a cardiologist because of the genetic nature of this disease.

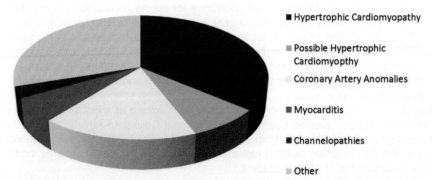

■ Hypertrophic Cardiomyopathy

■ Possible Hypertrophic Cardiomyopthy

Coronary Artery Anomalies

■ Myocarditis

■ Channelopathies

■ Other

Fig. 1. Causes of sudden cardiac death in young athletes. (*Data from* Maron BJ, Thompson PD, Ackerman MJ, et al. Recommendations and considerations related to preparticipation screening for cardiovascular abnormalities in competitive athletes: 2007 update. Circulation 2007;115:1643–55.)

Table 1
Common causes of SCA. Some of the most typical findings in diseases associated with SCA

Disorder	History	Physical Examination	ECG	Echocardiogram	Other
HCM	Syncope, presyncope, dyspnea, chest pain, fatigue with exercise, palpitations	LVOTO murmur, mitral regurgitation murmur	LVH, LAE, abnormal T waves, ventricular ectopy	LVH, SAM, LVOTO	FH: enlarged heart, sudden cardiac death
Coronary artery abnormalities	Syncope, presyncope, or chest pain during or immediately following exercise	Normal	LVH, evidence of prior infarct, arrhythmia; often resting ECG is normal	Abnormal origin or course of coronary arteries	May be difficult to appreciate on echocardiogram; additional imaging may be required
Myocarditis	Recent fever/illness, malaise. Syncope, presyncope, dyspnea with exercise. Palpitations, chest pain	Tachycardia, tachypnea, organomegaly, JVD, ectopic beats	Tachycardia, low voltage QRS, ST–T-wave changes, PR prolongation, arrhythmia	Left ventricular dilatation, valve regurgitation, depressed function, pericardial effusion	CXR: cardiomegaly, increased pulmonary vascular markings
Channelopathies (LQTS)	Syncope, presyncope with exercise or trigger, seizure, cardiac arrest, palpitations	Normal	Prolonged QTc, abnormal T waves, bradycardia	Normal	FH: sudden cardiac death, syncope, seizures, sensorineural deafness

Abbreviations: CXR, chest radiograph; FH, family history; JVD, jugular venous distension; LAE, left atrial enlargement; LVH, left ventricular outflow tract obstruction; QTc, corrected QT interval; SAM, systolic anterior motion of the mitral valve.

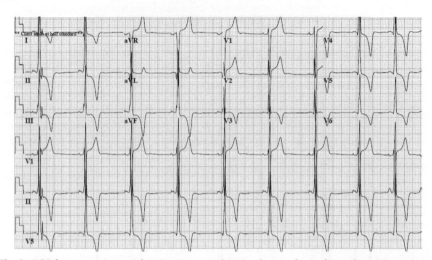

Fig. 2. ECG from a patient with HCM. Increased QRS voltages throughout the ECG consistent with LVH. T-wave inversion in inferior and lateral leads showed abnormal repolarization. Note that the precordial leads are obtained at half standard. (*Courtesy of* H. Singh, MD, Detroit, MI.)

Coronary Artery Abnormalities

Coronary artery abnormalities placing athletes at risk for SCA include abnormal origin and intramural course of the coronary artery. These coronary artery configurations (**Fig. 3**) compromise myocardial blood supply and can lead to ischemia under certain physiologic conditions. Symptoms of syncope or chest pain may occur with exercise, although the initial presentation may be SCA.[35] Physical examination is unremarkable. ECG may show LVH, evidence of prior infarction, or arrhythmia, but is often normal at rest.[35] Q waves in leads I and aVL can be seen in anomalous coronary artery from the pulmonary artery, but this entity most commonly presents in infancy. Exercise stress test can sometimes show evidence of ischemia and reproduce symptoms, although it may be normal, particularly if maximal exertion is not achieved. Vigilant

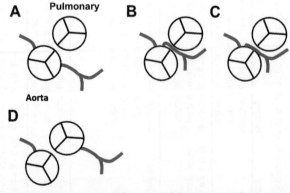

Fig. 3. Coronary artery arrangements. (*A*) Normal. (*B*) Interarterial course with left main coronary artery from the right sinus. (*C*) Intraluminal course with left main coronary artery from the right sinus. (*D*) Anomalous origin of the left coronary artery from the pulmonary artery.

echocardiography may identify coronary artery anomalies. Poor acoustic windows in an individual can make visualization of the coronary arteries challenging and another form of cross-sectional imaging is recommended. Treatment of coronary abnormalities consists of sports restriction and surgical repair.

Myocarditis

Myocarditis consists of inflammation of the heart muscle, most often as a consequence of prior or current infection. Antecedent viral prodrome followed by fatigue, arthralgia, and malaise are classic findings.[63] Diaphoresis, pallor, and syncope with activity provide evidence of poor cardiac function and inability to meet increased metabolic needs. Physical examination findings are those of congestive heart failure: jugular venous distension, pulmonary crackles, and hepatomegaly. A high-frequency, systolic regurgitant murmur at the cardiac apex from mitral regurgitation may be present as well. Tachycardia out of proportion to fever and irregular rhythms may occur. Atrial or ventricular ectopy can also be seen on ECG. If pericardial inflammation is present, increased voltages may be present throughout the precordial leads.[63] Cardiomegaly with increased pulmonary vascular markings is common on chest radiograph. The echocardiogram often reveals ventricular dilatation with poor systolic function and mitral regurgitation. Treatment of myocarditis is primarily supportive, with anticongestive therapy. Cardiac transplantation may be indicated when cardiac function fails to normalize after the acute illness.

Channelopathies

LQTS is an abnormality in cardiac repolarization manifested by prolongation of the QT interval on the ECG, often with other abnormalities of the T-wave morphology (**Fig. 4**). The inheritance pattern can be either autosomal dominant or recessive, allowing family history of channelopathy to raise suspicion for LQTS in an individual. Symptoms usually manifest by the teenage years, and include presyncope or syncope, seizure, palpitations, or SCA. Sensorineural deafness is a manifestation of Jervell and Lange-Nielsen syndrome, a specific form of LQTS type I.[64] Physical examination is often unremarkable, unless associated with a specific syndrome. ECG is the primary diagnostic tool, showing a corrected QT interval (QTc) greater than normal limits, and

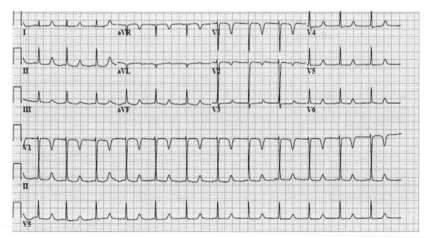

Fig. 4. ECG from a patient LQTS. Prolonged QTc with abnormal T-wave morphology. (*Courtesy of* H. Singh, MD, Detroit, MI.)

often greater than 470 to 480 milliseconds.[65] Significant overlap in the values of the QTc exists between individuals with a channelopathy and healthy subjects.[66] For this reason, a positive history of cardiac events or symptoms may be crucial in making the diagnosis. Genetic testing, additional ECG findings, and composite scoring systems have also been used to assist in diagnosis.[65] Echocardiogram is not helpful. Management may include activity restriction, medical therapy, possible defibrillator or pacemaker implantation, or left cervicothoracic stellectomy.

Key message

- The goal of preparticipation screening is to identify those at risk for sudden cardiac events
- General practitioners benefit by becoming familiar with the most common cardiac disorders responsible for sudden cardiac events and their presentations
- The most common causes of sudden cardiac events in adolescents include HCM, coronary anomalies, myocarditis, arrhythmias, certain connective tissue disorders, and congenital cardiac lesions like aortic stenosis
- Cardiac trauma including commotio cordis can be a cause of sudden death in adolescents

---

SUMMARY

Although primary prevention of SCA through screening is desirable, the ability to do so in a practical, reproducible, and comprehensive manner in the United States remains elusive. As a result, the AAP and AHA recommend the use of patient history, family history, physical examination, and additional testing depending on clinical suspicion as the mainstay of preparticipation screening. Knowledge of signs and symptoms of cardiac diseases can alert practitioners to those who may be at risk for SCA. Evidence is growing for the effective implementation of secondary preventative measures such as early access to CPR and defibrillation.

REFERENCES

1. 2010-11 High school athletics participation survey conducted by The National Federation of State High School Associations. Based on competition at the high school level in 2010-11 school year.
2. Corrado D, Biffi A, Migliore F, et al. Primary prevention of sudden death in young competitive athletes by preparticipation screening. Card Electrophysiol Clin 2013;5:13–21.
3. Baggish A, Hutter A Jr, Wang F. Cardiovascular screening in college athletes with and without electrocardiography. Ann Intern Med 2010;152:269–75.
4. Myerburg RJ, Vetter VL. Electrocardiograms should be included in preparticipation screening of athletes. Circulation 2007;116:2616–26.
5. Corrado D, Basso C, Pavei A, et al. Trends in sudden cardiovascular death in young competitive athletes after implementation of a preparticipation screening program. JAMA 2006;296:1593–601.
6. Maron BJ, Haas TS, Doerer JJ, et al. Comparison of U.S. and Italian experiences with sudden cardiac death in young competitive athletes and implications for preparticipation screening strategies. Am J Cardiol 2009;104:276–80.
7. Weiner RB, Wang F, Hutter A Jr, et al. The feasibility, diagnostic yield, and learning curve of portable echocardiography for out-of hospital cardiovascular disease screening. J Am Soc Echocardiogr 2012;25:568–75.

8. Lai WW, Geva T, Shirali GS. Guidelines and standards for performance of a pediatric echocardiogram: a report from the Task Force of the Pediatric Council of the American Society of Echocardiography. J Am Soc Echocardiogr 2006;19: 1413–30.

9. Halkin A, Steinvil A, Rosso R, et al. Preventing sudden death of athletes with electrocardiographic screening: what is the absolute benefit and how much will it cost? J Am Coll Cardiol 2012;60(22):2271–6.

10. Roberts WO, Stovitz SD. Incidence of sudden cardiac death in Minnesota high school athletes 1993-2012 screened with a standardized preparticipation evaluation. J Am Coll Cardiol 2013. http://dx.doi.org/10.1016/j.jacc.2013.05.080.

11. Harmon KG, Asif IM, Klossner D, et al. Incidence of sudden cardiac death in national collegiate athletic association athletes. Circulation 2011;123:1594–600.

12. Maron BJ, Doerer JJ, Haas TS, et al. Sudden deaths in young competitive athletes: analysis of 1866 deaths in the United States, 1980-2006. Circulation 2009; 119:1085–92.

13. Maron BJ, Thompson PD, Ackerman MJ, et al. Recommendations and considerations related to preparticipation screening for cardiovascular abnormalities in competitive athletes: 2007 update. Circulation 2007;115:1643–55.

14. Rodday MS, Treidman JK, Alexander ME, et al. Electrocardiogram screening for disorders that cause sudden cardiac death in asymptomatic children: a meta-analysis. Pediatrics 2012;129:e999–1010.

15. Section on Cardiology and Cardiac Surgery. Pediatric sudden cardiac arrest. Pediatrics 2012;129:e1094.

16. Campbell RM, Berger S. Preventing pediatric sudden cardiac death: where do we start? Pediatrics 2006;118:802.

17. Kovach J, Berger S. Automated external defibrillators and secondary prevention of sudden cardiac death among children and adolescents. Pediatr Cardiol 2012;33:402–6.

18. Hulkower S, Fagan B, Watts J, et al. Clinical inquiries: do preparticipation clinical exams reduce morbidity and mortality for athletes? J Fam Pract 2005;54:628–32.

19. Bernhardt DT, Roberts WO, American Academy of Family Physicians, American Academy of Pediatrics. PPE: preparticipation physical evaluation. 4th edition. Elk Grove Village (IL): American Academy of Pediatrics; 2010.

20. Behera S, Pattnaik T, Luke A. Practical recommendations and perspectives on cardiac screening for healthy pediatric athletes. Curr Sports Med Rep 2011; 10(2):90–8.

21. Veeram Reddy SR, Singh HR. Chest pain in children and adolescents. Pediatr Rev 2010;31:e1.

22. Venes D, editor. Taber's cyclopedic medical dictionary. 19th edition. Philadelphia: FA Davis; 1997.

23. Nadas AS, Daeschner CW, Roth A, et al. Paroxysmal tachycardia in infants and children: study of 41 cases. Pediatrics 1952;9:167.

24. Johnsrude CL. Current approach to pediatric syncope. Pediatr Cardiol 2000;21: 522–31.

25. Colman N, Bakker A, Linzer M, et al. Value of history-taking in syncope patients: in whom to suspect long QT. Europace 2009;11:937–43.

26. Martin WH III, Coyle EF, Bloomfield SA, et al. Effects of physical deconditioning after intense endurance training on left ventricular dimensions and stroke volume. J Am Coll Cardiol 1986;7:982–9.

27. Cooper WO, Habel LA, Sox CM, et al. ADHD drugs and serious cardiovascular events in children and young adults. N Engl J Med 2011;365:1896–904.

28. Dhar R, Stout CW, Link MS, et al. Cardiovascular toxicities of performance-enhancing substances in sports. Mayo Clin Proc 2005;80(10):1307–15.
29. Ghuran A, Nolan J. Recreational drug misuse: issues for the cardiologist. Heart 2000;83:627–33.
30. Mir A, Obafemi A, Young A, et al. Myocardial infarction associated with use of the synthetic cannabinoid K2. Pediatrics 2011;128:e1622.
31. Tan HL, Hoffman N, van Langen IM, et al. Sudden unexplained death: heritability and diagnostic yield of cardiological and genetic examination in surviving relatives. Circulation 2005;112:207–13.
32. Loeys BL, Deitz HC, Braveman AC, et al. The revised Ghent nosology for the Marfan syndrome. J Med Genet 2010;47(7):476–85.
33. Salerno JC, Seslar SP. Supraventricular tachycardia. Arch Pediatr Adolesc Med 2009;163(3):268–74.
34. Hershberger RE, Lindenfeld J, Mestroni L, et al. Genetic evaluation of cardiomyopathy – a Heart Failure Society of America practice guideline. J Card Fail 2009; 15:83–97.
35. Basso C, Maron BJ, Corrado D, et al. Clinical profile of congenital coronary artery anomalies with origin from the wrong aortic sinus leading to sudden death in young competitive athletes. J Am Coll Cardiol 2000;35:1493–501.
36. Maron BJ, Zipes DP. 36th Bethesda Conference: eligibility recommendations for competitive athletes with cardiovascular abnormalities. J Am Coll Cardiol 2005; 45(8):1318–75.
37. Corrado D, Pelliccia A, Heidbuchel H, et al. Recommendation for interpretation of the 12-lead electrocardiogram in the athlete. Eur Heart J 2010;31: 243–59.
38. Pelliccia A, Maron BJ, Culasso F, et al. Clinical significance of abnormal electrocardiographic patterns in trained athletes. Circulation 2000;102:278–84.
39. Spirito P, Pelliccia A, Proschan MA, et al. Morphology of the "Athlete's Heart" assessed by echocardiography in 947 elite athletes representing 27 sports. Am J Cardiol 1994;74:802–6.
40. Henschen S. Skilanglauf und Skiwettlauf. Eine medizinische Sportstudie. Mitt Med Klin Upsala (Jena) 1899;2:15–8.
41. Sharma S, Whyte G, Elliot P, et al. Electrocardiographic changes in 1000 highly trained junior elite athletes. Br J Sports Med 1999;33:319–24.
42. Myetes I, Kaplinsky E, Yahini J, et al. Wenkebach A-V block: a frequent feature following heavy physical training. Am Heart J 1975;990:426–30.
43. Brady WJ, Chan TC. Electrocardiographic manifestations: benign early repolarization. J Emerg Med 1999;17:473–8.
44. Pluim BM, Zwinderman AH, van dre Laarse A, et al. The athlete's heart: a meta-analysis of cardiac structure and function. Circulation 2000;101:336–44.
45. Pelliccia A, Maron MS, Maron BJ. Assessment of left ventricular hypertrophy in a trained athlete: differential diagnosis of physiological athlete's heart from pathologic hypertrophy. Prog Cardiovasc Dis 2012;54:387–96.
46. Barbier J, Ville N, Kervio G, et al. Sports-specific features of athlete's heart and their relation to echocardiographic parameters. Herz 2006;31:531–43.
47. Pellicia A, Culasso F, Di Paolo F, et al. Physiologic left ventricular cavity dilatation in elite athletes. Ann Intern Med 1999;130:23–31.
48. Maron BJ, Pelliccia A. The heart of trained athletes: cardiac remodeling and the risks of sports, including sudden death. Circulation 2006;114:1633–44.
49. Pelliccia A, Maron BJ, Sparato A, et al. The upper limit of physiologic cardiac hypertrophy in highly trained elite athletes. N Engl J Med 1991;324:295–301.

50. Csandy M, Forster T, Hogye M, et al. Three-year echocardiographic follow-up study on canoeist boys. Acta Cardiol 1986;41:213–5.
51. Griffet V, Finet G, Di Filippo S, et al. Athlete's heart in the young: electrocardiographic and echocardiographic adolescents. Ann Cardiol Angeiol 2013;62(2): 116–21.
52. Pavlick G, Olexo O, Osvath P, et al. Echocardiographic characteristics of male athletes of different age. Br J Sports Med 2001;35:95–9.
53. Maron BJ, Pelliccia A, Sparato A, et al. Reduction in left ventricular wall thickness after deconditioning in highly trained Olympic athletes. Br Heart J 1993; 69:125–8.
54. Kung HC, Hoyert DL, Xu J, et al. Deaths: final data for 2005. Natl Vital Stat Rep 2008;56(10):1–20.
55. Van Camp SP, Bloor CM, Mueller FO, et al. Nontraumatic sports death in high school and college athletes. Med Sci Sports Exerc 1995;27:641–7.
56. Maron BJ, Shirani J, Poliac LC, et al. Sudden death in young competitive athletes: clinical, demographic, and pathological profiles. JAMA 1996;276: 199–204.
57. Maron BJ, Carney KP, Lever HM, et al. Relationship of race to sudden cardiac death in competitive athletes with hypertrophic cardiomyopathy. J Am Coll Cardiol 2003;41:974–80.
58. Varnava AM, Elliott PM, Sharma S, et al. Hypertrophic cardiomyopathy: the interrelation of disarray, fibrosis, and small vessel disease. Heart 2000;84:476–82.
59. Spirito P, Autore C, Rapezzi C, et al. Syncope and risk of sudden death in hypertrophic cardiomyopathy. Circulation 2009;119:1703–10.
60. Savage DD, Seides SF, Clark CE. Electrocardiographic findings in patients with obstructive and nonobstructive hypertrophic cardiomyopathy. Circulation 1978; 58:402–8.
61. Klues HG, Schiffers A, Maron BJ. Phenotypic spectrum and patterns of left ventricular hypertrophy in hypertrophic cardiomyopathy: morphologic observations and significance as assessed by two-dimensional echocardiography in 600 patients. J Am Coll Cardiol 1995;26(7):1699–708.
62. Maron BJ, Olivotto I, Spirito P. Epidemiology of hypertrophic cardiomyopathy-related death: revisited in a large non-referral-based patient population. Circulation 2000;102:858–64.
63. Feldman AM, McNamara D. Myocarditis. N Engl J Med 2000;343:1388–98.
64. Schulze-Bahr E, Haverkamp W, Wedekind H, et al. Autosomal recessive long-QT syndrome (Jervell Lange-Nielsen syndrome) is genetically heterozygous. Hum Genet 1997;100:573–6.
65. Schwartz PJ, Moss AJ, Vincent GM, et al. Diagnostic criteria for the long QT syndrome: an update. Circulation 1993;88:782–4.
66. Taggart NW, Haglund CM, Tester DJ, et al. Diagnostic miscues in congenital long-QT syndrome. Circulation 2007;115:2613–20.

Cardiac Trauma During Teenage Years

Peep Talving, MD, PhD, Demetrios Demetriades, MD, PhD*

KEYWORDS

- Cardiac injury • Teenagers • Epidemiology • Diagnosis • Treatment • Outcomes

KEY POINTS

- Blunt cardiac trauma includes a wide spectrum of conditions, ranging from asymptomatic myocardial contusion to fatal cardiac arrhythmias and/or cardiac rupture.
- Blunt cardiac rupture is a common cause of instant death in traffic injuries.
- The role of cardiac biomarkers remains controversial; however, normal electrocardiogram and troponin levels may rule out a significant blunt cardiac trauma in most cases.
- Significant chest trauma, especially in the presence of multiple rib or sternal fractures or lung contusions, is associated with a high incidence of cardiac involvement.
- Insignificant blunt cardiac injury during sports may cause fatal arrhythmia in teens.
- The diagnosis of penetrating cardiac injury is usually clinical. The Focused Assessment with Sonography in Trauma examination is the most useful and reliable bedside investigation.
- Patients with penetrating cardiac trauma or blunt cardiac rupture presenting with cardiac arrest or imminent cardiac arrest should be managed with an emergency-room resuscitative thoracotomy.
- Survivors of penetrating cardiac injuries should be evaluated with early and late echocardiography to detect anatomic or functional cardiac sequelae.

INTRODUCTION

Trauma is overall the fourth most common cause of death and the leading cause of death in individuals younger than 40 years, accounting for 5 million fatalities worldwide on an annual basis.[1] Thoracic trauma is directly responsible for 25% of trauma deaths, and contributes indirectly to another 25% of trauma-related mortalities.[2]

Thoracic trauma may result in a wide spectrum of cardiac lesions, ranging from an asymptomatic myocardial contusion to a rapidly fatal cardiac tamponade or exsanguination caused by a transmural laceration. The reported incidence of cardiac injuries

Division of Acute Care Surgery (Trauma, Emergency Surgery and Surgical Critical Care), Department of Surgery, Keck School of Medicine, LAC+USC Medical Center, University of Southern California, 2051 Marengo Street, IPT – C5L100, Los Angeles, CA 90033-4525, USA
* Corresponding author.
E-mail address: demetria@usc.edu

Pediatr Clin N Am 61 (2014) 111–130
http://dx.doi.org/10.1016/j.pcl.2013.09.016
0031-3955/14/$ – see front matter © 2014 Elsevier Inc. All rights reserved.

varies widely, with 15% to 76% of patients sustaining major chest injury depending on whether the diagnosis has been made clinically or on autopsy.[3–7] Nevertheless, in penetrating trauma and in victims who die at the scene of the injury, the incidence of cardiac involvement is much higher.[8,9]

Cardiac trauma is uncommon in the pediatric population in the United States. Kaptein and colleagues,[10] in a National Trauma Data Bank (NTDB) review, reported that only 0.03% of all pediatric trauma cases (age <8 years) had a documented cardiac injury. The vast majority of cardiac lesions in this population, however, occurred in teenagers (73%). The American Association for the Surgery of Trauma (AAST) has defined the severity of cardiac injuries in their organ injury scale for standardization purposes (**Table 1**).[11] This article reviews the management of cardiac trauma under the following categories:

1. Blunt cardiac injury (BCI)
2. Penetrating cardiac injury (PCI)

BLUNT CARDIAC INJURY
Background

Borch described the very first myocardial contusion in 1676, and Akenside elucidated the first autopsy-verified BCI in 1764.[12,13] Since the Borch and Akenside reports BCI

Table 1
American Association for the Surgery of Trauma organ injury scale: heart

Grade	Description of Injury
I	Blunt injury with minor electrographic abnormalities Blunt or penetrating pericardial wound without cardiac injury, tamponade, or herniation
II	Blunt cardiac injury with heart block or ischemic changes without heart failure Penetrating tangential myocardial wound up to, but not extending through, endocardium without tamponade
III	Blunt cardiac injury with sustained ($\geq$6 beats/min) or multifocal ventricular contractions Blunt or penetrating injury with septal rupture, pulmonary or tricuspid valvular incompetence, papillary muscle dysfunction, or distal coronary artery occlusion without cardiac failure Blunt pericardial laceration with cardiac herniation Blunt cardiac injury with cardiac failure Penetrating tangential myocardial wound up to, but not extending through, endocardium, with tamponade
IV	Blunt or penetrating injury with septal rupture, pulmonary or tricuspid valve incompetence, papillary muscle dysfunction, or distal coronary artery arterial occlusion with cardiac failure Blunt or penetrating injury with aortic or mitral valve incompetence Blunt or penetrating injury of the right ventricle, right atrium, or left atrium
V	Blunt or penetrating injury with proximal coronary artery occlusion Blunt or penetrating injury of the left ventricle Stellate wound with <50% tissue loss of the right ventricle, right atrium, or left atrium
VI	Blunt avulsion of the heart; penetrating wound producing >50% tissue loss of a chamber

From Moore EE, Cogbill TH, Malangoni MA, et al. Organ injury scaling. Surg Clin North Am 1995;75:293; with permission.

has been a subject of debate, and the injury is still poorly defined. In the past, BCI has had a variety of diagnostic descriptions including myocardial contusion, cardiac contusion, or commotio cordis, to mention a few. To consolidate the terminology, Mattox and colleagues[14] in 1992 suggested defining nonpenetrating or blunt cardiac lesions in a standardized manner.

In the teenage population, the most common mechanism of traumatic cardiac injury is blunt, accounting for 60% of cases. Kaptein and colleagues,[10] in their NTDB review, noted that rib fractures, hemothorax, and pulmonary contusions served as markers of BCI in pediatric patients, possibly because a pliable chest wall allows transfer of the energy to the heart. Overall, 10% of all teenagers in this study required a resuscitative thoracotomy. The overall mortality in teenagers sustaining cardiac injuries was noted to be 42%.

Sports-related cardiac injuries among young athletes are rare. A recent study in National Collegiate Athletic Association student-athletes reported 273 sudden cardiac deaths over a 5-year study period, with an incidence of 1 per 43,770 participants per year. The majority of deaths (68%) was nonmedical, and occurred outside of the playing field. The medical causes of sudden death were cardiovascular-related incidents in 56% (n = 45), and represented 75% of deaths occurring during exertion. Basketball was by far the highest-risk sport, with an overall annual sudden cardiac death rate of 1 in 11,394 participants per year.[15] Whereas the coronary artery disease as a cause of sudden cardiac death prevails in athletes older than 45 years, electrical conduction abnormalities or cardiac channelopathies have risen in prominence as a cause of cardiac deaths in younger individuals during sports activities.[16]

In general, BCI can be subclassified as electrical or structural in nature, with a clinical presentation ranging from asymptomatic alterations in the electrocardiogram (ECG) or elevation of cardiac enzymes to lesions involving the septal wall, valvular apparatus, coronary artery, or instantly fatal rupture of the cardiac wall.[17,18] Sinus tachycardia or nonspecific T- and ST-segment changes may be the only manifestation in the vast majority of BCI cases.

The mechanisms of BCI include motor vehicle crashes, auto-versus-pedestrian impacts, crush injuries, falls, assaults, or sports and recreational injuries (**Fig. 1**).[19] However, in recent decades there have been numerous reports describing instantaneous cardiac arrest following very modest blunt chest injuries either in a domestic setting or during sports-related activities in young individuals without cardiovascular preconditions.[20] It has been postulated that these fatal BCIs are due to a pliable chest wall in young individuals, allowing direct transfer of the impact from the precordium to the myocardium.[17] Another determinant of fatal blunt injury is the timing of the impact during the electrical cardiac cycle. In an experimental model, blunt impact to the anterior chest occurring in a 30- to 15-millisecond window before the T-wave peak produced fatal ventricular fibrillation, which resembled the catastrophic events described in young individuals as commotio cordis (**Fig. 2**).[21] The incidence of commotio cordis, and its role in sudden cardiac deaths and fatality rates, have been undetermined and underreported. Recently, however, Maron and colleagues[22] investigated the incidence and mortality rates of commotio cordis based on the unique US Commotio Cordis Registry data set. Of a total of 216 cases reported to the registry since 1970, 161 (75%) were younger than 18 years and 77% of victims were engaged in sporting activities during the cardiac event. The overall reported mortality was 72%. Of interest, these investigators noted a progressive 5-fold increase in survival following commotio cordis–related cardiac events, from 10% to 15% before the year 2000 to greater than 50% during the recent 5-year period.

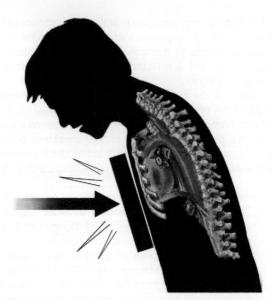

Fig. 1. Typical mechanism of blunt cardiac injury in a motor vehicle crash. (*Courtesy of* A. Demetriades, BS, Los Angeles, CA; with permission.)

There is no reliable correlation between electrical abnormalities and structural lesions in BCI. The observed structural lesions following BCI range from subendocardial or subepicardial to full-thickness bruising of the myocardium that may result in the spectrum of injuries mentioned in **Table 1**. An autopsy study by Parmley and

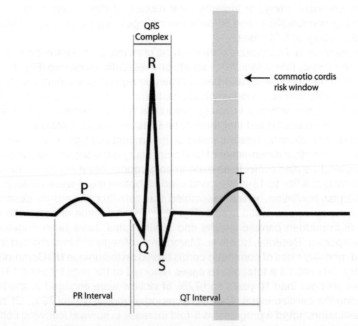

Fig. 2. Electrical cardiac cycle with vulnerable window for ventricular fibrillation in direct blunt injury. (*Courtesy of* A. Demetriades, BS, Los Angeles, CA; with permission.)

colleagues[23] noted that the most common structural lesion was multichamber cardiac wall rupture, followed by partial lacerations and severe contusions of the myocardium. Valvular lesions in this study were almost nonexistent. In another recent coroner's study, Teixeira and colleagues[18] from Los Angeles noted that 32% of all deaths following blunt trauma had a BCI, with 64% involving multiple cardiac chambers (**Fig. 3**). In the contemporary clinical setting, the most common pathologic features following BCI consist of contusions that are asymptomatic and require no workup, unless they are associated with significant dysrhythmias or cardiac failure.

Screening and Diagnosis

There is a lack of a gold standard in the diagnosis of BCI, and there is no single test that can diagnose cellular, electrical, and/or structural lesions. For this reason, the diagnosis of BCI relies on a combination of history, clinical examination, ECG, cardiac enzyme assays, computed tomography (CT) for associated injuries, echocardiography, and nuclear studies. Diagnostic modalities in the workup of BCI and its complications are listed in **Box 1**. In many cases, the injury is clinically insignificant and requires observation but no treatment. However, it is of paramount importance to recognize and treat those injuries that are clinically significant and require aggressive management so as to avoid fatal arrhythmias or cardiogenic shock. Many trauma providers define BCI when there is blunt thoracic trauma accompanied by cardiogenic shock, arrhythmias requiring treatment, or structural lesions related to cardiac insult. The recent evidence-based guidelines by the Eastern Association for Surgery on Trauma state that all patients who have a significant mechanism of injury or those who respond poorly to resuscitative efforts should be screened for BCI (**Box 2**).[24]

Chest Radiography

A chest radiograph is frequently the initial screening modality obtained following blunt chest injury. This investigation is nonspecific for BCI. The most specific pathologic chest-radiographic findings indicating severe BCI are pulmonary congestion and a widened mediastinum owing to cardiac failure or tamponade, respectively. However, a widened mediastinum is more frequently seen with sternal fracture and an associated retrosternal hematoma, thoracic spine fracture with hematoma in the posterior mediastinum, or thoracic aortic injury. Moreover, chest radiography reliably reveals concomitant injuries to the lung and the chest wall.

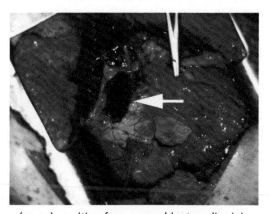

Fig. 3. Atrial rupture (*arrow*) resulting from severe blunt cardiac injury.

Box 1
The spectrum of diagnostic modalities in workup of blunt cardiac injury

History and physical examination

Chest radiograph

Electrocardiogram

Cardiac enzymes

   Creatine phosphokinase myocardial band

   Cardiac troponin I

   Cardiac troponin T

Echocardiography

   Transthoracic echocardiography

   Transesophageal echocardiography

Nuclear imaging studies

   Gated radionuclide angiography

   Multiple gated acquisition angiography

   Technetium pyrophosphate scanning

   Single-photon emission computed tomography

   Thallium-201 scanning

   Antimyosin scintigraphy

Pulmonary artery catheterization

Electrocardiogram

The 12-lead ECG should be performed in all patients sustaining a significant chest trauma, and they should receive continuous cardiac monitoring. Overall, an abnormal ECG can be noted in 40% to 83% of BCI patients within the first 24 to 48 hours following injury. There is a variety of rhythm abnormalities associated with BCI (**Box 3**). The most frequently observed electrical abnormalities on ECG are sinus tachycardia, followed by nonspecific ST-T wave changes, atrial fibrillation, premature ventricular contractions, and right bundle branch block.[25–27] The presence of sinus tachycardia should lead to a search for active hemorrhage. Atrial fibrillation, albeit rare in this setting, has been associated with poor outcomes. The most common fatal arrhythmia following BCI is ventricular fibrillation, even in the absence of major structural abnormality (see **Box 3**).

Cardiac Enzymes

Many studies have looked at the diagnostic value of cardiac enzymes, such as myocardial band of creatine phosphokinase (CK-MB), cardiac troponin T (cTnT), or cardiac troponin I (cTnI) in BCI settings. In a prospective study by Salim and colleagues,[26] it was noted that the ECG and cTnI had positive predictive values of 28% and 48% in diagnosing a BCI, respectively. However, with normal ECG and enzyme assay on admission, these markers uncombined had a negative predictive value of 95% and 93%, respectively. When both tests (ECG + cTnI) were abnormal or normal, the positive and negative predictive values increased to 62% and 100%, respectively. Another study by Walsh and colleagues[28] noted that combination of

---

Box 2
Evidence-based recommendations for the management of blunt cardiac injury (BCI)

Level I

An admission electrocardiogram (ECG) should be performed on all patients in whom there is suspected BCI.

Level II

1. If the admission ECG is abnormal (arrhythmia, ST-segment changes, ischemia, heart block, unexplained sinus tachycardia), the patient should be admitted for continuous ECG monitoring for 24 to 48 hours. Conversely, if the admission ECG is normal, the risk of having a BCI that requires treatment is insignificant, and the pursuit of diagnosis should be terminated.

2. If the patient is hemodynamically unstable, an imaging study (echocardiogram) should be obtained. If an optimal transthoracic echocardiogram cannot be performed, the patient should have a transesophageal echocardiogram.

3. Nuclear medicine studies add little when compared with echocardiography, and thus are not useful if an echocardiogram has been performed.

Level III

1. Elderly patients with known cardiac disease, unstable patients, and those with an abnormal admission ECG can be safely operated on provided they are appropriately monitored. Consideration should be given to placement of a pulmonary artery catheter in such cases.

2. The presence of a sternal fracture does not predict the presence of BCI, and thus does not necessarily indicate that monitoring should be performed.

3. Neither creatinine phosphokinase with isoenzyme analysis nor measurement of circulating cardiac troponin T are useful in predicting which patients have or will have complications related to BCI.

From Clancy K, Velopulos C, Bilaniuk JW, et al. Screening for blunt cardiac injury: an Eastern Association for the Surgery of Trauma practice management guideline. J Trauma Acute Care Surg 2012;73(5 Suppl 4);S301–6; with permission.

Box 3
Cardiac arrhythmias associated with blunt cardiac injury

Sinus tachycardia

Atrial fibrillation

ST-segment elevations/depressions

T-wave abnormalities

Atrioventricular blocks

Right bundle branch block

Bradycardia

Ventricular tachycardia

Ventricular fibrillation

ECG and cardiac cTnI reliably diagnosed significant BCI. Likewise, Rajan and Zell-weger[29] observed that a cTnI value of less than 1.05 μg/L on admission and within 6 hours ruled out BCI. However, there are no studies that correlate cardiac biomarkers to the extent of BCI or outcomes.[6,30,31] Some trauma care providers do not perform routine troponin assays unless evaluating for coronary artery involvement following BCI.[32] Accepting the ambiguity of the currently available data, the authors' current practice is to obtain a 12-lead ECG and cTnI assays on admission, at 4 hours, and at 8 hours in all patients sustaining significant BCI.

Echocardiography

Echocardiography is not a useful screening tool following BCI, and should be reserved for patients with hemodynamic compromise or arrhythmias. Echocardiography provides direct visualization of ventricular contusions, cardiac chamber size, wall motion, valvular function, cardiac tamponade, septal defects, and/or intracardiac thrombi. In many instances, transthoracic echocardiography (TTE) may be limited by chest wall injuries, pain, chest tubes, and chest-wall emphysema following severe chest trauma.

Karalis and colleagues[33] performed a TTE on 105 patients following severe thoracic injury. Twenty patients (19%) required a transesophageal echocardiogram (TEE) owing to suboptimal TTE images. These investigators reported myocardial contusion in 30% of patients, infrequently requiring interventions and associated with favorable outcome. TEE was found to be of value when TTE images were suboptimal and in cases of suspected aortic injury. Bromberg and colleagues[34] demonstrated the role of TTE in children with hemodynamic compromise in the setting of BCI. Based on these reports, TTE may be a good choice as the initial study, with TEE being of use in cases with suboptimal TTE images or suspected aortic injury.

Treatment

Asymptomatic patients with abnormal ECG or cardiac enzymes should be observed in a monitored intensive care unit until findings return to normal. There is no need for any specific treatment in this group of patients. Echocardiography should be performed to evaluate for any underlying functional or anatomic abnormalities. The treatment of symptomatic patients with cardiogenic shock or arrhythmias is similar to that for non-traumatic conditions, and may include replacement of intravascular volume, inotropic agents, and occasional placement of an intra-aortic balloon pump.[35] Serial echocardiography should be performed to rule out delayed tamponade or other structural complications. Treatment of coronary artery injury includes medical management, percutaneous intervention, and/or operative revascularization. Fibrinolytic therapy is usually contraindicated because of associated injuries, although it may be an option in isolated cardiac trauma.[36] Treatment of any BCI with pericardial tamponade and hypotension requires immediate surgical exploration. Operative repair is preferably performed off bypass, to avoid the risks associated with systemic anticoagulation and the risks of inducing arrest in a severely contused heart.[36,37]

Cardiac ruptures following severe blunt impact are universally fatal. Multiple coroner's studies have revealed that approximately 30% of all deaths following blunt trauma are due to cardiac rupture.[18,23] Large myocardial contusions following BCI are associated with arrhythmias, late rupture, aneurysm formation, congestive heart failure, and/or intracavitary thrombus formation, and hence require careful clinical and sonographic follow-up.[38] Asymptomatic patients with an absence of BCI structural abnormalities have a good prognosis.

Key message

- Trauma is the leading cause of death in individuals younger than 40 years
- Cardiac trauma in the pediatric population is rare
- Blunt trauma is the most common mechanism in the teenage population
- Commotio cordis refers to a rare catastrophic event caused by ventricular fibrillation as a result of a BCI
- Most common abnormality following a BCI is asymptomatic myocardial contusion
- Diagnosis is established with a combination of history, physical examination, ECG, cardiac enzymes, echocardiography, and/or CT for associated injuries
- Clinical presentation includes a wide spectrum ranging from asymptomatic to catastrophic events
- Based on the clinical presentation, treatment may involve observation only or management of cardiogenic shock, arrhythmias, and/or coronary injuries
- Careful clinical and sonographic follow-up is recommended

PENETRATING CARDIAC INJURY
Background

Cardiac injuries have been described since Homer's *Iliad*. The first successful attempt to repair a penetrating cardiac wound was performed by Dr Ansel Cappelen of Norway in 1895. Unfortunately, this patient expired 3 days later because of sepsis. The first cardiac repair resulting in survival was performed by Ludwig Rehn of Germany who, in 1896, repaired a right ventricular stab wound in a 22-year-old man.[39] In 1907, Duval of France described median sternotomy as the universal access to cardiac wounds, a technique that is still in use today. Dr Hill of Montgomery, Alabama, reported the first repair of cardiac injury in the United States, involving a wound to the left ventricle in a 13-year-old teenager. A detailed and thorough history of penetrating cardiac wounds has been described by contemporary investigators.[40]

Cardiac injuries constitute the most lethal lesion following a traumatic event. Campbell and colleagues[41] conducted a population-based study over 2 consecutive years in South Africa, and observed that 1198 patients incurred cardiac injury during the study period. The survival data of all cardiac injuries reviewed at their emergency medical facilities and mortuaries yielded a prehospital case fatality rate of 94%. Of note, in this examination 50% of those reaching hospital with signs of life also expired, comprising an overall mortality of 97%. Likewise, Rhee and colleagues[42] performed a population-based retrospective cohort analysis of 20,181 victims of penetrating cardiac injuries over a 7-year time interval, and noted an overall case fatality rate of 80.7%. When stratified according to the trauma mechanism, stab wounds and gunshot wounds to the heart resulted in mortality rates of 67.4% and 90.3%, respectively. Clarke and colleagues[43] conducted another population-based investigation of cardiac injuries in South Africa, noting an overall case fatality of 76%. These 3 studies included both adults and adolescents.

There are few data on outcomes of pediatric penetrating cardiac injuries. Lustenberger and colleagues from Los Angeles reported their 11-year in-hospital outcomes of penetrating cardiac involvement, specifically in teenagers. Of all 4569 pediatric trauma admissions during the study period, penetrating cardiac injuries were diagnosed in 32 patients (0.7%); 81.2% had sustained a stab wound to the heart (**Fig. 4**). The cardiac chambers involved were the right ventricle, left ventricle, right

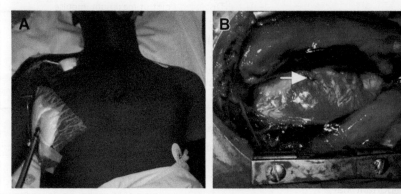

Fig. 4. (*A*) A teenager who sustained a stab wound to the anterior chest. The wound resulted in right ventricular injury and cardiac tamponade. (*B*) The repaired cardiac stab wound to the right ventricle (*arrow*) of the same patient.

atrium, and multiple chambers in 46.9%, 43.8%, 18.8%, and 9.4%, respectively. Overall, only 28.1% survived to discharge. Nonsurvivors had a significantly higher incidence of transmural cardiac wounds. When survival was stratified according to location of cardiac injury, patients with a wound to the right atrium, left ventricle, right ventricle, and multiple chambers had mortality rates of 83.3%, 78.6%, 66.7%, and 100%, respectively.[44] Many investigators have attempted to determine predictors of survival following PCI. Asensio and colleagues[45] prospectively studied 60 patients who sustained a cardiac injury and noted an overall survival of 37%. Survival was predicted in this study by the presence of sinus rhythm and trauma mechanism: 68% and 14% following stab wounds and gunshot wounds, respectively. The location of the injury to any particular cardiac chamber or the presence of tamponade, however, did not predict outcomes. Tyburski and colleagues[46] retrospectively studied predictors of outcomes following cardiac injuries in 302 patients, and noted that hemodynamic stability and trauma mechanism predicted survival: 58% and 23% following stab wounds and gunshot wounds, respectively. A future meta-analysis of all available investigations may identify reliable predictors of outcomes in these instances.

Screening and Clinical Diagnosis

Any stab wound or gunshot wound to the chest has a potential for cardiac injury. A majority of individuals with gunshot wounds to the heart expire on the field. By contrast, cardiac injuries following stab wounds are more likely to reach hospital care. Most cardiac stab wounds (84%) involve the "cardiac box," defined as an area inferior to clavicles, superior to costal margins, and medial to midclavicular lines.[47] Nevertheless, any gunshot wound to the torso can potentially traverse the mediastinum and reach the heart. Likewise, stab wounds to the deltoid area, upper abdomen, or posterior chest may cause cardiac injury. Of interest, Degiannis and colleagues[48] from South Africa noted that mortality in patients arriving at the emergency department with precordial in comparison with extraprecordial stab wounds resulted in 96% versus 75% survival. This finding indicates the seriousness of penetrating injury to any location in the chest or in proximity to the chest.

Patients with PCI may present in shock. Some cases with small superficial injuries or short prehospital times may be hemodynamically stable on admission. Distended neck veins, as expected in patients with cardiac tamponade, may not be seen in the presence of significant blood loss. On the other hand, neck-vein distention can also be seen in tension pneumothorax and sometimes with restlessness. The classic Beck's triad includes muffled heart sounds, distended neck veins, and hypotension, and occurs in 90% of cases of cardiac tamponade. It is important for health care providers to be vigilant, as some of these findings of tamponade or impending tamponade may be missed in an emergency setting. Another clinical sign, present in about 10% of cases of cardiac tamponade, is pulsus paradoxus (a decrease in systolic blood pressure >10 mm Hg during inspiration). An interesting and common clinical sign of cardiac injury is severe agitation, frequently misinterpreted as intoxication. The reason for the agitation may be related to increased intracranial pressure and venous outflow stasis from the brain caused by the increased intrapericardial pressure. Because of the lack of valves in the internal jugular veins, the elevated intrapericardial pressure is transmitted directly in a retrograde fashion to the brain.

It is important that any penetrating injury in proximity to the chest, especially in the presence of hypotension or agitation, should be presumed to be due to cardiac trauma until proved otherwise.

Investigations

Timely management is of critical importance for the survival of victims with cardiac trauma. Patients with major hemodynamic instability should promptly undergo emergency-room resuscitative thoracotomy or should be rushed to the operating room without waiting for any investigations. Diagnostic studies should be reserved only for stable patients with no clear evidence of cardiac trauma.

Focused Assessment With Sonography in Trauma

The Focused Assessment with Sonography in Trauma (FAST) examination is a quick, useful, and reliable bedside investigation in the emergency room (**Fig. 5**). Bedside FAST performed by a surgeon or emergency medicine provider assesses for free fluid in 4 areas: the perisplenic area, pelvis, hepatorenal space, and pericardium. There are multiple prospective and retrospective investigations depicting the diagnostic accuracy of FAST in cardiac injuries.[49–52] In summary, the pericardial FAST has an overall pooled sensitivity of 100% and specificity of 99%, and the international consensus conference described the FAST examination as "an expeditious focused interrogation of pericardial and peritoneal space looking for free fluid as a marker of injury."[53] In

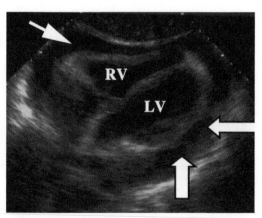

Fig. 5. Focused Assessment with Sonography in Trauma depicts pericardial effusion consistent with cardiac tamponade (*arrows*). LV, left ventricle; RV, right ventricle.

some clinical settings a false-negative study can occur, which may obscure a potentially fatal cardiac injury.[49,50,54–56] These scenarios include pericardial effusion decompressing into the chest, massive hemothorax precluding a reliable sonographic window, mediastinal hemorrhage, or extensive emphysema of the anterior chest wall, frequently associated with pneumothoraces. If there is high suspicion of a cardiac injury and a negative FAST, further steps must be urgently taken, including immediate insertion of a chest tube and a repeat FAST examination.[50,56]

Chest Radiography

Chest radiography should be performed based on the stability of the patient. Radiologic findings suspicious for cardiac involvement may be found in about half of the patients, and include a globular heart (**Fig. 6**), widened upper mediastinum, and pneumopericardium. In a series of 70 cases, Demetriades[37] reported an incidence of 47% of radiologic findings suggestive of cardiac trauma. However, chest radiographs may not be useful early in the course of the process, because a minimum of 200 mL of pericardial fluid is necessary for it to cause enlargement of the cardiac silhouette. The superior vena cava may become distended because of increased pericardial pressure as a result of tamponade, and may be evident on the chest radiograph as a widened upper mediastinum. Pneumopericardium itself does not suggest pericardial tamponade, although its presence supports pericardial violation (**Fig. 7**).

Electrocardiogram

The ECG has been widely used in the initial evaluation of patients with potential cardiac injury, but holds only moderate diagnostic accuracy in this setting. ECG findings may reflect either tamponade or ischemia. The classic findings of tamponade consist of low-voltage QRS complexes, alternating magnitude of QRS complexes (known as electrical alternans), sinus tachycardia, and tachyarrhythmia. Ischemic changes are reflected by ST-segment depressions or elevations.[57,58]

Pericardiocentesis

Emergent pericardiocentesis as a management strategy in cases of PCI has been abandoned in high-level trauma centers around the world for the following reasons. First, the blood in the pericardial cavity may clot, rendering false-negative results on

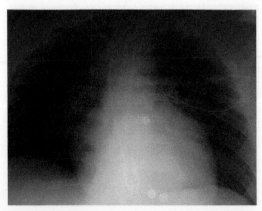

Fig. 6. Chest radiograph demonstrating a "globular heart" caused by cardiac tamponade following penetrating cardiac injury.

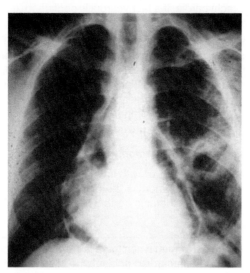

Fig. 7. Chest radiograph showing extensive pneumoperitoneum caused by a pericardial stab wound.

aspiration in 50% to 60% of cases of cardiac tamponade. Second, cardiac wall injury, coronary artery injuries, hemothorax, pneumothorax, and mediastinal hematoma can occur as a result of the procedure.[59] Hence, pericardiocentesis can be used only as a temporizing measure if surgical expertise is not immediately available.

Subxiphoid Pericardial Window

Because of the inherent limitations in diagnostic modalities in diagnosing cardiac injury, the subxiphoid pericardial window (SPW) has been historically considered as the gold-standard diagnostic procedure. Hemodynamic compromise with suspicion of cardiac injury requiring immediate sternotomy is a clear contraindication for the SPW. However, some centers have continued to investigate this modality because of the limitations of FAST in their experience.[8,60,61] In a recent prospective, randomized, single-center study from South Africa, the SPW was not inferior to sternotomy as a diagnostic and treatment option for stable patients with pericardial tamponade.[61]

Central Venous Pressure

The diagnostic value of central venous pressure (CVP) in the management of PCI has been abandoned in the era of echocardiography. In a retrospective study, Symbas and colleagues[62] noted that CVP values beyond 12 mm Hg with precordial stab wounds were strongly suggestive of cardiac tamponade. Other investigators, however, have not observed reliable associations between elevated CVP and cardiac tamponade.[63]

Computed Tomography

CT has become an integral part of evaluation of a stable trauma victim. CT is readily available and is usually a second-tier diagnostic modality in stable patients with penetrating chest injuries. CT may reveal the triad of high-attenuation pericardial effusion, distention of the inferior vena cava and renal veins, and periportal low-attenuation fluid suggestive of increased venous pressure.[64,65] The experienced clinician, however, avoids any time-consuming diagnostic modality in patients with suspected cardiac injury.

SURGICAL MANAGEMENT

All penetrating injuries to the mediastinum with positive pericardial FAST and hemodynamic compromise should undergo surgical exploration. In the emergency room, stabilize the patient with intravenous fluids. No time should be wasted, including awaiting response to fluids or bladder catheterization or any other procedures. The only useful investigation besides FAST may be a chest radiograph, provided it does not delay the surgical treatment. In cardiac arrest or impending cardiac arrest, resuscitative thoracotomy in the emergency department provides the best chance for survival.

Emergency-Room Resuscitative Thoracotomy

All trauma patients in cardiac arrest or with imminent cardiac arrest should undergo resuscitative thoracotomy to decompress the pericardial cavity, with bleeding controlled by cross-clamping of the thoracic aorta when warranted (**Fig. 8**).

Open-Heart Resuscitation

Cardiac massage must be performed when there is cardiac arrest, in addition to aortic cross-clamp placement and intracardiac epinephrine injection (1 mg), which may be repeated. In an asystolic arrest or in a severe bradycardia, 0.5 mg atropine is administered. In ventricular fibrillation (VF) an open-heart defibrillation is performed at 20 J, escalated to 30 J if warranted. Other cardiac resuscitation drugs can be used, including amiodarone when defibrillation is unsuccessful in VF, and bicarbonate is used to mitigate acidosis.[66] Bicarbonate may be very useful, as noted by Schnuriger and colleagues,[67] in patients subjected to open cardiopulmonary resuscitation following trauma with severe acidosis.

Operating-Room Management

Patients with evidence of PCI who are not in cardiac arrest or with imminent cardiac arrest should be transferred to the operating room for immediate exploration. The decision to transfuse blood components is a crucial part of management. A median sternotomy provides universal access, and is the incision of choice for the majority of patients with suspected cardiac injuries (**Fig. 9**). The incision does not require special positioning of the patient, is rapid, bloodless, provides good exposure to the heart and

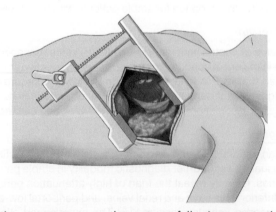

Fig. 8. Resuscitative emergency-room thoracotomy following penetrating cardiac injury. Cardiac wound to the left ventricle is repaired with figure-of-8 sutures. (*Courtesy of* A. Demetriades, BS, Los Angeles, CA; with permission.)

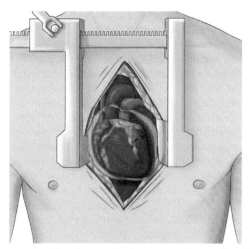

Fig. 9. Median sternotomy incision for repair of a penetrating cardiac injury. Cardiac wound to the right ventricle is repaired with figure-of-8 sutures. (*Courtesy of* A. Demetriades, BS, Los Angeles, CA; with permission.)

both lungs, and is associated with less postoperative pain and pulmonary complications than a lateral thoracotomy. The vast majority of cardiac wounds can be repaired with a nonabsorbable figure-of-8 suture. In complex lacerations, pledgeted repairs may be warranted (**Fig. 10**). Cardiopulmonary bypass is almost never required during the acute stage. The priority is to stabilize the patient quickly, and any other intracardiac defects should be repaired electively at a later time.

Postoperative Complications

The most frequent complications that may occur immediately after operation include hypothermia, acidosis, and/or coagulopathy attributable to cardiac tamponade, hypoperfusion, exsanguination, and extensive fluid resuscitation. Cardiac arrhythmias are usually seen in patients undergoing coronary artery ligation and in those who have suffered profound hypothermia.

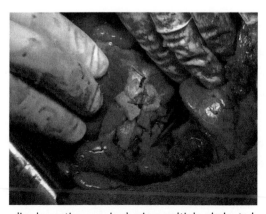

Fig. 10. Complex cardiac laceration repaired using multiple pledgeted sutures.

Delayed complications may occur weeks to years after injury, and include ventricular hypokinesia, atrial and/or ventricular septal defects, valvular lesions, injury to chordae tendinae or papillary muscles, or pseudoaneurysm formation. All survivors should undergo routine early and late clinical, ECG, and echocardiographic evaluation to look for evidence of cardiac injury. Even if postoperative evaluation is normal, follow-up a few weeks after the injury is valuable. In a study of 54 patients who survived a PCI, late follow-up (mean 23 months) showed ECG abnormalities in 31% and echocardiographic abnormalities in 31%, including valvular or septal defects, pericardial effusion, and dilatation.[9] More recently, Tang and colleagues[68] performed a retrospective review of all cardiac injuries treated at Los Angeles County General hospital over a 10-year period. Rate of survival to discharge was 26.9% and postdischarge follow-up was available for 42% of survivors, with a mean follow-up of 1.9 months. Follow-up revealed abnormal findings in 17.4% of patients. The disorders seen, in decreasing order, were pericardial effusion (47%), hypokinesia (42%), decreased ejection fraction (42%), intramural thrombus (21%), valvular injury (21%), cardiac enlargement (11%), conduction abnormality (11%), pseudoaneurysm (5%), aneurysm (5%), and septal defect (5%). However, in this review none of the structural lesions found after discharge required surgical correction, and the investigators reported no benefit of follow-up echocardiography performed beyond hospital discharge.

Retained Cardiac Missiles

Retained cardiac missiles may lead to complications including embolization, endocarditis, coronary artery thrombosis, septic pericarditis, and transmural erosion.[69,70] The risk of surgical removal of the intracardiac foreign body must be carefully weighed against the risks of complications of the procedure. In some reports, retained missiles have been tolerated well.[71]

Prognosis

The mechanism of injury, injured cardiac structure, coronary vessel involvement, presence of tamponade, associated injuries, length of prehospital time, and the experience of the trauma team determine survival after penetrating cardiac trauma. As previously described, the overall case-fatality rates of penetrating cardiac injuries are high, ranging from 80% to 97%.[41–43] The vast majority of deaths occur in the prehospital setting. For those who reach the hospital with signs of life, the in-hospital mortality rates range between 4% and 71% in clinical series over recent decades.[44–46,72–77]

Key message

- PCI in children and adolescents is rare
- Penetrating injury may involve gunshot wound or stab injury to the chest
- Stab wound is more common in this age group, although gunshot wound is more likely to be fatal
- Prompt initiation of treatment in an emergency setting is crucial
- FAST examination is a quick and reliable bedside investigation
- Patients in cardiac arrest or with impending cardiac arrest should undergo emergency-room resuscitative thoracotomy and open-heart resuscitation
- Long-term follow-up may include echocardiography in addition to clinical assessment based on cardiac involvement

SUMMARY

Estimates for incidence of cardiac trauma during adolescence vary widely. PCI is rare, but lethal. BCI includes a wide spectrum of cardiac involvement, ranging from asymptomatic myocardial contusion to instantly fatal cardiac rupture. Any significant chest trauma, especially in the presence of multiple rib or sternal fractures or lung contusions, is associated with a high incidence of cardiac trauma. Insignificant blunt cardiac trauma can result in fatal arrhythmia in teens, leading to sudden cardiac death in many instances. Initial normal ECG and troponin levels rule out significant blunt cardiac trauma. The diagnosis of penetrating cardiac trauma is mostly clinical. The FAST examination is the most useful and reliable bedside investigation in the emergency room. Patients admitted with penetrating cardiac trauma or blunt cardiac rupture in cardiac arrest or with imminent cardiac arrest should be managed with an emergency-room resuscitative thoracotomy. Survivors of PCI should be evaluated clinically and with early and late echocardiography, to evaluate for anatomic or functional cardiac sequelae.

REFERENCES

1. Murray CJ, Lopez AD. Mortality by cause for eight regions of the world: global burden of disease study. Lancet 1997;349(9061):1269–76.
2. Jones KW. Thoracic trauma. Surg Clin North Am 1980;60(4):957–81.
3. Doty DB, Anderson AE, Rose EF, et al. Cardiac trauma: clinical and experimental correlations of myocardial contusion. Ann Surg 1974;180(4):452–60.
4. Demetriades D, van der Veen BW. Penetrating injuries of the heart: experience over two years in South Africa. J Trauma 1983;23(12):1034–41.
5. Rothstein RJ. Myocardial contusion. JAMA 1983;250(16):2189–91.
6. Adams JE 3rd, Davila-Roman von G, Bessey PQ, et al. Improved detection of cardiac contusion with cardiac troponin I. Am Heart J 1996;131(2):308–12.
7. Turk EE, Tsang YW, Champaneri A, et al. Cardiac injuries in car occupants in fatal motor vehicle collisions–an autopsy-based study. J Forensic Leg Med 2010;17(6):339–43.
8. Brewster SA, Thirlby RC, Snyder WH 3rd. Subxiphoid pericardial window and penetrating cardiac trauma. Arch Surg 1988;123(8):937–41.
9. Demetriades D, Charalambides C, Sareli P, et al. Late sequelae of penetrating cardiac injuries. Br J Surg 1990;77(7):813–4.
10. Kaptein YE, Talving P, Konstantinidis A, et al. Epidemiology of pediatric cardiac injuries: a National Trauma Data Bank analysis. J Pediatr Surg 2011;46(8): 1564–71.
11. Moore EE, Malangoni MA, Cogbill TH, et al. Organ injury scaling. IV: thoracic vascular, lung, cardiac, and diaphragm. J Trauma 1994;36(3):299–300.
12. Akenside M. Account of blow upon heart and its effects. Philos Trans R Soc Lond Biol 1764;353.
13. Borch O. cited by Warburg E. Subacute and chronic pericardial and myocardial lesions due to nonpenetrating traumatic injuries: a clinical study. London: Oxford University Press; 1938.
14. Mattox KL, Flint LM, Carrico CJ, et al. Blunt cardiac injury. J Trauma 1992;33(5): 649–50.
15. Harmon KG, Asif IM, Klossner D, et al. Incidence of sudden cardiac death in national collegiate athletic association athletes. Circulation 2011;123(15):1594–600.
16. Sheppard MN. Aetiology of sudden cardiac death in sport: a histopathologist's perspective. Br J Sports Med 2012;46(Suppl 1):i15–21.

17. Maron BJ, Gohman TE, Kyle SB, et al. Clinical profile and spectrum of commotio cordis. JAMA 2002;287(9):1142–6.
18. Teixeira PG, Georgiou C, Inaba K, et al. Blunt cardiac trauma: lessons learned from the medical examiner. J Trauma 2009;67(6):1259–64.
19. Maron BJ, Link MS, Wang PJ, et al. Clinical profile of commotio cordis: an under appreciated cause of sudden death in the young during sports and other activities. J Cardiovasc Electrophysiol 1999;10(1):114–20.
20. Maron BJ, Poliac LC, Kaplan JA, et al. Blunt impact to the chest leading to sudden death from cardiac arrest during sports activities. N Engl J Med 1995; 333(6):337–42.
21. Link MS, Wang PJ, Pandian NG, et al. An experimental model of sudden death due to low-energy chest-wall impact (commotio cordis). N Engl J Med 1998; 338(25):1805–11.
22. Maron BJ, Haas TS, Ahluwalia A, et al. Increasing survival rate from commotio cordis. Heart Rhythm 2013;10(2):219–23.
23. Parmley LF, Manion WC, Mattingly TW. Nonpenetrating traumatic injury of the heart. Circulation 1958;18(3):371–96.
24. Clancy K, Velopulos C, Bilaniuk JW, et al. Screening for blunt cardiac injury: an Eastern Association for the Surgery of Trauma practice management guideline. J Trauma Acute Care Surg 2012;73(5 Suppl 4):S301–6.
25. Lindstaedt M, Germing A, Lawo T, et al. Acute and long-term clinical significance of myocardial contusion following blunt thoracic trauma: results of a prospective study. J Trauma 2002;52(3):479–85.
26. Salim A, Velmahos GC, Jindal A, et al. Clinically significant blunt cardiac trauma: role of serum troponin levels combined with electrocardiographic findings. J Trauma 2001;50(2):237–43.
27. Snow N, Richardson JD, Flint LM Jr. Myocardial contusion: implications for patients with multiple traumatic injuries. Surgery 1982;92(4):744–50.
28. Walsh P, Marks G, Aranguri C, et al. Use of V4R in patients who sustain blunt chest trauma. J Trauma 2001;51(1):60–3.
29. Rajan GP, Zellweger R. Cardiac troponin I as a predictor of arrhythmia and ventricular dysfunction in trauma patients with myocardial contusion. J Trauma 2004;57(4):801–8 [discussion: 808].
30. Feliciano D, Rozycki GS. Advances in the diagnosis and treatment of thoracic trauma. Surg Clin North Am 1999;79(6):1417–29.
31. Ferjani M, Droc G, Dreux S, et al. Circulating cardiac troponin T in myocardial contusion. Chest 1997;111(2):427–33.
32. Mattox KL, Estrera AL, Wall MJ. Traumatic heart disease. In: Bonow RO, Mann DL, Zipes DP, et al, editors. Braunwald's heart disease. 7th edition. Philadelphia: Elsevier Saunders; 2005. p. 1672–8.
33. Karalis DG, Victor MF, Davis GA, et al. The role of echocardiography in blunt chest trauma: a transthoracic and transesophageal echocardiographic study. J Trauma 1994;36(1):53–8.
34. Bromberg BI, Mazziotti von M, Canter CE, et al. Recognition and management of nonpenetrating cardiac trauma in children. J Pediatr 1996;128(4):536–41.
35. Elie MC. Blunt cardiac injury. Mt Sinai J Med 2006;73(2):542–52.
36. Bjornstad JL, Pillgram-Larsen J, Tonnessen T. Coronary artery dissection and acute myocardial infarction following blunt chest trauma. World J Emerg Surg 2009;4:14.
37. Demetriades D. Cardiac wounds. Experience with 70 patients. Ann Surg 1986; 203(3):315–7.

38. Schick EC Jr. Nonpenetrating cardiac trauma. Cardiol Clin 1995;13(2):241–7.
39. Blatchford JW 3rd. Ludwig Rehn: the first successful cardiorrhaphy. Ann Thorac Surg 1985;39(5):492–5.
40. Asensio JA, Petrone P, Pereira B, et al. Penetrating cardiac injuries: a historic perspective and fascinating trip through time. J Am Coll Surg 2009;208(3): 462–72.
41. Campbell NC, Thomson SR, Muckart DJ, et al. Review of 1198 cases of penetrating cardiac trauma. Br J Surg 1997;84(12):1737–40.
42. Rhee PM, Foy H, Kaufmann C, et al. Penetrating cardiac injuries: a population-based study. J Trauma 1998;45(2):366–70.
43. Clarke DL, Quazi MA, Reddy K, et al. Emergency operation for penetrating thoracic trauma in a metropolitan surgical service in South Africa. J Thorac Cardiovasc Surg 2011;142(3):563–8.
44. Lustenberger T, Talving P, Lam L, et al. Penetrating cardiac trauma in adolescents: a rare injury with excessive mortality. J Pediatr Surg 2013;48(4):745–9.
45. Asensio JA, Petrone P, Karsidag T, et al. Penetrating cardiac injuries. Complex injuries and difficult challenges. Ulus Travma Acil Cerrahi Derg 2003;9(1):1–16.
46. Tyburski JG, Astra L, Wilson RF, et al. Factors affecting prognosis with penetrating wounds of the heart. J Trauma 2000;48(4):587–90 [discussion: 590–1].
47. Oppell von UO, Bautz P, de Groot M. Penetrating thoracic injuries: what we have learnt. Thorac Cardiovasc Surg 2000;48(1):55–61.
48. Degiannis E, Loogna P, Doll D, et al. Penetrating cardiac injuries: recent experience in South Africa. World J Surg 2006;30(7):1258–64.
49. Rozycki GS, Feliciano D, Schmidt JA, et al. The role of surgeon-performed ultrasound in patients with possible cardiac wounds. Ann Surg 1996;223(6):737–44.
50. Rozycki GS, Feliciano D, Ochsner MG, et al. The role of ultrasound in patients with possible penetrating cardiac wounds: a prospective multicenter study. J Trauma 1999;46(4):543–51.
51. Rozycki GS, Ballard RB, Feliciano D, et al. Surgeon-performed ultrasound for the assessment of truncal injuries: lessons learned from 1540 patients. Ann Surg 1998;228(4):557–67.
52. Patel AN, Brennig C, Cotner J, et al. Successful diagnosis of penetrating cardiac injury using surgeon-performed sonography. Ann Thorac Surg 2003;76(6): 2043–6.
53. Scalea TM, Rodriguez A, Chiu WC, et al. Focused Assessment with Sonography for Trauma (FAST): results from an international consensus conference. J Trauma 1999;46(3):466–72.
54. Simmons JD, Haraway AN, Schmieg RE, et al. Is there a role for secondary thoracic ultrasound in patients with penetrating injuries to the anterior mediastinum? Am Surg 2008;74(1):11–4.
55. Harris DG, Papagiannopoulos KA, Pretorius J, et al. Current evaluation of cardiac stab wounds. Ann Thorac Surg 1999;68(6):2119–22.
56. Ball CG, Williams BH, Wyrzykowski AD, et al. A caveat to the performance of pericardial ultrasound in patients with penetrating cardiac wounds. J Trauma 2009;67(5):1123–4.
57. Spodick DH. Acute cardiac tamponade. Pathologic physiology, diagnosis and management. Prog Cardiovasc Dis 1967;10(1):64–96.
58. Spodick DH. Acute cardiac tamponade. N Engl J Med 2003;349(7):684–90.
59. Prior JP, Asensio JA. Thoracic vascular injury. In: Peitzman A, Rhodes M, Schwab CW, et al, editors. The trauma manual: trauma and acute care surgery. Philadelphia: Lippincott Williams & Wilkins; 2008. p. 230–42.

60. Miller FB, Bond SJ, Shumate CR, et al. Diagnostic pericardial window. A safe alternative to exploratory thoracotomy for suspected heart injuries. Arch Surg 1987;122(5):605–9.

61. Nicol AJ, Navsaria PH, Hommes M, et al. Sternotomy or drainage for a hemopericardium after penetrating trauma: a randomized controlled trial. Ann Surg 2013. [Epub ahead of print].

62. Symbas PN, Harlaftis N, Waldo WJ. Penetrating cardiac wounds: a comparison of different therapeutic methods. Ann Surg 1976;183(4):377–81.

63. Meyer DM, Jessen ME, Grayburn PA. Use of echocardiography to detect occult cardiac injury after penetrating thoracic trauma: a prospective study. J Trauma 1995;39(5):902–7.

64. Goldstein L, Mirvis SE, Kostrubiak IS, et al. CT diagnosis of acute pericardial tamponade after blunt chest trauma. AJR Am J Roentgenol 1989;152(4): 739–41.

65. Restrepo CS, Lemos DF, Lemos JA, et al. Imaging findings in cardiac tamponade with emphasis on CT. Radiographics 2007;27(6):1595–610.

66. Neumar RW, Otto CW, Link MS, et al. Part 8: adult advanced cardiovascular life support: 2010 American Heart Association guidelines for cardiopulmonary resuscitation and emergency cardiovascular care. Circulation 2010;122(18 Suppl 3):S729–67.

67. Schnuriger B, Talving P, Inaba K, et al. Biochemical profile and outcomes in trauma patients subjected to open cardiopulmonary resuscitation: a prospective observational pilot study. World J Surg 2012;36(8):1772–8.

68. Tang AL, Inaba K, Branco BC, et al. Postdischarge complications after penetrating cardiac injury: a survivable injury with a high postdischarge complication rate. Arch Surg 2011;146(9):1061–6.

69. Jemielity M, Perek B, Buczkowski P. Benign presentation of cardiac injury: a case report. Journal Trauma 2006;61(6):1540–2.

70. Saadia R, Levy RD, Degiannis E, et al. Penetrating cardiac injuries: clinical classification and management strategy. Br J Surg 1994;81(11):1572–5.

71. Symbas PN, Picone AL, Hatcher CR, et al. Cardiac missiles. A review of the literature and personal experience. Ann Surg 1990;211(5):639–47.

72. Mattox KL, Koch von L, Beall AC Jr, et al. Logistic and technical considerations in the treatment of the wounded heart. Circulation 1975;52(Suppl 2):I210–4.

73. Feliciano D, Bitondo CG, Mattox KL, et al. Civilian trauma in the 1980s. A 1-year experience with 456 vascular and cardiac injuries. Ann Surg 1984;199(6): 717–24.

74. Knott-Craig CJ, Dalton RP, Rossouw GJ, et al. Penetrating cardiac trauma: management strategy based on 129 surgical emergencies over 2 years. Ann Thorac Surg 1992;53(6):1006–9.

75. Buckman RF Jr, Badellino MM, Mauro LH, et al. Penetrating cardiac wounds: prospective study of factors influencing initial resuscitation. J Trauma 1993; 34(5):717–25.

76. Johnson SB, Nielsen JL, Sako EY, et al. Penetrating intrapericardial wounds: clinical experience with a surgical protocol. Ann Thorac Surg 1995;60(1): 117–20.

77. Gao JM, Gao YH, Wei GB, et al. Penetrating cardiac wounds: principles for surgical management. World J Surg 2004;28(10):1025–9.

Hypertension in the Teenager

Elizabeth I. Anyaegbu, MD, MSCI[a],
Vikas R. Dharnidharka, MD, MPH[b],*

KEYWORDS

- Hypertension • Obesity • Adolescents • Antihypertensive medications
- Cardiovascular mortality

KEY POINTS

- Over the last two decades, essential hypertension has become common in children and adolescents, and it is related to the obesity epidemic.
- Hypertension is underrecognized in children and diagnosis is based on specific normative standards, including sex, age, and height.
- Modifiable risk factors for essential hypertension in children, such as obesity and sodium consumption, should be addressed during treatment.
- Primary care physicians may play an important role in reduction of cardiovascular mortality by early detection, appropriate management, and referral when needed.

INTRODUCTION

The current prevalence of hypertension in children is estimated at about 1% to 5%, with higher rates among minority adolescents.[1–3] Primary hypertension (PH), also referred to as essential hypertension, previously considered a disease of adulthood, has now become increasingly common in the pediatric population largely due to the obesity epidemic.[4,5] Obese children are three times more likely to develop hypertension than their nonobese counterparts.[6,7] Therefore, this article focuses on obesity-related teenage hypertension. The article also discusses hypertension in nonobese teenagers, for which significant data exist.

The relationship between obesity and hypertension has been clearly defined in multiple studies across different ethnic and gender groups.[1,7–12] The cause of obesity-related hypertension has been linked to sympathetic hyperactivity, insulin resistance, and vascular structure changes.[13,14] Sorof and colleagues[7] demonstrated the presence of sympathetic nervous system hyperactivity in obese school-age children,

Disclosures: The authors have no relevant financial disclosures.
a Division of Pediatric Nephrology, Driscoll Children's Hospital, College of Medicine, Texas A&M University, 3533 South Alameda Street, Corpus Christi, TX 78411, USA; b Division of Pediatric Nephrology, St Louis Children's Hospital, Washington University School of Medicine in St Louis, 660 South Euclid Avenue, St Louis, MO 63110, USA
* Corresponding author.
E-mail address: Dharnidharka_V@kids.wustl.edu

Pediatr Clin N Am 61 (2014) 131–151
http://dx.doi.org/10.1016/j.pcl.2013.09.011
0031-3955/14/$ – see front matter © 2014 Elsevier Inc. All rights reserved.

evidenced by increased heart rate and blood pressure (BP) variability, which contributed to the pathogenesis of isolated systolic hypertension in this cohort. Increased sodium content of the cerebrospinal fluid has been shown to increase sympathetic nervous system activity through activation of the renin-angiotensin-aldosterone pathway in the brain.[13,14] Obese individuals have selective insulin resistance, which leads to increased sympathetic activity and alteration of vascular reactivity. The resultant sodium retention is evidenced by decreased urinary sodium excretion.[15] The lessons learned from the study of obese hypertensive individuals can be largely applied to the diverse population of hypertensive children.

DEFINITION AND CLASSIFICATION OF PEDIATRIC HYPERTENSION

Pediatric hypertension is usually asymptomatic and can easily be missed by healthcare professionals. The National Heart, Lung, and Blood Institute (NHLBI) of the National Institute of Health (NIH) commissioned the Task Force on Blood Pressure Control in Children to develop normative standards for BP. These standards were derived from the survey of more than 83,000 person-visits of infants and children. The percentile curves describe age-specific and gender-specific distributions of systolic and diastolic BP in infants and children adjusted for height[16]; these have been updated periodically.

Hypertension in children and adolescents is diagnosed based on specific references, including age, gender, and height. Hypertension is defined as systolic and/or diastolic BP greater than the 95th percentile for age, gender, and height on three or more separate occasions. BP greater than 90th percentile but less than the 95th percentile for age, sex, and height defines prehypertension, representing a category of patients at high risk for developing hypertension.[2,3,17–19] It is crucial that healthcare providers be aware that the BP at the 90th percentile for an older child often exceeds the adult threshold for prehypertension of 120/80 mm Hg. As a result, beginning at 12 years of age, the BP range that defines prehypertension includes any BP reading of greater than 120/80 mm Hg, even if it is less than the 90th percentile.[16] We now know that prehypertension may not be completely benign and the rate of progression to hypertension was reported at 7% per year over a 2-year interval.[18] Stage I hypertension refers to systolic and/or diastolic BP greater than the 95th percentile but less than or equal to the 99th percentile plus 5 mm Hg. There are no data on the progression from stage I to stage II hypertension in children.

Stage II hypertension is defined as systolic and/or diastolic BP greater than the 99th percentile plus 5 mm Hg. This represents a more severe form of hypertension, commonly associated with target organ damage. An analysis by the National High Blood Pressure Education Program Working Group on High Blood Pressure in Children and Adolescents revealed an increased risk for left ventricular hypertrophy (LVH)[20] in participants with stage II hypertension. Surprisingly, in some studies, children and adolescents with prehypertension also had a substantially increased left ventricular mass index with a twofold higher prevalence of LVH than their normotensive counterparts.[21–23] Classification of hypertension is summarized in **Table 1**.

Primary and Secondary Hypertension

Based on the cause, hypertension can be categorized as PH or essential hypertension when there is no identifiable cause and as secondary hypertension (SH) when there is an underlying cause for hypertension. PH is now the most common cause of hypertension in adolescents and young adults. It is usually characterized by stage I (mild) hypertension and associated with a positive family history of hypertension.[24] SH

Table 1
Definition and classification of hypertension in children

Normotensive children	Systolic and/or diastolic BP <90th percentile for sex, age, and height
Prehypertension	Systolic and/or diastolic BP greater than the 90th but less than the 95th percentile or BP >120/80 mm Hg but less than the 95th percentile
Stage I Hypertension	Systolic and/or diastolic BP greater than the 95th but less than the 99th percentile plus 5 mm Hg
Stage II Hypertension	Systolic and/or diastolic BP greater than the 99th percentile plus 5 mm Hg for sex, age, and height

Adapted from Lurbe E, Alvarez J, Redon J. Diagnosis and treatment of hypertension in children. Curr Hypertens Rep 2010;12:480–6; with permission.

should be considered in very young children, those with stage II hypertension, and children with clinical features that suggest systemic diseases associated with hypertension. SH may be due to

- An underlying renal parenchymal disease
- Endocrine disease
- Vascular
- Neurologic condition.

Key message

- Diagnosis of pediatric hypertension is often missed due to the absence of symptoms.
- Hypertension is diagnosed based on specific references, including age, gender, and height.
- Three stages of hypertension are
  - Prehypertension
  - Stage I hypertension
  - Stage II hypertension.
- Based on cause, hypertension can be either primary (no identifiable cause) or secondary (underlying cause present).

RISK FACTORS FOR ESSENTIAL HYPERTENSION

A parental family history of hypertension is linked to a twofold-increased risk of developing essential hypertension in children and young adults.[24–27] This association led to extensive research to elucidate the underlying genetic cause of PH. Family studies have shown that 20% to 40% of cases seen are genetically determined. Different monogenic causes of PH have been established, including mutations in the corticosteroidogenic genes, CYP11B1 and HSD11B2[28–30]; mutations in the epithelial sodium channel (SCNN1B, SCNN1G); in the WNK serine-threonine kinase[31,32]; and polymorphisms in the renin-angiotensin-aldosterone system.[30,33,34] However, pure monogenic causes of PH are still rare.

In a 10-year longitudinal study, African American children were shown to have a significantly greater elevation in systolic BP compared with white children from childhood to adulthood, even after adjusting for height, body mass index (BMI), and socioeconomic status.[35–38] Recently, mutations in the apolipoprotein-L1 gene in chromosome 22 were discovered that seem to explain the increased prevalence of hypertension-associated nephropathy in the African American population.[39,40] These mutations are thought to have an autosomal recessive pattern of inheritance and patients who are homozygous for the mutations have a higher likelihood for developing hypertension-associated nephropathy, focal segmental glomerulosclerosis, and HIV-associated nephropathy.[40–43]

Increasing age and BMI have also been significantly associated with the development of hypertension[44] with a higher prevalence in African Americans and Asians.[45] There is a growing body of evidence on the inverse relationship between birth weight and hypertension in children and adolescents. A strong association has been observed among patients with a history of low birth weight and intrauterine growth retardation. A more significant relationship is seen when adjustments are made for current body weight.[46–50]

In a recent study by Yang and colleagues,[51] children were found to consume between 1300 mg and 8100 mg of sodium a day (mean of 3387 mg). Children with the highest sodium intake were twice as likely to have elevated BP compared with those with lower sodium intake. This effect was more pronounced in the overweight and obese children. Overweight or obese children in the highest quartile of sodium consumption had more than three times the risk of elevated or high BP compared with overweight children in the lowest quartile of sodium consumption.[51]

Key message

- Risk factors for developing PH
  - Family history has been linked to increased risk
  - Racial predilection has been seen; the African American population is at higher risk
  - Increasing age and BMI
  - Low birth weight and intrauterine growth retardation
  - Increased sodium consumption.

DIAGNOSIS OF HYPERTENSION
Clinical Evaluation of a Hypertensive Teen

History
A thorough history is essential in guiding the evaluation and management of a hypertensive adolescent. Detailed information regarding the timing when elevated BP was first noted and the presence of comorbid conditions are crucial for establishing the diagnosis. For this age group, the clinical history should include questions about the use of anabolic steroids, stimulants, and caffeine-containing energy drinks, which can elevate the BP.[52] A history of snoring in an obese individual should prompt the evaluation for obstructive sleep apnea. History suggestive of renal disease or an endocrine tumor should be elicited.

Physical examination
A comprehensive physical examination could suggest the underlying cause of hypertension in children and the presence of target organ damage. Attention to the BMI is essential to identify overweight and obese patients. **Table 2** summarizes the physical

Table 2
Physical findings and diagnostic evaluation of a hypertensive adolescent

Physical Examination	Causes	Investigation
General: overweight, obese, acanthosis nigricans	PH or metabolic syndrome	Urinalysis, fasting blood sugar, lipid panel. Obtain ambulatory BP monitoring to rule out white coat hypertension
Edema, pallor, palpable kidneys on abdominal examination (polycystic kidney disease), rash, arthralgia, growth retardation	Renal parenchymal disease	Urinalysis, serum creatinine, electrolytes, complete blood count, urine protein to creatinine ratio, antinuclear antibodies, dsDNAse, complements C3 or C4, renal ultrasound
Tachycardia, widened pulse pressure, enlarged thyroid, weight loss, tremor	Hyperthyroidism	Thyroid function test: free T4 and thyroid-stimulating hormone
Moon facies, acne, hirsutism, truncal obesity, striae	Cushing's syndrome, steroid therapy, Liddle syndrome	Serum electrolytes, cortisol level, serum renin and aldosterone
Weak lower extremity pulses, BP in upper limbs more than 10 mm Hg greater than lower extremity BP	Coarctation of the aorta	Echocardiography
Abdominal bruit	Renal artery stenosis	Renal artery angiography, captopril scintigraphy
Tachycardia, flushing, visual disturbances, episodic hypertension	Pheochromocytoma	24-h urine metanephrine I^{131} or I^{123} metaiodobenzylguanidine scan
Café au lait spots, axillary or inguinal freckling	Neurofibromatosis	CT scan or MRI
Bradycardia, widened pulse pressure	Central nervous system lesion: tumor, bleed	CT scan or MRI

findings and laboratory investigations used to look for common causes of SH in the adolescent.

BP measurement

To obtain an accurate resting BP, patients should be allowed to sit for at least 5 minutes with the back supported and both feet on the ground.[16] A study of 390 children evaluated at 580 visits by Podoll and colleagues[53] revealed that 74% of BP readings were predominantly higher at the vital sign station using oscillometric devices compared with readings taken by auscultation in the examination room by personnel trained according to the Fourth Task Force recommendations.[16] Mean differences of 13.2 plus or minus 8.9 mm Hg for systolic and 9.6 plus or minus 7.6 mm Hg for diastolic BP were seen. This highlights the importance of proper technique and the need to reevaluate initial elevated BP readings carefully.[53]

BP should be measured with an appropriate-sized cuff in an upper extremity. The preferred method of measurement is by auscultation, especially because the normative BP tables for children are based on similar measurements. An appropriate-sized cuff should have an inflatable bladder width that spans at least 40% of the patient's arm circumference measured at the midpoint between the olecranon (elbow) and the acromion (shoulder). The bladder length should cover 80% to 100% of the arm circumference.[16] Although previous recommendations to determine cuff adequacy included cuff length, current recommendations are based on the cuff width only. Previous recommendations from the Task Force on High Blood Pressure in Children and Adolescents were that the width of the BP cuff should cover at least three-quarters of the length of the arm measured from the acromion to the olecranon.[54] However, this was found to result in an exaggeration in pediatric cuff choice. A review by Arafat and Mattoo[55] evaluated the appropriateness of this recommendation and reported that if three-quarters of the arm length is used to determine cuff size, there would be an overestimation in pediatric cuff selection. An update on the Task Force recommendations in 1996 included recommendations for a cuff width of 40% of the mid-upper arm circumference; there was no reference to cuff length or the reason for the change in recommendations.[54] It is thought that the updated recommendation is based on the idea that the bladder width should be 40% to 50% of the mid-upper arm circumference, supported by evidence that the correct ratio of bladder width to arm circumference is 0.4.[55]

BP readings are overestimated when the cuff size is too small, which increases the possibility of a wrong diagnosis of hypertension. Elevated BP readings obtained by oscillometric devices that exceed the 90th percentile should be confirmed by auscultation.

In the outpatient setting, documented elevations in BP on three separate occasions at least 1 week apart are essential to confirm the diagnosis. Alternatively, ambulatory BP monitoring (ABPM) could be performed to arrive at the diagnosis of hypertension.[56–58]

ABPM

ABPM forms the basis for the diagnosis when there is discordance in BP readings between daytime ambulatory BP measurements and office BP readings. It is particularly useful in patients with white coat or isolated clinic hypertension and masked hypertension. White coat hypertension is defined as office hypertension and ambulatory normotension, whereas masked hypertension, the opposite, refers to ambulatory hypertension and office normotension.

ABPM uses oscillometric measures to obtain BP measurements. BP is measured every 20 to 30 minutes in the patient's home environment over a 24-hour period. Patients are advised to continue their routine activities but avoid rigorous activities during this monitoring period. A record of the actual sleep and wake times is maintained by the patients to enable evaluation of nocturnal dipping patterns and nocturnal hypertension. In the authors' practice, we measure BP every 30 minutes during the day and every hour at night. An adequate ABPM report should have at least 40 to 50 BP readings with at least one reading every hour including at nighttime.[59] BP load is the percent of BP above the 95th percentile for age, gender, and height in the 24-hour period. Based on the ABPM, hypertension is defined as elevated mean systolic BP above the 95th percentile and/or an elevated BP load above 25%. Normative standards have been established and are available for ambulatory BP measurements.[60]

Twenty-four hour ABPM has become commonplace in pediatric nephrology clinics for diagnosing white coat hypertension and masked hypertension. There is growing evidence supporting its use in the pediatric population.[57,58,60–64] Nephrology groups own and perform ABPM; it is less commonly performed by the cardiologist and rarely by the endocrinologist. Recently, Davis and Davis[65] recommended incorporating ABPM in the primary care setting to increase diagnostic accuracy of hypertension and avoid unnecessary treatment. This makes it important that primary care providers be familiar with the role of ABPM for their patients with discordant BP readings or other diagnostic challenges.

The prevalence of white coat hypertension and masked hypertension in the general population are reported at 1% and 10%, respectively.[66] Patients with white coat hypertension have a lower risk for cardiovascular mortality than those with masked or sustained hypertension, although they have a greater risk for developing sustained hypertension later.[67–69] White coat hypertension in children is not associated with the development of LVH or hypertension-related kidney damage, unlike PH, which has been linked to microalbuminuria.[70–72] However, it has been related to a slight increase in left ventricular mass index, intermediate in range between normotensive and hypertensive subjects. This finding was highlighted in a study by Lande and colleagues[73] in which 81 subjects were divided in three groups matched for age and BMI. They were studied and found to have mean left ventricular mass indices of 29.2, 32.3, and 25.1 g/m^2 in the normotensive, white coat hypertensive, and sustained hypertensive groups, respectively. White coat hypertension has been associated with increased pulse wave velocity, which is a marker of increased arterial stiffness and it might signify a greater cardiovascular risk than previously thought.[74]

Masked hypertension has also been associated with increased cardiovascular mortality and other target organ damage in adults.[75] In a study of 592 children aged between 5 and 18 years, Lurbe and colleagues[66] showed that subjects with masked hypertension were likely to be obese and to have a family history of hypertension and were at an increased risk of developing sustained hypertension. Masked hypertension is a precursor of sustained hypertension and LVH in young children and adolescents. The risk for LVH is similar between participants with stage I hypertension and masked hypertension.[72]

ABPM has been closely associated with target organ damage and increased left ventricular mass index, leading to increased cerebrovascular events and a concomitant increase in cardiovascular mortality risk.[73,76,77] White coat hypertension is linked to a low risk for stroke, a finding by Verdecchia and colleagues[78] who reported a hazard ratio for stroke of 1.15 and 2.01 in patients with white coat hypertension and sustained hypertension, respectively. Researchers from the Dublin outcome study proposed ambulatory arterial stiffness index as a novel marker of cardiovascular mortality.[79–81]

Investigations in a Hypertensive Adolescent

Initial investigations
Initial evaluation should include a urinalysis, serum creatinine, and echocardiography to evaluate for LVH. Renal sonography need not be routinely performed in the obese adolescent with a normal physical examination and normal urinalysis results. This was confirmed in a retrospective study by Tuli and Dharnidharka[82] in which routine renal imaging in 50 children did not provide any additional diagnostic information to the initial evaluation. These recommendations are similar to the evaluation of an adult hypertensive patient.

Subsequent investigations
Subsequent investigations include fasting blood sugar and lipid profile in the obese teenager to rule out comorbid conditions.

Selected tests in unusual cases
Further investigations should be guided by the history, risk factors, and symptoms identified as outlined in **Table 2**.

> **Key message**
>
> - Detailed history and comprehensive physical examination are important for indentifying an underlying cause of hypertension and other comorbid conditions.
> - BP estimation by proper technique is crucial.
> - Elevated BP readings above the 90th percentile obtained by oscillometric devices should be confirmed by auscultation.
> - BP readings are overestimated when the cuff size is small.
> - Elevated BP on three separate occasions at least 1 week apart is essential to confirm the diagnosis.
> - ABPM may be performed to diagnose hypertension in cases of discordance between ambulatory BP and office BP readings.

MANAGEMENT OF A HYPERTENSIVE TEEN

After the diagnosis of hypertension is reached, management should be tailored to the individual patient.[52] **Fig. 1** shows an algorithm for the management of teenage hypertension according to the severity.

Therapeutic Lifestyle Modification

Therapeutic lifestyle modification is the first line of management of pediatric hypertension and can be the sole modality of therapy in patients diagnosed with

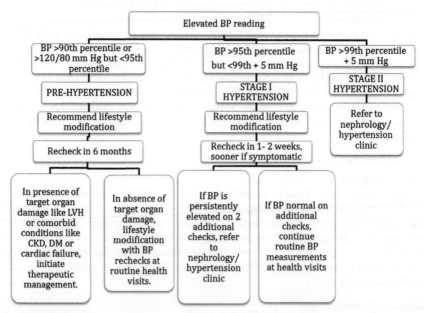

Fig. 1. Management of hypertension based on severity. CKD, chronic kidney disease; DM, diabetes mellitus. (*Data from* National High Blood Pressure Education Program Working Group on High Blood Pressure in Children and Adolescents. The fourth report on the diagnosis, evaluation, and treatment of high blood pressure in children and adolescents. Pediatrics 2004;114:555–76; and Lande MB, Flynn JT. Treatment of hypertension in children and adolescents. Pediatr Nephrol 2009;24:1939–49.)

prehypertension and stage I hypertension. It focuses on dietary management, increased physical activity, stress reduction, and avoidance of illicit drug and tobacco use.[83–85] Dietary management should include an age-appropriate, salt-restricted diet with emphasis on weight loss in overweight or obese children. To have a better chance of success, the entire family should adopt these lifestyle modifications; a primary provider can be instrumental in this endeavor.

Pharmacologic Therapy

The available evidence on the therapeutic management of pediatric hypertension is based on available evidence and consensus expert opinion when such evidence is lacking. The Fourth Task Force report on High Blood Pressure in Children and Adolescents include the following indications for pharmacologic therapy[16]:

- Symptomatic hypertension
- Persistent hypertension despite lifestyle modification
- SH
- Presence of hypertensive target organ damage, such as LVH, hypertensive retinopathy, and microalbuminuria
- Presence of comorbid conditions that increase cardiovascular risk, such as diabetes mellitus.[16]

For patients with uncomplicated PH, the target BP is less than the 95th percentile for age, gender, and height; whereas it is less than the 90th percentile for patients with comorbid conditions such as diabetes, chronic kidney disease, or evidence of target organ damage.[16]

Choice of antihypertensive medications

There are no specific recommendations on the optimal first-line agent for the treatment of pediatric hypertension.[52,86] The classes of antihypertensive medications that can be used in the pediatric hypertensive patient include:

- Calcium channel blockers (CCBs)
- Angiotensin-converting enzyme inhibitors (ACEI)
- Angiotensin receptor blockers (ARBs)
- Diuretics, beta-blockers (BBs)
- Alpha-blockers
- Centrally acting agents, vasodilators
- Combined alpha-adrenergic and beta-adrenergic antagonists
- Renin inhibitors
- Aldosterone receptor blockers.[87,88]

Commonly used formulations from the different classes are shown in **Table 3**.

The general practice is to choose an agent from one of these classes and to titrate the dosage to achieve therapeutic effect while monitoring for side effects.[52,89] Combination therapy is recommended if BP control is not achieved with a single drug.[16,90] Home BP measurements can be obtained to monitor the patient's response to therapy.

Less than a quarter of all drugs are approved by the Food and Drug Administration (FDA) for use in children. Despite this, almost all the antihypertensive agents available in the United States have been used in pediatric patients. The Food and Drug Administration Modernization Act (FDAMA) in 1997, resulted in companies being incentivized to conduct clinical trials in pediatrics and has resulted in wider availability of pediatric-approved antihypertensive agents and dosing recommendations.[91] The drugs initially

Table 3	
Classes of antihypertensive medications available in the market	
CCBs	Amlodipine, felodipine, isradipine, nifedipine, diltiazem, and verapamil
ACEIs	Enalapril, fosinopril, lisinopril, quinapril, captopril, benazepril, and ramipril
ARBs	Valsartan losartan candesartan, azilsartan, olmesartan, and irbesartan
Diuretics	Chlorothiazide, hydrochlorothiazide, chlorthalidone, amiloride, spironolactone,[a] and triamterene
Beta-adrenergic antagonists	Atenolol, metoprolol, propranolol, labetalol, timolol, nadolol, and nebivolol
Peripheral alpha-antagonists	Doxazosin,[b] prazosin, terazosin, phentolamine, and phenoxybenzamine
Centrally acting agents	Clonidine, methyl dopa, guanfacine, and guanethidine
Vasodilators	Hydralazine, minoxidil, and reserpine
Aldosterone antagonists	Eplerenone, spirinolactone[a]
Combination drugs	Amlodipine-benazepril, lisinopril-hydrochlorothiazide, losartan-hydrochlorothiazide, bisoprolol-hydrochlorothiazide, olmesartan-hydrochlorothiazide, olmesartan, amlodipine, olmesartan-hydrochlorothiazide-amlodipine

[a] Spirinolatone is not routinely used as a chronic antihypertensive drug.
[b] Among alpha-antagonists, doxazosin is commonly used for PH, whereas the others are not routinely used for PH.

approved and the current FDA-approved antihypertensive agents in children are outlined in **Table 4**.

Knowledge of the underlying cause can provide a pathophysiologic approach to guide therapy.[85] For instance, patients with hypertension secondary to steroid use would benefit from diuretic therapy with hydrochlorothiazide given that the underlying mechanism for hypertension in this setting is sodium and water retention.

Treatment with an ACEI or an ARB would be the appropriate therapy for a patient with diabetes to help prevent the progression of diabetic nephropathy.

BBs are beneficial in treatment of hypertension associated with hyperthyroidism. BBs are indicated after effective alpha-blockade in the preoperative treatment of pheochromocytoma to control the tachycardia associated with high circulating catecholamine levels and alpha-blockade. They should be administered only after adequate alpha-blockade, to prevent unopposed alpha-adrenergic activity. BBs should be avoided in patients with asthma and diabetes. They are associated with weight gain and should be used with caution in the obese patient.

There is no ideal first-line agent for the treatment of PH in the teenager. Among the different antihypertensive classes, ACEIs, ARBs, CCBs, BBs, or diuretics are frequently used as first-line agents. There is no evidence in pediatric hypertension that one agent is superior to another. An ideal first-line agent should be effective; have short-term and long-term safety; be readily available, palatable, and affordable; have long-acting formulations; and be easy to administer.[86] Pediatricians should be familiar with one or two agents from each class and their side-effect profile.

It is recommended that a single agent be used at the minimum dose during initiation of pharmacologic therapy. **Table 5** shows the initial doses of commonly used agents.

Table 4 FDA-approved antihypertensives	
Before FDAMA	**After FDAMA**
Propranolol	Children age >1 mo • Enalapril
Propranolol (long acting)	Children age >1 y • Candesartan
Oral clonidine	Children age >6 y • Lisinopril • Losartan • Valsartan • Amlodipine
Transdermal clonidine	Children age >12 y • Guanfacine
Hydralazine	—
Minoxidil	—
Hydrochlorothiazide	—

Abbreviation: FDAMA, Food and Drug Administration Modernization Act.

Data from Welch WP, Yang W, Taylor-Zapata P, et al. Antihypertensive drug use by children: are the drugs labeled and indicated? J Clin Hypertens (Greenwich) 2012;14:388–95.

Table 5 Doses of common antihypertensive agents for out patient treatment of hypertension		
Class	**Drug**	**Dose**
ACEIs	Captopril	Initial: 0.3–0.5 mg/kg/dose Maximum: 6 mg/kg/d
	Enalapril	Initial: 0.08 mg/kg/d up to 5 mg/d Maximum: 0.6 mg/kg/d up to 40 mg/d
	Lisinopril	Initial: 0.07 mg/kg/d up to 5 mg/d Maximum: 0.6 mg/kg/d up to 40 mg/d
ARBs	Losartan	Initial: 0.7 mg/kg/d up to 50 mg/d Maximum: 1.4 mg/kg/d up to 100 mg/d
Alpha-blockers and BBs	Labetalol	Initial: 1–3 mg/kg/d Maximum: 10–12 mg/kg/d up to 1200 mg/d
BBs	Atenolol	Initial: 0.5–1 mg/kg/d Maximum: 2 mg/kg/d up to 100 mg/d
	Metoprolol	Initial: 1–2 mg/kg/d Maximum: 6 mg/kg/d up to 200 mg/d
	Propranolol	Initial: 1–2 mg/kg/d Maximum: 4 mg/kg/d up to 640 mg/d
CCBs	Amlodipine	6 to 17 y: 2.5–5 mg once daily
Diuretics	Hydrochlorothiazide	<6 mo: 2–4 mg/kg/d 6 mo to 2 y: 1–2 mg/kg/d; maximum 37.5 mg 2–12 y: 1–2 mg/kg/d; maximum 100 mg/d

In VRD's practice, treatment of a hypertensive teenager begins with amlodipine, lisinopril, or hydrochlorothiazide, not in any particular order.

Data from National High Blood Pressure Education Program Working Group on High Blood Pressure in Children and Adolescents. The fourth report on the diagnosis, evaluation, and treatment of high blood pressure in children and adolescents. Pediatrics 2004;114:555–7.

The dosage can be titrated every 2 weeks to achieve control, sooner if the patient is symptomatic. A second agent should be added when the maximum dose is reached or if the patient develops side effects.

Following documentation of elevated BP on three consecutive occasions, at least 1 week apart, hypertensive patients should receive nonpharmacologic therapy, including lifestyle modification. Pharmacologic therapy should be instituted in symptomatic patients and stage II hypertension and prompt referral should be made to the nephrologist.

Benefits of antihypertensive therapy

There are reports showing the reversal of target organ damage following the institution of antihypertensive therapy in children.[92–94] Seeman and colleagues[93] reported a regression in LVH in a small pediatric cohort treated with ramipril monotherapy over a 6-month period.

Other forms of therapy

Bariatric surgery has a role in the treatment of hypertension in the morbidly obese adult and might become an option in the obese pediatric adolescent in the future. A recent study by Visockiene and colleagues[95] demonstrated an improvement in metabolic syndrome including hypertension with up to 30% reduction in weight.

Renal nerve denervation is a therapeutic option in adults with resistant hypertension, which refers to uncontrolled hypertension despite therapy with three or more antihypertensives. Studies in animals and humans have shown that the renal nerves play a role in BP regulation. The efficacy of renal nerve denervation was demonstrated in the Symplicity HTN-2 trial in which participants with resistant hypertension were randomized to either a treatment arm, managed with renal denervation and baseline antihypertensives, or to the control arm, managed with only baseline antihypertensives. A significant change of −32/−12 mm Hg in BP in the treatment arm compared with a +1/0 mm Hg change in the control arm was observed 6 months after intervention. These BP changes persisted at 2 years in a follow-up study.[96–98] Although renal nerve denervation has not yet been performed in the pediatric population, it might have a role in the future for the treatment of resistant hypertension in the adolescent hypertensive patient.

Key message

- Life-style modification can be the sole modality of treatment in many adolescents with hypertension.
- Indications for pharmacotherapy include
  - Symptomatic hypertension
  - SH
  - Persistent hypertension despite life-style modification
  - Presence of target organ damage (LVH, retinopathy, microalbuminuria)
  - Presence of comorbid conditions.
- Target BP is less than 95th percentile for uncomplicated PH and less than 90th percentile for patients with comorbid conditions (diabetes, kidney disease, evidence of target organ damage).
- No specific recommendations exist regarding optimal first-line agent for treatment of pediatric hypertension.
- Knowledge of underlying cause and comorbid conditions may guide therapy.

SPORTS PARTICIPATION FOR THE HYPERTENSIVE ADOLESCENT

There is no evidence to support restricting the hypertensive youth from sports participation. There are no reports of sudden cardiac death associated with sports in hypertensive athletes in the absence of underlying cardiovascular disease, such as hypertrophic cardiomyopathy.[52,99]

The American Academy of Pediatrics (AAP) recommendations for sports participation in the hypertensive individual include unrestricted competitive sports participation for individuals with prehypertension or stage I hypertension without end organ damage such as LVH.[100] A regular exercise routine and dietary change should be encouraged to promote weight management and BP control as part of lifestyle modification. Individuals with stage II hypertension without evidence of end organ damage should be restricted from isometric exercises such as weight-lifting and push-ups, which can result in an acute rise in BP. This restriction should be in place until BP control is achieved with lifestyle modification and or drug therapy. With attendant cardiovascular disease, eligibility for sports participation should be based on the nature and severity of the coexistent cardiovascular disease.[100]

Recommendations from the American College of Sports Medicine include developing a training regimen for the hypertensive athlete, which consists of dynamic and resistance exercises.[101] Expert opinion recommendations include limiting competitive and highly static sports only in the athlete with uncontrolled stage II hypertension or in the presence of target organ damage.[16]

Key message

- Do not restrict competitive sports participation for adolescents with prehypertension, stage I hypertension, and well-controlled stage II hypertension with no target organ damage.
- Limit competitive and highly static sports for athletes with uncontrolled stage II hypertension or with target organ damage.

SCREENING CHILDREN FOR HYPERTENSION
AAP Recommendations

The AAP, the European Society of Hypertension, and the European Society of Cardiology recommend regular BP screening in children older than age 3 years at routine health visits. Despite these recommendations, hypertension in children is still underdiagnosed by clinicians.[102,103] The presence of elevated BP is more often overlooked in children with normal weight and those without a family history of cardiovascular disease. Children whose BP is less than 120/80 mm Hg (a measurement which is viewed as normal in adults but which could portend problems in children depending on age, gender, and height) were eight times more likely to have their elevated BP missed. This underscores the need for better BP monitoring in children and adolescents in an attempt to prevent the long-term complications of hypertension.[104]

On the contrary, a recent review by Thompson and colleagues[105] found that there is limited direct evidence supporting hypertension screening for prevention of cardiovascular diseases. Further study is needed to address the gaps identified on the usefulness of aggressive hypertension screening in children.

> **Key message**
>
> - Regular BP screening is recommended in children older than 3 years of age.
> - Hypertension is underdiagnosed in children.
> - Elevated BP is more likely missed in those with normal body weight and negative family history.

COMPLICATIONS OF HYPERTENSION IN ADOLESCENTS

Although the long-term complications of hypertension, such as stroke, cardiac failure, myocardial infarction, and kidney disease, are rare in the pediatric population, hypertension in children has been predictive of hypertension in adulthood.[106–111]

Childhood hypertension has been associated with risk factors of cardiovascular disease, including LVH and increased arterial wall thickness.[22,72,112–119] LVH is the most frequently reported form of end organ damage in hypertensive children and adolescents with a prevalence of 14% to 26%.[120] Hypertensive children have an increased left ventricular mass index even after adjustments for age, sex, and BMI, which is associated with an increased risk of cardiovascular mortality.[23] This risk is amplified by arterial stiffening, a cardinal feature in hypertensive individuals.

A correlation between hypertension and lower neurocognitive test scores was seen in the third National Health and Nutrition Examination Survey (NHANES III).[121] This association was further highlighted in a study conducted by Lande and colleagues[122] of 32 newly diagnosed hypertensive children and adolescents aged between 10 and 18 enrolled from a hypertension clinic. These patients were found to have significantly reduced cognitive function compared with the normotensive controls matched for age, sex, weight, race, IQ, and socioeconomic status. This cognitive impairment might represent an early manifestation of hypertensive damage to the brain that may precede more overt complications such as stroke.[108,123,124] A follow-up study showed that treatment of these hypertensive children resulted in an improvement of their cognitive executive function.[125] This highlights the role of early diagnosis and optimal treatment.

Renal dysfunction represents a form of hypertension-related end organ damage, which manifests as a reduction in glomerular filtration rate and an elevated urine microalbumin excretion. Microalbuminuria correlates well with progression of nephropathy and is a surrogate of increased cardiovascular mortality.[120] The usefulness of routine screening for microalbuminuria in the hypertensive child has not been proven.

Uncontrolled hypertension can cause damage to the retinal vasculature[126] and the report from the National High Blood Pressure Education Program (NHBPEP) recommends that hypertensive children undergo a retinal examination for evidence of target organ damage.[54] Retinopathy is very rare in teenagers with isolated hypertension. A study of 83 hypertensive children found just mild abnormalities on retinal examination in only three children.[127]

There is growing evidence that there is increased mortality risk with childhood obesity related to an increased incidence of hypertension, ischemic heart disease, diabetes, and stroke.[128] This further highlights the importance of advocating lifestyle modification in the treatment of the overweight or obese individual to reduce the risk of premature mortality.

Key message

- Long-term cardiovascular complications may not be seen in pediatric ages.
- Hypertension in childhood and adolescence predict hypertension as adults.
- Childhood hypertension is associated with LVH and increased arterial wall thickness.
- Lower neurocognitive scores and renal injury have been described with hypertension.

SUMMARY

With the advent of the obesity epidemic, PH has become an important cause of pediatric hypertension. In concert with obesity, diseases such as diabetes mellitus, metabolic syndrome, obstructive sleep apnea, dyslipidemia, orthopedic complications, and psychosocial issues have emerged as common pediatric issues. Insulin resistance, sympathetic overactivity, and vascular structure abnormalities explain the association between obesity and hypertension in the pediatric population. Complications of uncontrolled hypertension, including LVH and renal dysfunction, have become more prevalent in this population as a result. Early diagnosis and management of hypertension is important in preventing long-term complications. The value of weight loss in BP control has been demonstrated in clinical studies and remains the first line of therapy in the pediatric patient who presents with hypertension. Pharmacologic therapy is necessary for treatment of symptomatic hypertension and in the presence of target organ damage to prevent and, in some cases, reverse established complications.

REFERENCES

1. Sorof JM, Lai D, Turner J, et al. Overweight, ethnicity, and the prevalence of hypertension in school-aged children. Pediatrics 2004;113:475–82.
2. McNiece KL, Poffenbarger TS, Turner JL, et al. Prevalence of hypertension and pre-hypertension among adolescents. J Pediatr 2007;150:640–4, 644.e1.
3. Acosta AA, Samuels JA, Portman RJ, et al. Prevalence of persistent prehypertension in adolescents. J Pediatr 2012;160:757–61.
4. Falkner B, Gidding SS, Ramirez-Garnica G, et al. The relationship of body mass index and blood pressure in primary care pediatric patients. J Pediatr 2006;148: 195–200.
5. Flynn JT, Falkner BE. Obesity hypertension in adolescents: epidemiology, evaluation, and management. J Clin Hypertens (Greenwich) 2011;13:323–31.
6. Sorof J, Daniels S. Obesity hypertension in children: a problem of epidemic proportions. Hypertension 2002;40:441–7.
7. Sorof JM, Poffenbarger T, Franco K, et al. Isolated systolic hypertension, obesity, and hyperkinetic hemodynamic states in children. J Pediatr 2002;140:660–6.
8. Macedo ME, Trigueiros D, de Freitas F. Prevalence of high blood pressure in children and adolescents. Influence of obesity. Rev Port Cardiol 1997;16: 27–30, 7–8.
9. Morrison JA, Barton BA, Biro FM, et al. Overweight, fat patterning, and cardiovascular disease risk factors in black and white boys. J Pediatr 1999;135: 451–7.
10. Tu W, Eckert GJ, DiMeglio LA, et al. Intensified effect of adiposity on blood pressure in overweight and obese children. Hypertension 2011;58:818–24.

11. Rosner B, Cook N, Portman R, et al. Blood pressure differences by ethnic group among United States children and adolescents. Hypertension 2009;54:502–8.

12. Brady TM, Fivush B, Parekh RS, et al. Racial differences among children with primary hypertension. Pediatrics 2010;126:931–7.

13. Julius S, Nesbitt S. Sympathetic overactivity in hypertension. A moving target. Am J Hypertens 1996;9:113S–20S.

14. Palatini P. Sympathetic overactivity in hypertension: a risk factor for cardiovascular disease. Curr Hypertens Rep 2001;3(Suppl 1):S3–9.

15. Rocchini AP. Insulin resistance, obesity and hypertension. J Nutr 1995;125: 1718S–24S.

16. National High Blood Pressure Education Program Working Group on High Blood Pressure in Children and Adolescents. The fourth report on the diagnosis, evaluation, and treatment of high blood pressure in children and adolescents. Pediatrics 2004;114:555–76.

17. Redwine KM, Falkner B. Progression of prehypertension to hypertension in adolescents. Curr Hypertens Rep 2012;14:619–25.

18. Redwine KM, Acosta AA, Poffenbarger T, et al. Development of hypertension in adolescents with pre-hypertension. J Pediatr 2012;160:98–103.

19. Redwine KM, Daniels SR. Prehypertension in adolescents: risk and progression. J Clin Hypertens (Greenwich) 2012;14:360–4.

20. Basiratnia M, Esteghamati M, Ajami GH, et al. Blood pressure profile in renal transplant recipients and its relation to diastolic function: tissue Doppler echocardiographic study. Pediatr Nephrol 2011;26:449–57.

21. Richey PA, Disessa TG, Hastings MC, et al. Ambulatory blood pressure and increased left ventricular mass in children at risk for hypertension. J Pediatr 2008;152:343–8.

22. Drukteinis JS, Roman MJ, Fabsitz RR, et al. Cardiac and systemic hemodynamic characteristics of hypertension and prehypertension in adolescents and young adults: the Strong Heart Study. Circulation 2007;115:221–7.

23. Stabouli S, Kotsis V, Rizos Z, et al. Left ventricular mass in normotensive, prehypertensive and hypertensive children and adolescents. Pediatr Nephrol 2009; 24:1545–51.

24. Goldstein IB, Shapiro D, Weiss RE. How family history and risk factors for hypertension relate to ambulatory blood pressure in healthy adults. J Hypertens 2008; 26:276–83.

25. Alpay H, Ozdemir N, Wuhl E, et al. Ambulatory blood pressure monitoring in healthy children with parental hypertension. Pediatr Nephrol 2009;24:155–61.

26. Giussani M, Antolini L, Brambilla P, et al. Cardiovascular risk assessment in children: role of physical activity, family history and parental smoking on BMI and blood pressure. J Hypertens 2013;31(5):983–92.

27. Zhou L, Chen Y, Sun N, et al. Family history of hypertension and arterial elasticity characteristics in healthy young people. Hypertens Res 2008;31:833–9.

28. Mongia A, Vecker R, George M, et al. Role of 11betaHSD type 2 enzyme activity in essential hypertension and children with chronic kidney disease (CKD). J Clin Endocrinol Metab 2012;97:3622–9.

29. Nguyen KD, Pihur V, Ganesh SK, et al. Effects of rare and common blood pressure gene variants on essential hypertension: results from the Family Blood Pressure Program, CLUE, and Atherosclerosis Risk in Communities studies. Circ Res 2013;112:318–26.

30. Corvol P, Soubrier F, Jeunemaitre X. Molecular genetics of the renin-angiotensin-aldosterone system in human hypertension. Pathol Biol (Paris) 1997;45:229–39.

31. Luft FC. Mendelian forms of human hypertension and mechanisms of disease. Clin Med Res 2003;1:291–300.
32. Toka HR, Luft FC. Monogenic forms of human hypertension. Semin Nephrol 2002;22:81–8.
33. Poch E, Gonzalez D, Giner V, et al. Molecular basis of salt sensitivity in human hypertension. Evaluation of renin-angiotensin-aldosterone system gene polymorphisms. Hypertension 2001;38:1204–9.
34. Giner V, Poch E, Bragulat E, et al. Renin-angiotensin system genetic polymorphisms and salt sensitivity in essential hypertension. Hypertension 2000;35:512–7.
35. Dekkers JC, Snieder H, Van Den Oord EJ, et al. Moderators of blood pressure development from childhood to adulthood: a 10-year longitudinal study. J Pediatr 2002;141:770–9.
36. Wang X, Poole JC, Treiber FA, et al. Ethnic and gender differences in ambulatory blood pressure trajectories: results from a 15-year longitudinal study in youth and young adults. Circulation 2006;114:2780–7.
37. Harshfield GA, Treiber FA, Wilson ME, et al. A longitudinal study of ethnic differences in ambulatory blood pressure patterns in youth. Am J Hypertens 2002;15:525–30.
38. Manatunga AK, Jones JJ, Pratt JH. Longitudinal assessment of blood pressures in black and white children. Hypertension 1993;22:84–9.
39. Freedman BI, Murea M. Target organ damage in African American hypertension: role of APOL1. Curr Hypertens Rep 2012;14:21–8.
40. Freedman BI, Kopp JB, Langefeld CD, et al. The apolipoprotein L1 (APOL1) gene and nondiabetic nephropathy in African Americans. J Am Soc Nephrol 2010;21:1422–6.
41. Freedman BI, Langefeld CD. The new era of APOL1-associated glomerulosclerosis. Nephrol Dial Transplant 2012;27:1288–91.
42. Kopp JB, Nelson GW, Sampath K, et al. APOL1 genetic variants in focal segmental glomerulosclerosis and HIV-associated nephropathy. J Am Soc Nephrol 2011;22:2129–37.
43. Papeta N, Kiryluk K, Patel A, et al. APOL1 variants increase risk for FSGS and HIVAN but not IgA nephropathy. J Am Soc Nephrol 2011;22:1991–6.
44. He Q, Ding ZY, Fong DY, et al. Blood pressure is associated with body mass index in both normal and obese children. Hypertension 2000;36:165–70.
45. Lo JC, Sinaiko A, Chandra M, et al. Prehypertension and hypertension in community-based pediatric practice. Pediatrics 2013;131:e415–24.
46. Edvardsson VO, Steinthorsdottir SD, Eliasdottir SB, et al. Birth weight and childhood blood pressure. Curr Hypertens Rep 2012;14:596–602.
47. Primatesta P, Falaschetti E, Poulter NR. Birth weight and blood pressure in childhood: results from the Health Survey for England. Hypertension 2005;45:75–9.
48. Salgado CM, Jardim PC, Teles FB, et al. Influence of low birth weight on microalbuminuria and blood pressure of school children. Clin Nephrol 2009;71:367–74.
49. Martinez-Aguayo A, Aglony M, Bancalari R, et al. Birth weight is inversely associated with blood pressure and serum aldosterone and cortisol levels in children. Clin Endocrinol (Oxf) 2012;76:713–8.
50. Barker DJ. Birth weight and hypertension. Hypertension 2006;48:357–8.
51. Yang Q, Zhang Z, Kuklina EV, et al. Sodium intake and blood pressure among US children and adolescents. Pediatrics 2012;130:611–9.

52. Lande MB, Flynn JT. Treatment of hypertension in children and adolescents. Pediatr Nephrol 2009;24:1939–49.
53. Podoll A, Grenier M, Croix B, et al. Inaccuracy in pediatric outpatient blood pressure measurement. Pediatrics 2007;119:e538–43.
54. Update on the 1987 Task Force Report on High Blood Pressure in Children and Adolescents: a working group report from the National High Blood Pressure Education Program. National High Blood Pressure Education Program Working Group on Hypertension Control in Children and Adolescents. Pediatrics 1996; 98:649–58.
55. Arafat M, Mattoo TK. Measurement of blood pressure in children: recommendations and perceptions on cuff selection. Pediatrics 1999;104:e30.
56. Bald M. Ambulatory blood pressure monitoring in children and adolescents. Current insights into a new technique. Minerva Pediatr 2002;54:13–24.
57. Gavrilovici C, Goldsmith DJ, Reid C, et al. What is the role of ambulatory BP monitoring in pediatric nephrology? J Nephrol 2004;17:642–52.
58. Graves JW, Althaf MM. Utility of ambulatory blood pressure monitoring in children and adolescents. Pediatr Nephrol 2006;21:1640–52.
59. Flynn JT, Urbina EM. Pediatric ambulatory blood pressure monitoring: indications and interpretations. J Clin Hypertens (Greenwich) 2012;14:372–82.
60. Urbina E, Alpert B, Flynn J, et al. Ambulatory blood pressure monitoring in children and adolescents: recommendations for standard assessment: a scientific statement from the American Heart Association Atherosclerosis, Hypertension, and Obesity in Youth Committee of the council on cardiovascular disease in the young and the council for high blood pressure research. Hypertension 2008;52:433–51.
61. Lingens N, Dobos E, Witte K, et al. Twenty-four-hour ambulatory blood pressure profiles in pediatric patients after renal transplantation. Pediatr Nephrol 1997;11: 23–6.
62. Khan IA, Gajaria M, Stephens D, et al. Ambulatory blood pressure monitoring in children: a large center's experience. Pediatr Nephrol 2000;14:802–5.
63. Kanbay M, Turkmen K, Ecder T, et al. Ambulatory blood pressure monitoring: from old concepts to novel insights. Int Urol Nephrol 2012;44:173–82.
64. Flynn JT. Ambulatory blood pressure monitoring should be routinely performed after pediatric renal transplantation. Pediatr Transplant 2012;16:533–6.
65. Davis TK, Davis AJ. Ambulatory Blood Pressure Monitoring Should be used in the Primary Care Setting to Diagnose Hypertension. Am J Hypertens 2013; 26(9):1057–8.
66. Lurbe E, Torro I, Alvarez V, et al. Prevalence, persistence, and clinical significance of masked hypertension in youth. Hypertension 2005;45:493–8.
67. Bidlingmeyer I, Burnier M, Bidlingmeyer M, et al. Isolated office hypertension: a prehypertensive state? J Hypertens 1996;14:327–32.
68. Colombo F, Catarame S, Cossovich P, et al. Isolated office hypertension: are there any markers of future blood pressure status? Blood Press Monit 2000;5: 249–54.
69. Staessen JA, Asmar R, De Buyzere M, et al. Task Force II: blood pressure measurement and cardiovascular outcome. Blood Press Monit 2001;6:355–70.
70. Seeman T, Pohl M, Palyzova D, et al. Microalbuminuria in children with primary and white-coat hypertension. Pediatr Nephrol 2012;27:461–7.
71. Stabouli S, Kotsis V, Toumanidis S, et al. White-coat and masked hypertension in children: association with target-organ damage. Pediatr Nephrol 2005;20: 1151–5.

72. McNiece KL, Gupta-Malhotra M, Samuels J, et al. Left ventricular hypertrophy in hypertensive adolescents: analysis of risk by 2004 National High Blood Pressure Education Program Working Group staging criteria. Hypertension 2007;50: 392–5.
73. Lande MB, Meagher CC, Fisher SG, et al. Left ventricular mass index in children with white coat hypertension. J Pediatr 2008;153:50–4.
74. Sung SH, Cheng HM, Wang KL, et al. White coat hypertension is more risky than prehypertension: important role of arterial wave reflections. Hypertension 2013; 61(6):1346–53.
75. Shimbo D, Newman JD, Schwartz JE. Masked hypertension and prehypertension: diagnostic overlap and interrelationships with left ventricular mass: the Masked Hypertension Study. Am J Hypertens 2012;25:664–71.
76. Stabouli S, Kotsis V, Zakopoulos N. Ambulatory blood pressure monitoring and target organ damage in pediatrics. J Hypertens 2007;25:1979–86.
77. Nadar SK, Tayebjee MH, Messerli F, et al. Target organ damage in hypertension: pathophysiology and implications for drug therapy. Curr Pharm Des 2006;12: 1581–92.
78. Verdecchia P, Reboldi GP, Angeli F, et al. Short- and long-term incidence of stroke in white-coat hypertension. Hypertension 2005;45:203–8.
79. Dolan E, Thijs L, Li Y, et al. Ambulatory arterial stiffness index as a predictor of cardiovascular mortality in the Dublin Outcome Study. Hypertension 2006;47: 365–70.
80. Li Y, Wang JG, Dolan E, et al. Ambulatory arterial stiffness index derived from 24-hour ambulatory blood pressure monitoring. Hypertension 2006;47: 359–64.
81. Li Y, Dolan E, Wang JG, et al. Ambulatory arterial stiffness index: determinants and outcome. Blood Press Monit 2006;11:107–10.
82. Tuli SY, Dharnidharka VR. Utility of renal imaging in the diagnostic evaluation of obese childhood primary hypertension. Clin Pediatr 2005;44:589–92.
83. Batisky DL. Obesity and the role of lifestyle and dietary intervention in the management of pediatric hypertension. J Med Liban 2010;58:171–4.
84. Bacon SL, Sherwood A, Hinderliter A, et al. Effects of exercise, diet and weight loss on high blood pressure. Sports Med 2004;34:307–16.
85. Brierley J, Marks SD. Treating the causes of paediatric hypertension using non-invasive physiological parameters. Med Hypotheses 2010;75:439–41.
86. Batisky DL. What is the optimal first-line agent in children requiring antihypertensive medication? Curr Hypertens Rep 2012;14:603–7.
87. Blowey DL. Update on the pharmacologic treatment of hypertension in pediatrics. J Clin Hypertens (Greenwich) 2012;14:383–7.
88. Flynn JT. Management of hypertension in the young: role of antihypertensive medications. J Cardiovasc Pharmacol 2011;58:111–20.
89. Kavey RE, Daniels SR, Flynn JT. Management of high blood pressure in children and adolescents. Cardiol Clin 2010;28:597–607.
90. Flynn JT. Pharmacologic management of childhood hypertension: current status, future challenges. Am J Hypertens 2002;15:30S–3S.
91. Welch WP, Yang W, Taylor-Zapata P, et al. Antihypertensive drug use by children: are the drugs labeled and indicated? J Clin Hypertens (Greenwich) 2012;14:388–95.
92. Litwin M, Niemirska A, Sladowcka-Kozlowska J, et al. Regression of target organ damage in children and adolescents with primary hypertension. Pediatr Nephrol 2010;25:2489–99.

93. Seeman T, Gilik J, Vondrak K, et al. Regression of left-ventricular hypertrophy in children and adolescents with hypertension during ramipril monotherapy. Am J Hypertens 2007;20:990–6.
94. Sharma M, Kupferman JC, Brosgol Y, et al. The effects of hypertension on the paediatric brain: a justifiable concern. Lancet Neurol 2010;9:933–40.
95. Visockiene Z, Brimas G, Abaliksta T, et al. Metabolic changes one year after laparoscopic adjustable gastric banding operation in morbidly obese subjects. Wideochir Inne Tech Malo Inwazyjne 2013;8:13–21.
96. Esler MD, Krum H, Schlaich M, et al. Renal sympathetic denervation for treatment of drug-resistant hypertension: one-year results from the Symplicity HTN-2 randomized, controlled trial. Circulation 2012;126:2976–82.
97. Esler MD, Krum H, Sobotka PA, et al. Renal sympathetic denervation in patients with treatment-resistant hypertension (The Symplicity HTN-2 Trial): a randomised controlled trial. Lancet 2010;376:1903–9.
98. Kandzari DE, Bhatt DL, Sobotka PA, et al. Catheter-based renal denervation for resistant hypertension: rationale and design of the SYMPLICITY HTN-3 Trial. Clin Cardiol 2012;35:528–35.
99. Maron BJ, Haas TS, Ahluwalia A, et al. Incidence of cardiovascular sudden deaths in Minnesota high school athletes. Heart Rhythm 2013;10:374–7.
100. Graham L. AAP updates policy statement on athletic participation by children and adolescents with systemic hypertension. Am Fam Physician 2010;82:1285.
101. Pescatello LS, Franklin BA, Fagard R, et al. American College of Sports Medicine position stand. Exercise and hypertension. Med Sci Sports Exerc 2004;36:533–53.
102. Hansen ML, Gunn PW, Kaelber DC. Underdiagnosis of hypertension in children and adolescents. JAMA 2007;298:874–9.
103. Lurbe E, Cifkova R, Cruickshank JK, et al. Management of high blood pressure in children and adolescents: recommendations of the European Society of Hypertension. J Hypertens 2009;27:1719–42.
104. Brady TM, Solomon BS, Neu AM, et al. Patient-, provider-, and clinic-level predictors of unrecognized elevated blood pressure in children. Pediatrics 2010;125:e1286–93.
105. Thompson M, Dana T, Bougatsos C, et al. Screening for hypertension in children and adolescents to prevent cardiovascular disease. Pediatrics 2013;131(3):490–525.
106. Lauer RM, Clarke WR, Mahoney LT, et al. Childhood predictors for high adult blood pressure. The Muscatine Study. Pediatr Clin North Am 1993;40:23–40.
107. Lauer RM, Clarke WR. Childhood risk factors for high adult blood pressure: the Muscatine Study. Pediatrics 1989;84:633–41.
108. Mahoney LT, Clarke WR, Burns TL, et al. Childhood predictors of high blood pressure. Am J Hypertens 1991;4:608S–10S.
109. Bao W, Threefoot SA, Srinivasan SR, et al. Essential hypertension predicted by tracking of elevated blood pressure from childhood to adulthood: the Bogalusa Heart Study. Am J Hypertens 1995;8:657–65.
110. Chen W, Srinivasan SR, Ruan L, et al. Adult hypertension is associated with blood pressure variability in childhood in blacks and whites: the bogalusa heart study. Am J Hypertens 2011;24:77–82.
111. Beckett LA, Rosner B, Roche AF, et al. Serial changes in blood pressure from adolescence into adulthood. Am J Epidemiol 1992;135:1166–77.

112. Tolwinska J, Glowinska B, Urban M, et al. Ultrasonographic evaluation of athero-sclerotic changes in carotid and brachial arteries in obese and hypertensive children. Przegl Lek 2005;62:1346–51.
113. Sorof JM, Turner J, Martin DS, et al. Cardiovascular risk factors and sequelae in hypertensive children identified by referral versus school-based screening. Hypertension 2004;43:214–8.
114. Sorof JM, Alexandrov AV, Cardwell G, et al. Carotid artery intimal-medial thick-ness and left ventricular hypertrophy in children with elevated blood pressure. Pediatrics 2003;111:61–6.
115. Tracy RE, Newman WP 3rd, Wattigney WA, et al. Histologic features of athero-sclerosis and hypertension from autopsies of young individuals in a defined geographic population: the Bogalusa Heart Study. Atherosclerosis 1995;116: 163–79.
116. Berenson GS, Srinivasan SR, Bao W, et al. Association between multiple car-diovascular risk factors and atherosclerosis in children and young adults. The Bogalusa Heart Study. N Engl J Med 1998;338:1650–6.
117. Sorof JM, Alexandrov AV, Garami Z, et al. Carotid ultrasonography for detection of vascular abnormalities in hypertensive children. Pediatr Nephrol 2003;18: 1020–4.
118. Sorof JM, Cardwell G, Franco K, et al. Ambulatory blood pressure and left ven-tricular mass index in hypertensive children. Hypertension 2002;39:903–8.
119. Chamontin B, Amar J, Barthe P, et al. Blood pressure measurements and left ventricular mass in young adults with arterial hypertension screened at high school check-up. J Hum Hypertens 1994;8:357–61.
120. Lurbe E, Alvarez J, Redon J. Diagnosis and treatment of hypertension in chil-dren. Curr Hypertens Rep 2010;12:480–6.
121. Lande MB, Kaczorowski JM, Auinger P, et al. Elevated blood pressure and decreased cognitive function among school-age children and adolescents in the United States. J Pediatr 2003;143:720–4.
122. Lande MB, Adams H, Falkner B, et al. Parental assessments of internalizing and externalizing behavior and executive function in children with primary hyperten-sion. J Pediatr 2009;154:207–12.
123. Kupferman JC, Lande MB, Adams HR, et al. Primary hypertension and neuro-cognitive and executive functioning in school-age children. Pediatr Nephrol 2013;28:401–8.
124. Lande MB, Kupferman JC, Adams HR. Neurocognitive alterations in hyperten-sive children and adolescents. J Clin Hypertens (Greenwich) 2012;14:353–9.
125. Lande MB, Adams H, Falkner B, et al. Parental assessment of executive function and internalizing and externalizing behavior in primary hypertension after anti-hypertensive therapy. J Pediatr 2010;157:114–9.
126. Chatterjee S, Chattopadhyay S, Hope-Ross M, et al. Hypertension and the eye: changing perspectives. J Hum Hypertens 2002;16:667–75.
127. Foster BJ, Ali H, Mamber S, et al. Prevalence and severity of hypertensive retinopathy in children. Clin Pediatr 2009;48:926–30.
128. Reilly JJ, Kelly J. Long-term impact of overweight and obesity in childhood and adolescence on morbidity and premature mortality in adulthood: systematic review. Int J Obes (Lond) 2011;35:891–8.

Identification of Obesity and Cardiovascular Risk Factors in Childhood and Adolescence

Preetha L. Balakrishnan, MD

KEYWORDS

- Obesity • Risk factors • Cardiovascular • Childhood • Adolescence

KEY POINTS

- Overweight and obese youth are at increased risk for premature cardiovascular disease.
- Identification of obesity with the consistent use of body mass index and anthropometric measurements is necessary to identify children and adolescents with cardiovascular risk factors.
- The development of atherosclerosis begins in childhood and is accelerated in the presence of obesity.
- Screening for hyperlipidemia is of particular importance in the overweight and obese child and adolescent in order to implement interventions to prevent early cardiovascular events.

Excessive adiposity is increasing on both the national and international levels. Adults, adolescents, and children are all affected by the epidemic. Obesity in the child and adolescent population is a growing problem. Rates of obesity have risen dramatically in a short period of time. Between 1999 and 2000, the prevalence of US teenagers aged 12 to 19 years who were identified as overweight or obese was 30% ± 1.4%, and in 2003 to 2004 it increased significantly to 34.3% ± 2.6%.[1] Similar increases were seen in children, with the most dramatic increase seen in the 6-year-old to 11-year-old cohort. According to the 2013 Heart Disease and Stroke Statistics Update, 23.9 million (31.8%) children aged 2 to 19 years are overweight or obese and 12.7 million (16.9%) are obese.[2]

The primary goal of labeling adolescents as overweight or obese should be to identify a population that is at an increased risk for current or future disease related to their excess adiposity. Obesity has a strong association with cardiovascular disease and, specifically, accelerated atherosclerosis.[3] As a result, it is of the utmost importance that clinicians identify and risk stratify overweight and obese individuals in order to

Disclosures: None.

Division of Cardiology, The Carman and Ann Adams Department of Pediatrics, Wayne State University School of Medicine, 3901 Beaubien Boulevard, Detroit, MI 48201-2119, USA

E-mail address: pbalakri@dmc.org

Pediatr Clin N Am 61 (2014) 153–171
http://dx.doi.org/10.1016/j.pcl.2013.09.013   pediatric.theclinics.com
0031-3955/14/$ – see front matter © 2014 Elsevier Inc. All rights reserved.

institute primary prevention and/or treatment to reduce future cardiovascular morbidity and mortality in this vulnerable population.

This article (1) discusses the definition of child and adolescent obesity and the need for standardization, (2) discusses anthropometric measurements and the potential pitfalls and benefits of using additional measures when assessing the overweight and/or obese child, (3) reviews data to advocate for ethnic-specific cut-points and further research in minority populations, (4) reviews literature about the metabolic syndrome in children and current recommendations, (5) reviews literature concerning the cardiovascular effects of obesity, and (6) summarizes systematic reviews of obesity prevention studies. In conclusion, this article calls for a standardized definition of obesity and the measures of obesity in the child and adolescent; as well as increased awareness and screening of the cardiovascular complications of the obesity epidemic.

Key message

- Obesity is strongly associated with accelerated atherosclerosis
- Overweight and obese adolescents should be consistently identified
- Primary care providers can be instrumental in reducing future cardiovascular morbidity/mortality by identifying, screening, and instituting primary prevention

---

DEFINITIONS OF ADOLESCENT OBESITY

One of the first problems to arise when considering obesity in the pediatric population is how to define and identify it. The 2007 obesity guidelines by the American Academy of Pediatrics[4] recommends using body mass index (BMI), a measure of body weight relative to height. Unlike in adults, in whom absolute BMI cutoff points are used to define obesity, this article recommends the use of percentiles specific for age and gender to categorize children as underweight, normal weight, overweight, or obese. The expert panel advocates the use of 2 specific cutoff points to minimize overdiagnosis and prevent underdiagnosis, using the 85th and 95th percentiles for age and gender. If patients are between the 85th and 94th percentiles, they should be categorized as overweight, and if they are greater than or equal to the 95th percentile they are categorized as obese. This approach represents a change in terminology, but not in cutoff points, from the 1998 expert committee recommendations in which the term obese was avoided.[5]

This recommended cutoff point is in agreement with the US Centers for Disease Control and Prevention (CDC) growth standards of 2000.[6,7] However, in addition to this recommendation there are several other organizations with varying cutoff points. The World Health Organization (WHO) developed international standards for children 0 to 5[8] and 5 to 19 years of age,[9] as did the International Obesity Task Force (IOTF).[10] In addition, there are several country-specific references that are used in individual nations.

The lack of agreement about definitions and cutoff points has been attributed to the lack of strong evidence and the absence of a definite correlation between childhood weight and future health outcomes.[11] Although there is clearly no perfect measure or cutoff point, several studies have compared the different growth curves and cutoff points of different organizations.[12–15] The studies showed disagreement between growth curves and showed that usage of the WHO criteria yielded a higher prevalence of overweight/obesity. The most recent study[12] was conducted in Spain and classified participants as obese, overweight, or normal weight based on CDC, WHO, and the Spanish Reference Criteria. Forty-eight percent were categorized as obese by the

WHO criteria, 43% by the CDC criteria, and 16% by the Spanish Reference Criteria. The study also analyzed biochemical variables and vascular parameters in the participants. Of particular interest are the differences noted between the WHO and CDC criteria. Application of the WHO criteria showed that obese children had significantly higher insulin levels, homeostasis model assessment (HOMA) index, and vascular parameters (with the exception of intima media thickness), and lower high-density lipoprotein (HDL) levels than overweight children. Overweight children characterized by the WHO criteria had higher HOMA index and arterial compliance, and lower HDL levels compared with normal-weight individuals. The CDC criteria also identified significant differences between the obese participants and the normal-weight individuals; however, fewer biochemical differences and no vascular differences were found between the overweight and obese groups. These findings suggest that the WHO criteria may be more useful to identify individuals with biochemical and vascular derangements, and that these individuals may, as a result, be at higher risk for future poor health outcomes. Larger studies in a more heterogeneous population are needed to further validate these findings. A Canadian study[13] showed similar findings when comparing the WHO, IOTF, and CDC cut-points with a 2004 prevalence of overweight/obesity of 35% using the WHO criteria, 26% with IOTF criteria, and 28% with CDC data.

A recent review of multiple systematic reviews and clinical guidelines performed in the United Kingdom concluded that, among the various indices available to gauge body fatness in children and adolescents, subjective clinical assessment is the worst measure, and BMI-for-age percentiles using national reference data is the best means to diagnose/define obesity in children and adolescents.[16] The review also discusses the Cole[10]-IOTF reference data, which were intended to define child and adolescent obesity for international comparisons of the prevalence of obesity rather than for the clinical diagnosis of overweight and obesity.

Overall, the literature seems to support the use of BMI for age using national reference data to identify overweight and obese children and adolescents. Consistency in technique of measurement and application of criteria is likely of the utmost importance in clinical practice. It seems that, despite the ease of application of BMI for age, many practitioners are reluctant to use this powerful clinical tool (**Table 1**).[17]

Key message

- There is a lack of agreement between different organizations regarding the definition of obesity and cutoff points
- Use and consistency of method is likely of the utmost importance
- BMI is a powerful but underused tool

ANTHROPOMETRIC MEASURES OF OVERWEIGHT AND OBESITY

Although BMI is the most thoroughly researched and advocated tool to identify children and adolescents who are overweight/obese, it is not the only tool. Other measures of excess adiposity are available and the benefits and drawbacks of these measures have been discussed in the literature. Waist circumference, skinfold thickness, hip circumference, waist/hip ratio, and waist/height ratio are examples of the more commonly used alternative measurements. In addition, measurements that can be derived from those listed earlier include arm muscle area, arm fat area, the Rohrer index, and the conicity index. More direct methods of measuring increased adiposity include dual-energy x-ray absorptiometry (DXA), densitometry, underwater

Table 1 BMI cutoff points (AAP, CDC, WHO, IOTF criteria)	
AAP[4]	Use CDC 2000 BMI-for-age growth charts Overweight: 85th to 94th percentile for sex and age Obesity: ≥95th percentile or BMI ≥30 kg/m², whichever is lower
CDC[7]	Use CDC 2000 BMI-for-age growth charts Overweight: at or more than the sex-specific 85th percentile but less than the 95th percentile Obesity: at or more than the sex-specific 95th percentile
WHO (0–5 y)[8]	Percentile and z-score curves for boys and girls aged 0–60 mo Curves consist of weight for age, length/height for age, weight for length/height, and BMI for age
WHO (5–19 y)[9]	Percentile and z-score curves for boys and girls aged 5–19 y Overweight: >+1SD (equivalent to BMI 25 kg/m² at 19 y) Obese: >+2SD (equivalent to BMI 30 kg/m² at 19 y)
IOTF[10]	Designed for international comparisons of prevalence of overweight and obesity Based on adult cutoff points of BMI 25 kg/m² for overweight and 30 kg/m² for obese Organized by sex for ages 2–18 y and defined to pass through BMI of 25 and 30 kg/m² at age 18 y

Abbreviations: AAP, American Academy of Pediatrics; SD, standard deviation.
Data from Refs.[4,7–10]

weighing, computed tomography scan, and foot-to-foot bioelectrical impedance analysis; however, these methods are expensive and have not been found to be reliable in individual children.[18,19]

Studies have noted that skinfold thicknesses may be more strongly associated with body fatness in children,[20,21] although these studies were performed in specific ethnic groups. Other studies comparing the two have shown that skinfold measurement and BMI are both good measures of adiposity in adolescents.[22,23] In a recent study when triceps and subscapular skinfold thicknesses and BMI were compared with the reference standard percent body fat by DXA in a large multiethnic population, girls with increased percent body fat by DXA were identified equally well by BMI and skinfold thickness.[24] Boys were identified slightly more accurately by skinfold thickness, albeit not by a large margin. In contrast, skinfold thickness was superior to BMI when identifying children with low body fat. In addition, total fat mass was more strongly correlated with BMI than skinfold thickness. Skinfold thickness is an inexpensive and easy way to measure adiposity, but it is not as accurate or reproducible as other measurements. Although it is likely not of use in isolation, it may add some useful information when following a patient over time with several measurements once the operator has become familiar with the technique.

Waist circumference is an easy and inexpensive method that has been well researched in the adult population and has been shown to predict development of disease and to correlate strongly with body fat in adults. However, the measurement procedure has not been standardized and there are no validated reference data or substantial research in children. There are multiple ways to measure waist circumference including the midpoint between the lowest rib and the iliac crest, immediately below the lowest rib, at the umbilicus, at the narrowest and widest points, and immediately above the iliac crest.[25] Adult studies have shown that the site of measurement does not influence the risk of cardiovascular disease mortality in adults.[26] However, in pediatrics, single cutoff points are not reasonable because of the rapid somatic growth of children, so it may be more important to standardize the measurement as well as reference the measurement to a certain age and gender. A major obstacle in the use of waist circumference in the adolescent population is the lack of standardized cutoff points in the literature. A systematic review by de Moraes and colleagues[27] analyzed the various cutoff points used for waist circumference to evaluate abdominal obesity in the adolescent population and there was no consensus in the literature. A recent study of a large population of multiethnic school-aged children in the United States showed that DXA fat mass was highly correlated with BMI (Spearman rank correlation coefficient [rs] = 0.83) and sum of skinfolds (rs = 0.9), and DXA truncal fat was highly correlated with waist circumference (rs = 0.79).[28] Body fat distribution has been associated with obesity and not just total body fat. As a result, it has been suggested that combining BMI with an index of body fat distribution may increase the physician's ability to identify children with cardiovascular and metabolic risk factors.[29]

Because of the lack of universally accepted cutoff points for waist circumference, the use of waist/height ratio has been suggested, because it is independent of age and sex.[29] In adults, a waist/height ratio greater than 0.5 has been associated with increased cardiovascular risk and the investigators propose using this cutoff in children and adolescents as well. Other studies have shown that although waist circumference and BMI have strong correlations with percent body fat and a high probability of identifying children and adolescents as obese and overweight, the waist/hip ratio was not well correlated with percent body fat and was not significantly effective at identifying obese and overweight.[28,30,31]

In conjunction with BMI, waist circumference may be the most valuable tool in the arsenal of anthropometric measurements because of its ease of performance; however, a standardized method and cutoff points are necessary to make it a more powerful and effective screening tool. Cook and colleagues[32] proposed a series of growth curves for waist circumference that may be useful for clinical application but need to be validated in future longitudinal studies.

Key message

- In addition to BMI, anthropometric measurements may increase the clinician's ability to identify at-risk adolescents
- Waist circumference is easy to perform, but there is a need to standardize the method and cutoff points

---

RACIAL/ETHNIC DIFFERENCES IN OBESITY

In addition to the controversies regarding the definition and standardization of measures of obesity, there are complex differences in rates of obesity and predisposition to obesity among various ethnicities. Many large, longitudinal studies have been performed in predominantly white cohorts.[33–35] As a result, the current recommendations and data are most representative of the white population and therefore may not consistently identify at-risk youths of other ethnicities. Different ethnicities seem to be prone to the metabolic derangements associated with obesity at different levels. In the most recent National Health and Nutrition Examination Survey (NHANES), from 2009 to 2010, the prevalence of obesity in children and adolescents was 21.2% for Hispanic subjects, 24.3% for non-Hispanic black subjects, and 14% for non-Hispanic white subjects. There was also a racial/ethnic-specific trend identified among non-Hispanic black male subjects with a significant increasing trend of obesity (odds ratio, 1.10; 95% confidence interval, 1.03–1.17).[36] As a result, this cohort needs to be monitored even more carefully. The EPOCH (Evaluating Processes of Care and the Outcomes of Children in Hospital) study of fat distribution, prevalence of obesity, and the metabolic syndrome among a diverse group of Colorado youth found similar results.[37] Hispanic and African American youth had a higher prevalence of obesity and metabolic syndrome as well as more centralized fat distribution and larger abdominal subcutaneous fat deposition than their non-Hispanic white counterparts. In the CATCH (Child and Adolescent Trial for Cardiovascular Health) study, a large, multi-center, multiethnic, school-based intervention study, mean BMI and prevalence of overweight and obesity were higher for African American and Hispanic youth than for white youth.[38] The investigators discussed the importance of the effect of socio-economic status in the prevalence rates and cautioned that race-specific references are confounded by socioeconomic status.

It has been established in the adult population that people from south Asia have metabolic derangements at lower BMIs and anthropometric cut-points than their white counterparts.[39–41] These differences have been attributed to differences in body fat distribution and composition. A recent study in children showed that frac-tional body fat content was significantly greater at any BMI among subjects from south Asia.[42] In addition, ethnicity-specific differences in metabolic derangements were similar to those seen in adults.

These findings suggest that ethnicity-specific BMI and anthropometric cut-points are needed to properly identify high-risk minority children who may not be correctly identified by current standards. Longitudinal data in nonwhite Hispanic, Asian, and Native American populations are also needed to help establish ethnicity-specific recommendations in children.

Key message

- Different ethnicities are prone to metabolic derangements at different levels of obesity
- Ethnicity-specific parameters would likely enhance clinicians' ability to identify at-risk obese adolescents
- Longitudinal studies in ethnically diverse populations are necessary

---

IDENTIFICATION OF THE METABOLIC SYNDROME IN CHILDHOOD AND ADOLESCENCE

The metabolic syndrome in adults is a cluster of conditions consisting of at least 3 of the following: high waist circumference, increased systolic or diastolic blood pressure, increased serum fasting glucose and/or triglyceride levels, and a low HDL cholesterol level. In adults, the US National Cholesterol Education Program Adult Treatment Panel III and the International Diabetes Federation have established the 2 main sets of criteria and cutoffs for diagnosis.[43,44]

However, the metabolic syndrome in the pediatric population has been more difficult to define. As with the definition of obesity, there is a lack of consensus regarding the definition of the metabolic syndrome in youth. A review by Ford and Li[45] showed that 40 unique definitions of pediatric metabolic syndrome were used in 27 different publications. Cook and colleagues[46] chose 4 definitions and applied them to a population of adolescents from NHANES from 1999 to 2002 to determine the prevalence of the metabolic syndrome based on definition. The prev-alence of the metabolic syndrome varied from 2% to 9.4% of all teenagers in the United States and 12.4% to 44.2% in obese teenagers. The study also showed great variation between genders and ethnicities. Despite the lack of consensus, longitudinal studies have shown that pediatric metabolic syndrome predicts adult metabolic syndrome, diabetes mellitus (DM), and cardiovascular disease.[47–49] It is important to determine which definition would capture the largest number of at-risk children. Because interventions are both time and resource intensive, it is also important to identify those who are at risk.

Several studies have made efforts to determine which components of the definition are most effective and yield the highest statistical results. Huang and colleagues[33] found that the use of more stringent criteria yielded a higher specificity but sacrificed sensitivity, whereas the opposite was true when using only 1 component of the definition. Using multiple variables in childhood yielded a high positive predictive value and may be the most useful way to prognosticate future risk. Schubert and colleagues[50] analyzed the sensitivity, specificity, and positive and negative predictive values of components of childhood metabolic syndrome for adult metabolic syndrome and type 2 DM using data from 3 longitudinal studies. Multiple components were better at predicting metabolic syndrome in adulthood, as was shown by Huang and colleagues.[33] However, with regard to type 2 DM, the metabolic components were more effective at identifying children not at risk than identifying those who were at risk. The metabolic components seem to be able to screen out children who are not at risk in order to focus on those with the potential to develop disease. The EPOCH study showed that ethnic minorities might have an increased risk for early development of the metabolic syndrome compared with their non-Hispanic white counterparts, beyond their increased obesity risk.[37]

In light of the absence of a consensus definition, the most recent recommendations by the National Lung, Heart, and Blood Institute[51] are (1) to intensify therapy with an emphasis on lifestyle modification in the presence of any combination of multiple risk factors; (2) the presence of obesity should prompt specific evaluation of all other cardiovascular risk factors; and (3) in the setting of obesity with any other major risk factor, the clinician should initiate interventions such as intensive weight reduction and risk factor–specific interventions as well as prompt evaluation for DM, liver function abnormalities, left ventricular hypertrophy, and sleep apnea.

Key message

- Pediatric metabolic syndrome predicts adult metabolic syndrome, DM, and cardiovascular disease

- Presence of obesity should prompt specific evaluation of all other cardiovascular risk factors

---

THE CARDIOVASCULAR IMPACT OF OBESITY

There are compelling findings from a growing body of evidence that a high BMI in childhood is associated with an increased risk of coronary heart disease in adulthood.[3,52,53] A large, population-based cohort study in Denmark showed that the risk of an adult cardiac event increased significantly for each 1-unit increase in BMI z-score at each age from 7 to 13 years in boys and 10 to 13 years in girls.[53] This finding suggests that weight gain, even at less than the cutoff points for overweight and obesity, may increase the risk for cardiovascular events in adulthood.

HYPERLIPIDEMIA

Hyperlipidemia is a growing problem in overweight and obese children. In addition to obesity, additional risk factors for coronary artery disease have been identified. Hyperlipidemia, hypertension, hyperglycemia, and smoking are all major modifiable risk factors.

Some of the most compelling evidence comes from the Pathologic Determinants of Atherosclerosis in Youth study (PDAY), which analyzed the coronary arteries, aortas, and the cardiovascular risk factors of a large cohort of 15-year-olds to 34-year-olds post mortem who died of trauma.[54] Obesity in men (BMI >30 kg/m²) was associated with both fatty streaks and raised lesions in the right coronary artery (RCA) and with microscopic grade atherosclerosis and stenosis in the left anterior descending artery (LAD). The association was strongest in men with a central pattern of obesity. No significant association of BMI and atherosclerosis was seen in young women.[55] In addition to the strong association of obesity and coronary artery lesions, the major findings of the PDAY study, as summarized by McGill and colleagues,[3] were that the extent of fatty streaks and raised lesions in the RCA and American Heart Association (AHA) grade 4 and 5 lesions (lesions vulnerable to rupture) in the LAD increased with age. Men and women had the same extent of fatty streaks and raised lesions in the abdominal aorta, but women had raised lesions in the RCA that were half as extensive as men by age 30 to 34 years, regardless of risk factors.[56] The extent of fatty streaks and raised lesions were positively associated with non-HDL cholesterol concentration and hyperglycemia[57] and inversely associated with HDL concentration.[58,59] Hypertension was strongly associated with raised lesions in the RCA,[60,61] and nonlipid risk factors were associated with atherosclerosis even in the presence of a favorable lipid panel.[62] In addition, in 2009, Malcolm and colleagues[63] studied tissue lipids in the left circumflex artery and abdominal aorta and found supporting associations between coronary artery disease risk factors and accelerated atherosclerosis. This body of evidence suggests that the process of accelerated atherosclerosis begins in adolescence, and that risk factors present in youth predict adult cardiovascular disease.

Additional autopsy data are available from the Bogalusa Heart Study, a longitudinal, population-based study that also showed that BMI, blood pressure, smoking, and serum lipid levels were associated with the extent of atherosclerosis.[64] In addition, the study concluded that as the number of cardiovascular risk factors increases so does the severity of asymptomatic atherosclerosis in young people.

In addition to autopsy studies, there is a growing body of literature using noninvasive methods that evaluate endothelial dysfunction and carotid intimal media thickness (cIMT) to correlate cardiovascular risk factors with the presence and increased risk of atherosclerotic disease.[65,66] The Bogalusa Heart Study has shown a strong relationship between cardiovascular risk factors in youth, particularly BMI and increased lipid levels, and increased cIMT in adulthood.[67,68] A more recent study from the Bogalusa Heart Study evaluated the ability of different measures of childhood lipid levels to predict increased cIMT in adulthood.[69] Non-HDL cholesterol, low-density lipoprotein (LDL) cholesterol, total cholesterol/HDL ratio, apolipoprotein B, and apolipoprotein B/apolipoprotein A-I levels were significant predictors. Non-HDL cholesterol level was as good as other lipid measures at predicting increased cIMT in adulthood. In the Muscatine Study, another long-term, population-based study, electron beam computed tomography was used to show coronary artery calcification in young adults with childhood coronary risk factors.[70] High BMI, high blood pressure, and low HDL levels in adolescence were strongly associated with coronary artery calcification, particularly in young men.

A prospective study combining 3 large longitudinal studies (Cardiovascular Risk in Young Finns, Bogalusa, and Childhood Determinants of Adult Health) showed that adolescents with dyslipidemia (National Cholesterol Education Program and NHANES criteria) were at significantly increased risk of having high cIMT in adulthood.[71] A recent study showed the triglyceride/HDL-C ratio is an independent predictor of arterial stiffness in youth, and particularly in obese youth.[72] Those adolescents who had the highest ratios also had the stiffest vessels. This finding was not seen when HDL or triglycerides were evaluated independently. The investigators concluded that triglyceride/HDL-C ratio may be a useful tool to identify obese children and adolescents who are at risk for accelerated atherosclerosis. A recent large, multinational population study of young adults analyzed the 7 metrics of cardiovascular health (blood pressure, cholesterol, glucose, BMI, physical activity, nonsmoking, and healthy diet) according to the AHA in 2010 and its association with cIMT.[73] An inverse relationship was found between the number of ideal health metrics and cIMT. Only 1% of the subjects met all 7 health metrics, suggesting that an international effort to improve cardiovascular health is warranted.

Expert committees have recommended control of modifiable risk factors since 1972.[74] Since that time many organizations have published guidelines and recommendations for the recognition and management of cardiovascular risk factors in pediatrics. The National Heart, Lung, and Blood Institute (NHLBI) has recently published one of the most comprehensive guidelines.[51] One of the most controversial recommendations is for universal screening of all youth from 9 to 11 years and 17 to 21 years of age with a nonfasting lipid panel in order to calculate the non-HD cholesterol level (**Box 1**). The triglyceride and LDL levels cannot be used in the nonfasting specimen. If the non-HDL level is more than 145 mg/dL or the HDL level is less than 40 mg/dL, an algorithm for further screening with fasting lipid panel has been recommended. In the other age groups, there are special situations in which screening with a fasting lipid profile is recommended (see **Box 1**). By universally screening all children, the panel hopes to capture the large percentage of children who are missed when screening is based on family history alone. In addition to lipid screening and management, the report includes evidence-based recommendations addressing the other known risk factors for cardiovascular disease. It is a valuable and practical tool, intended to assist primary care providers in the identification and management of cardiovascular risk factors in childhood and adolescence.

Key message

- Obesity, hyperlipidemia, hypertension, hyperglycemia, and smoking are all major modifiable cardiovascular risk factors

- The process of accelerated atherosclerosis begins in adolescence, so there is an important role for primary providers to slow this process

- Universal screening of all youth from 9 to 11 years and 17 to 21 years of age with a nonfasting lipid panel (NHLBI)

INCREASED LEFT VENTRICULAR MASS

Metabolic and hemodynamic derangements are associated with obesity and the development of the metabolic syndrome, as discussed earlier. Changes in cardiac geometry have also been shown to occur in the setting of obesity, specifically increased left ventricular mass, left ventricular dilatation, and decreased systolic and diastolic function.[75,76] Increased left ventricular mass predicts a higher incidence of clinical events related to cardiovascular disease.[77] In children and adolescents there has been some controversy regarding the cardiovascular effects of obesity. The left ventricular hypertrophy seen in overweight and obese adolescents has been attributed to a compensatory response caused by increased cardiac workload. However, several studies have shown that obese adolescents show changes in cardiac geometry in excess of cardiac workload.

Box 1
Lipid screening in childhood and adolescence

Childhood (2–11 years old)

Lipid screening (fasting lipid profile) for select situations:

1. (+) Family history[a]
2. Parent with hyperlipidemia[b]
3. Child with obesity[c], hypertension, diabetes, or who smokes
4. Child has moderate-risk or high-risk medical condition[d]

Universal screening between 9 and 11 years of age (nonfasting lipid profile to determine non–HDL-C[e])

  If non–HDL-C is greater than or equal to 145 mg/dL or HDL less than 40 mg/dL, obtain fasting lipid profile

Adolescence (12–21 years old)

Lipid screening (fasting lipid profile) for select situations:

1. (+) Family history[a]
2. Parent with hyperlipidemia[b]
3. Child with overweight[f], hypertension, diabetes, or who smokes
4. Child has moderate-risk or high-risk medical condition[d]

Universal screening between 17 and 21 years of age (nonfasting lipid profile to determine non–HDL-C[e])

  If non–HDL-C is greater than or equal to 145 mg/dL or HDL less than 40 mg/dL, obtain fasting lipid profile

[a] Family history is first-degree relatives with history of myocardial infarction, stroke, angina, coronary bypass graft/stent/angioplasty at less than 65 years old for female or less than 55 years of age for men.
[b] Parent with total cholesterol (TC) more than 240 mg/dL or known cholesterol abnormality.
[c] Obesity defined as BMI greater than or equal to 95th percentile.
[d] High-risk medical conditions: DM, chronic kidney disease/end-stage renal disease/after renal transplant, after orthotopic heart transplant, Kawasaki disease with aneurysms. Moderate-risk medical conditions: Kawasaki disease with regressed aneurysms, chronic inflammatory disease, human immunodeficiency virus infection, nephrotic syndrome.
[e] Non–HDL-C = TC minus HDL-C.
[f] Overweight defined as BMI ≥85th percentile.

Data from Expert Panel on Integrated Guidelines for Cardiovascular Health and Risk Reduction in Children and Adolescents, National Heart, Lung, and Blood Institute. Expert panel on integrated guidelines for cardiovascular health and risk reduction in children and adolescents: summary report. Pediatrics 2011;128(Suppl 5):S213–56.

  The Bogalusa Heart Study, a longitudinal study performed in a biracial population, studied the effects of growth, blood pressure, and excess body weight on left ventricular mass, and found that excess weight is an important, independent cause of the acquisition of increased left ventricular mass.[78] It also discussed the finding that increased left ventricular mass may precede the development of increased blood pressure. The Bogalusa Heart Study has also shown that adiposity beginning in childhood predicts increased left ventricular mass in young adults.[79] In childhood, BMI was the only independent predictor of adult left ventricular mass index (LVMI). The Strong Heart Study analyzed left ventricular geometry in a large population of American Indian adolescents with varying degrees of abnormal body size and found that the severity of abnormality in body habitus affected cardiac geometry.[80] Individuals categorized as overweight had increased left ventricular mass related to increased cardiac workload; however, in obese individuals, the level of increased left ventricular mass was in excess of the cardiac workload and was associated with reduced left ventricular systolic function and myocardial performance. These findings suggest exogenous factors influencing cardiac geometry in addition to the known hemodynamic factors, which increase cardiac workload.

An increased LVMI has been shown in children and adolescents in the current era versus age-matched and sex-matched counterparts from 20 years earlier, and has been attributed at least in part to the increase in BMI over the last 20 years.[81] Increased left ventricular hypertrophy as well as left ventricular dilatation was observed and may predispose to future left ventricular failure.

With recent advances in echocardiography, several studies have analyzed the effect of obesity on myocardial deformation with the use of strain and strain rate imaging, a measure of myocardial contractility.[82,83] In the absence of hypertension, obesity was associated with a significant reduction in systolic myocardial deformation in childhood affecting both the right and left ventricles. In addition, the study observed that LVMI was significantly higher in obese children.[84] A pilot study was performed in obese children with lipid abnormalities to evaluate vascular and myocardial interactions.[85] Obese children with lipid abnormalities had decreased systolic and diastolic left ventricular deformation and increased arterial wall stiffness; however, this study was performed in a small sample with several technical limitations. Nonetheless, a need for further testing of this population for abnormal vascular and myocardial changes is evident from the findings. Obesity has not only been shown to affect ventricular contractility but has also been implicated in reduced bilateral atrial myocardial deformation.[86] Obesity in childhood is a risk factor for future poor cardiovascular outcomes and disease, but echocardiographic data show that myocardial changes occur early in the disease process and may manifest at younger ages in the current pediatric obesity epidemic.

In the setting of obesity, other than LVMI, measures involving echocardiography primarily have a role in a research capacity at this time. Future longitudinal studies may be able to identify the characteristics that place individuals at a significantly increased risk such that increased monitoring may be useful.

Key message

- Increased left ventricular mass has been shown to occur in the setting of obesity
- Increased left ventricular mass predicts a higher incidence of future cardiovascular events

---

OBESITY PREVENTION STUDIES

Obesity in childhood and adolescence negatively affects cardiovascular health. There is a need for effective interventions to prevent overweight and obesity in youth. Showell and colleagues[87] performed a systematic review of home-based childhood obesity prevention studies that assessed diet and physical activity intervention studies with at least 1 year of follow-up in high-income countries. Six randomized controlled trials from the United States were included, 4 of which were exclusively conducted in the home setting. None of the home-based interventions showed a statistically significant positive effect on weight-related outcomes. Three studies showed a positive effect of diet and physical activity outcomes. One study targeted all family members in the household, which may suggest that the family involvement was more important than the home-based setting alone. Overall, the review concluded that, at present, there is insufficient evidence to support the effectiveness of home-based interventions in isolation. The relatively number of included studies suggests that more high-quality research is necessary to further investigate the effectiveness of home-based interventions.

In 2012, the Institute of Medicine published a report with recommendations and strategies to "create synergies that can further accelerate progress in preventing obesity"[88] that emphasizes a comprehensive approach and one that includes the community. Bleich and colleagues[89] performed a systematic review of community-based childhood obesity prevention programs that studied adiposity and obesity-related outcomes. Nine studies were included in the review, one of which was exclusively in the community setting and the remaining 8 were implemented in the community in addition to other venues. Although the investigators concluded that more research with more consistent methods are needed to fully understand the effectiveness of the intervention, they found moderate evidence that community-based interventions that include a school component and use both diet and activity interventions effectively prevent obesity or overweight in children. Combination interventions in multiple settings seemed to be more effective than single-component interventions.

Several systematic reviews have been performed of obesity prevention programs in school settings and have shown encouraging findings. One review showed that long-term interventions combined with diet and exercise and family involvement are associated with significant weight reduction in children.[90] However, the investigators concluded that more high-quality research is necessary to fully validate these findings and identify specific program components predictive of success. Another review found that the use of social cognitive theory or social learning theory in the development of the intervention, long-term follow-up, high parental involvement, targeted physical activity, and dietary change, and focus on child and parent perceptions had significant favorable findings.[91]

A 2011 Cochrane Review of childhood obesity prevention research showed strong evidence to support beneficial effects of child obesity prevention programs, particularly in children aged 6 to 12 years. The review emphasized the need for a multidisciplinary approach to prevention incorporating school-based interventions, including an emphasis on education, nutrition and increased physical activity, parental support and home-based interventions including improved diet and exercise, and cultural practices that support changes in nutrition and exercise.[92]

Key message

- A need exists for immediate preventive action to control the obesity epidemic
- A multidisciplinary approach using home, school, and community resources is emphasized
- More high-quality research studies to identify successful strategies for obesity prevention are warranted

---

SUMMARY

The first step in the prevention of the cardiovascular complications of the obesity epidemic is the recognition and identification of overweight and obese children and adolescents. Without appropriate intervention and prevention the current obesity epidemic predicts a future epidemic of early onset clinical cardiovascular disease.[93] The development of effective programs for the prevention of overweight and obesity in youth is necessary to turn the tide of the obesity epidemic. This article updates pediatricians on the current literature regarding the identification of obesity and its associated cardiovascular risk factors, as follows:

- BMI is an important and powerful tool to identify overweight and obese adolescents.
- Regardless of the chosen criteria use, consistency in techniques of measurement and application is likely of utmost importance.
- In conjunction with BMI, the addition of at least one anthropometric measurement likely enhances the clinicians' ability to recognize at-risk individuals as well as to monitor progress.
- Rates of obesity are highest among African American and Hispanic youth. As a result, screening for cardiovascular risk factors and prevention is particularly important in these populations.
- There is a need for a standardized pediatric definition of the metabolic syndrome. The metabolic syndrome in childhood seems to track into adulthood. At present, in the presence of obesity, practitioners should initiate intensive lifestyle modification, screening, and intervention for cardiovascular risk factors as well as evaluation for DM, liver function abnormalities, left ventricular hypertrophy, and sleep apnea.
- The development of atherosclerosis begins in childhood and is accelerated in the presence of obesity.
- Screening for hyperlipidemia is of particular importance in the overweight and obese child and adolescent in order to implement interventions to prevent early cardiovascular events.
- Obesity causes changes in cardiac geometry in excess of the cardiac workload and predicts an increased incidence of cardiac events.
- Although an ideal obesity prevention program has yet to be developed, a multidisciplinary approach with a combination of school, community, and parental involvement is most likely to yield successful results.

REFERENCES

1. Ogden CL, Carroll MD, Curtin LR, et al. Prevalence of overweight and obesity in the United States, 1999-2004. JAMA 2006;295(13):1549–55.
2. Go AS, Mozaffarian D, Roger VL, et al. Heart disease and stroke statistics–2013 update: a report from the American Heart Association. Circulation 2013;127(1):e6–245.
3. McGill HC Jr, McMahan CA, Gidding SS. Preventing heart disease in the 21st century: implications of the Pathobiological Determinants of Atherosclerosis in Youth (PDAY) study. Circulation 2008;117(9):1216–27.
4. Barlow SE, Expert C. Expert committee recommendations regarding the prevention, assessment, and treatment of child and adolescent overweight and obesity: summary report. Pediatrics 2007;120(Suppl 4):S164–92.
5. Barlow SE, Dietz WH. Obesity evaluation and treatment: Expert Committee recommendations. The Maternal and Child Health Bureau, Health Resources and Services Administration and the Department of Health and Human Services. Pediatrics 1998;102(3):E29.
6. Ogden CL, Kuczmarski RJ, Flegal KM, et al. Centers for Disease Control and Prevention 2000 growth charts for the United States: improvements to the 1977 National Center for Health Statistics version. Pediatrics 2002;109(1):45–60.

7. Ogden CL, Flegal KM. Changes in terminology for childhood overweight and obesity. Natl Health Stat Report 2010;(25):1–5.
8. WHO Multicentre Growth Reference Study Group. WHO child growth standards based on length/height, weight and age. Acta Paediatr 2006;450:76–85.
9. WHO 5-19 yo reference World Health Organization (WHO). 2007. Available at: http://www.who.int/growthref/en/. Accessed July 29, 2013.
10. Cole TJ, Bellizzi MC, Flegal KM, et al. Establishing a standard definition for child overweight and obesity worldwide: international survey. BMJ 2000;320(7244): 1240–3.
11. Flegal KM, Ogden CL. Childhood obesity: are we all speaking the same language? Adv Nutr 2011;2(2):159S–66S.
12. Martinez-Costa C, Nunez F, Montal A, et al. Relationship between childhood obesity cut-offs and metabolic and vascular comorbidities: comparative analysis of three growth standards. J Hum Nutr Diet 2013. [Epub ahead of print].
13. Shields M, Tremblay MS. Canadian childhood obesity estimates based on WHO, IOTF and CDC cut-points. Int J Pediatr Obes 2010;5(3):265–73.
14. Reilly JJ, Kelly J, Wilson DC. Accuracy of simple clinical and epidemiological definitions of childhood obesity: systematic review and evidence appraisal. Obes Rev 2010;11(9):645–55.
15. Wijnhoven TM, van Raaij JM, Spinelli A, et al. WHO European Childhood Obesity Surveillance Initiative 2008: weight, height and body mass index in 6–9-year-old children. Pediatr Obes 2013;8(2):79–97.
16. Reilly JJ. Assessment of obesity in children and adolescents: synthesis of recent systematic reviews and clinical guidelines. J Hum Nutr Diet 2010;23(3):205–11.
17. Voelker R. Improved use of BMI needed to screen children for overweight. JAMA 2007;297(24):2684–5.
18. Reilly JJ, Gerasimidis K, Paparacleous N, et al. Validation of dual-energy x-ray absorptiometry and foot-foot impedance against deuterium dilution measures of fatness in children. Int J Pediatr Obes 2010;5(1):111–5.
19. Radley D, Cooke CB, Fuller NJ, et al. Validity of foot-to-foot bio-electrical impedance analysis body composition estimates in overweight and obese children. Int J Body Compos Res 2009;7(1):15–20.
20. Sarria A, Garcia-Llop LA, Moreno LA, et al. Skinfold thickness measurements are better predictors of body fat percentage than body mass index in male Spanish children and adolescents. Eur J Clin Nutr 1998;52(8):573–6.
21. Sardinha LB, Going SB, Teixeira PJ, et al. Receiver operating characteristic analysis of body mass index, triceps skinfold thickness, and arm girth for obesity screening in children and adolescents. Am J Clin Nutr 1999;70(6): 1090–5.
22. Freedman DS, Wang J, Ogden CL, et al. The prediction of body fatness by BMI and skinfold thicknesses among children and adolescents. Ann Hum Biol 2007; 34(2):183–94.
23. Steinberger J, Jacobs DR, Raatz S, et al. Comparison of body fatness measurements by BMI and skinfolds vs dual energy X-ray absorptiometry and their relation to cardiovascular risk factors in adolescents. Int J Obes 2005;29(11): 1346–52.
24. Freedman DS, Ogden CL, Blanck HM, et al. The abilities of body mass index and skinfold thicknesses to identify children with low or elevated levels of dual-energy x-ray absorptiometry-determined body fatness. J Pediatr 2013;163(1):160–6.e1.
25. Ness-Abramof R, Apovian CM. Waist circumference measurement in clinical practice. Nutr Clin Pract 2008;23(4):397–404.

26. Ross R, Berentzen T, Bradshaw AJ, et al. Does the relationship between waist circumference, morbidity and mortality depend on measurement protocol for waist circumference? Obes Rev 2008;9(4):312–25.
27. de Moraes AC, Fadoni RP, Ricardi LM, et al. Prevalence of abdominal obesity in adolescents: a systematic review. Obes Rev 2011;12(2):69–77.
28. Boeke CE, Oken E, Kleinman KP, et al. Correlations among adiposity measures in school-aged children. BMC Pediatr 2013;13:99.
29. Maffeis C, Banzato C, Talamini G, et al. Waist-to-height ratio, a useful index to identify high metabolic risk in overweight children. J Pediatr 2008;152(2):207–13.
30. Neovius M, Linne Y, Rossner S. BMI, waist-circumference and waist-hip-ratio as diagnostic tests for fatness in adolescents. Int J Obes 2005;29(2):163–9.
31. Freedman DS, Khan LK, Serdula MK, et al. Inter-relationships among childhood BMI, childhood height, and adult obesity: the Bogalusa Heart Study. Int J Obes Relat Metab Disord 2004;28(1):10–6.
32. Cook S, Auinger P, Huang TT. Growth curves for cardio-metabolic risk factors in children and adolescents. J Pediatr 2009;155(3):S6.e15–26.
33. Huang TT, Nansel TR, Belsheim AR, et al. Sensitivity, specificity, and predictive values of pediatric metabolic syndrome components in relation to adult metabolic syndrome: the Princeton LRC follow-up study. J Pediatr 2008;152(2):185–90.
34. Lauer RM, Connor WE, Leaverton PE, et al. Coronary heart disease risk factors in school children: the Muscatine study. J Pediatr 1975;86(5):697–706.
35. Roche AF. Growth, maturation, and body composition: the FELS longitudinal study 1929-1991. Cambridge (United Kingdom): Cambridge University Press; 1992.
36. Ogden CL, Carroll MD, Kit BK, et al. Prevalence of obesity and trends in body mass index among US children and adolescents, 1999-2010. JAMA 2012;307(5):483–90.
37. Maligie M, Crume T, Scherzinger A, et al. Adiposity, fat patterning, and the metabolic syndrome among diverse youth: the EPOCH study. J Pediatr 2012;161(5):875–80.
38. Dwyer JT, Stone EJ, Yang M, et al. Prevalence of marked overweight and obesity in a multiethnic pediatric population: findings from the Child and Adolescent Trial for Cardiovascular Health (CATCH) study. J Am Diet Assoc 2000;100(10):1149–56.
39. Wulan SN, Westerterp KR, Plasqui G. Ethnic differences in body composition and the associated metabolic profile: a comparative study between Asians and Caucasians. Maturitas 2010;65(4):315–9.
40. Chandalia M, Lin P, Seenivasan T, et al. Insulin resistance and body fat distribution in South Asian men compared to Caucasian men. PLoS One 2007;2(8):e812.
41. Balakrishnan P, Grundy SM, Islam A, et al. Influence of upper and lower body adipose tissue on insulin sensitivity in South Asian men. J Investig Med 2012;60(7):999–1004.
42. Rosenbaum M, Fennoy I, Accacha S, et al. Racial/ethnic differences in clinical and biochemical type 2 diabetes mellitus risk factors in children. Obesity (Silver Spring) 2013;21(10):2081–90.
43. Alberti KG, Zimmet P, Shaw J. Metabolic syndrome–a new world-wide definition. A consensus statement from the International Diabetes Federation. Diabet Med 2006;23(5):469–80.

44. Expert Panel on Detection, Evaluation, and Treatment of High Blood Cholesterol in Adults. Executive summary of The Third Report of The National Cholesterol Education Program (NCEP) Expert Panel on Detection, Evaluation, and Treatment of High Blood Cholesterol in Adults (Adult Treatment Panel III). JAMA 2001;285(19):2486–97.
45. Ford ES, Li C. Defining the metabolic syndrome in children and adolescents: will the real definition please stand up? J Pediatr 2008;152(2):160–4.
46. Cook S, Auinger P, Li C, et al. Metabolic syndrome rates in United States adolescents, from the National Health and Nutrition Examination Survey, 1999-2002. J Pediatr 2008;152(2):165–70.
47. Morrison JA, Friedman LA, Gray-McGuire C. Metabolic syndrome in childhood predicts adult cardiovascular disease 25 years later: the Princeton Lipid Research Clinics Follow-up Study. Pediatrics 2007;120(2):340–5.
48. Morrison JA, Friedman LA, Wang P, et al. Metabolic syndrome in childhood predicts adult metabolic syndrome and type 2 diabetes mellitus 25 to 30 years later. J Pediatr 2008;152(2):201–6.
49. Ventura AK, Loken E, Birch LL. Risk profiles for metabolic syndrome in a nonclinical sample of adolescent girls. Pediatrics 2006;118(6):2434–42.
50. Schubert CM, Sun SS, Burns TL, et al. Predictive ability of childhood metabolic components for adult metabolic syndrome and type 2 diabetes. J Pediatr 2009; 155(3):S6.e1–7.
51. Expert Panel on Integrated Guidelines for Cardiovascular Health and Risk Reduction in Children and Adolescents, National Heart, Lung, and Blood Institute. Expert Panel on Integrated Guidelines for Cardiovascular Health and Risk Reduction in Children and Adolescents: summary report. Pediatrics 2011; 128(Suppl 5):S213–56.
52. Friedemann C, Heneghan C, Mahtani K, et al. Cardiovascular disease risk in healthy children and its association with body mass index: systematic review and meta-analysis. BMJ 2012;345:e4759.
53. Baker JL, Olsen LW, Sorensen TI. Childhood body-mass index and the risk of coronary heart disease in adulthood. N Engl J Med 2007;357(23): 2329–37.
54. McGill HC Jr, McMahan CA, Zieske AW, et al. Associations of coronary heart disease risk factors with the intermediate lesion of atherosclerosis in youth. The Pathobiological Determinants of Atherosclerosis in Youth (PDAY) research group. Arterioscler Thromb Vasc Biol 2000;20(8):1998–2004.
55. McGill HC Jr, McMahan CA, Herderick EE, et al. Obesity accelerates the progression of coronary atherosclerosis in young men. Circulation 2002;105(23): 2712–8.
56. McGill HC Jr, McMahan CA, Malcom GT, et al. Effects of serum lipoproteins and smoking on atherosclerosis in young men and women. The PDAY Research Group. Pathobiological Determinants of Atherosclerosis in Youth. Arterioscler Thromb Vasc Biol 1997;17(1):95–106.
57. McGill HC Jr, McMahan CA, Malcom GT, et al. Relation of glycohemoglobin and adiposity to atherosclerosis in youth. Pathobiological Determinants of Atherosclerosis in Youth (PDAY) Research Group. Arterioscler Thromb Vasc Biol 1995;15(4):431–40.
58. Relationship of atherosclerosis in young men to serum lipoprotein cholesterol concentrations and smoking. A preliminary report from the Pathobiological Determinants of Atherosclerosis in Youth (PDAY) Research Group. JAMA 1990;264(23):3018–24.

59. McGill HC Jr, McMahan CA, Zieske AW, et al. Association of coronary heart disease risk factors with microscopic qualities of coronary atherosclerosis in youth. Circulation 2000;102(4):374–9.
60. McGill HC Jr, Strong JP, Tracy RE, et al. Relation of a postmortem renal index of hypertension to atherosclerosis in youth. The Pathobiological Determinants of Atherosclerosis in Youth (PDAY) Research Group. Arterioscler Thromb Vasc Biol 1995;15(12):2222–8.
61. McGill HC Jr, McMahan CA, Tracy RE, et al. Relation of a postmortem renal index of hypertension to atherosclerosis and coronary artery size in young men and women. Pathobiological Determinants of Atherosclerosis in Youth (PDAY) Research Group. Arterioscler Thromb Vasc Biol 1998;18(7):1108–18.
62. McGill HC Jr, McMahan CA, Zieske AW, et al. Effects of nonlipid risk factors on atherosclerosis in youth with a favorable lipoprotein profile. Circulation 2001; 103(11):1546–50.
63. Malcom GT, McMahan CA, McGill HC Jr, et al. Associations of arterial tissue lipids with coronary heart disease risk factors in young people. Atherosclerosis 2009;203(2):515–21.
64. Berenson GS, Srinivasan SR, Bao W, et al. Association between multiple cardiovascular risk factors and atherosclerosis in children and young adults. The Bogalusa Heart Study. N Engl J Med 1998;338(23):1650–6.
65. Heiss G, Sharrett AR, Barnes R, et al. Carotid atherosclerosis measured by B-mode ultrasound in populations: associations with cardiovascular risk factors in the ARIC study. Am J Epidemiol 1991;134(3):250–6.
66. Brouwers MC, Reesink KD, van Greevenbroek MM, et al. Increased arterial stiffness in familial combined hyperlipidemia. J Hypertens 2009;27(5):1009–16.
67. Freedman DS, Dietz WH, Tang R, et al. The relation of obesity throughout life to carotid intima-media thickness in adulthood: the Bogalusa Heart Study. Int J Obes Relat Metab Disord 2004;28(1):159–66.
68. Li S, Chen W, Srinivasan SR, et al. Childhood cardiovascular risk factors and carotid vascular changes in adulthood: the Bogalusa Heart Study. JAMA 2003; 290(17):2271–6.
69. Frontini MG, Srinivasan SR, Xu J, et al. Usefulness of childhood non-high density lipoprotein cholesterol levels versus other lipoprotein measures in predicting adult subclinical atherosclerosis: the Bogalusa Heart Study. Pediatrics 2008; 121(5):924–9.
70. Mahoney LT, Burns TL, Stanford W, et al. Coronary risk factors measured in childhood and young adult life are associated with coronary artery calcification in young adults: the Muscatine Study. J Am Coll Cardiol 1996;27(2):277–84.
71. Magnussen CG, Venn A, Thomson R, et al. The association of pediatric low- and high-density lipoprotein cholesterol dyslipidemia classifications and change in dyslipidemia status with carotid intima-media thickness in adulthood evidence from the Cardiovascular Risk in Young Finns study, the Bogalusa Heart Study, and the CDAH (Childhood Determinants of Adult Health) study. J Am Coll Cardiol 2009;53(10):860–9.
72. Urbina EM, Khoury PR, McCoy CE, et al. Triglyceride to HDL-C ratio and increased arterial stiffness in children, adolescents, and young adults. Pediatrics 2013;131(4):e1082–90.
73. Oikonen M, Laitinen TT, Magnussen CG, et al. Ideal cardiovascular health in young adult populations from the United States, Finland, and Australia and its association with cIMT: The International Childhood Cardiovascular Cohort Consortium. J Am Heart Assoc 2013;2(3):e000244.

74. American Academy of Pediatrics. Committee on Nutrition: childhood diet and coronary heart disease. Pediatrics 1972;49(2):305–7.
75. Alpert MA. Obesity cardiomyopathy: pathophysiology and evolution of the clinical syndrome. Am J Med Sci 2001;321(4):225–36.
76. Pascual M, Pascual DA, Soria F, et al. Effects of isolated obesity on systolic and diastolic left ventricular function. Heart 2003;89(10):1152–6.
77. Levy D, Garrison RJ, Savage DD, et al. Prognostic implications of echocardiographically determined left ventricular mass in the Framingham Heart Study. N Engl J Med 1990;322(22):1561–6.
78. Urbina EM, Gidding SS, Bao W, et al. Effect of body size, ponderosity, and blood pressure on left ventricular growth in children and young adults in the Bogalusa Heart Study. Circulation 1995;91(9):2400–6.
79. Li X, Li S, Ulusoy E, et al. Childhood adiposity as a predictor of cardiac mass in adulthood: the Bogalusa Heart Study. Circulation 2004;110(22):3488–92.
80. Chinali M, de Simone G, Roman MJ, et al. Impact of obesity on cardiac geometry and function in a population of adolescents: the Strong Heart Study. J Am Coll Cardiol 2006;47(11):2267–73.
81. Crowley DI, Khoury PR, Urbina EM, et al. Cardiovascular impact of the pediatric obesity epidemic: higher left ventricular mass is related to higher body mass index. J Pediatr 2011;158(5):709–14.e1.
82. Sutherland GR, Di Salvo G, Claus P, et al. Strain and strain rate imaging: a new clinical approach to quantifying regional myocardial function. J Am Soc Echocardiogr 2004;17(7):788–802.
83. Greenberg NL, Firstenberg MS, Castro PL, et al. Doppler-derived myocardial systolic strain rate is a strong index of left ventricular contractility. Circulation 2002;105(1):99–105.
84. Di Salvo G, Pacileo G, Del Giudice EM, et al. Abnormal myocardial deformation properties in obese, non-hypertensive children: an ambulatory blood pressure monitoring, standard echocardiographic, and strain rate imaging study. Eur Heart J 2006;27(22):2689–95.
85. Koopman LP, McCrindle BW, Slorach C, et al. Interaction between myocardial and vascular changes in obese children: a pilot study. J Am Soc Echocardiogr 2012;25(4):401–10.e1.
86. Di Salvo G, Pacileo G, Del Giudice EM, et al. Atrial myocardial deformation properties in obese nonhypertensive children. J Am Soc Echocardiogr 2008; 21(2):151–6.
87. Showell NN, Fawole O, Segal J, et al. A systematic review of home-based childhood obesity prevention studies. Pediatrics 2013;132(1):e193–200.
88. Institute of Medicine. Accelerating progress in obesity prevention: solving the weight of the nation. Washington, DC: National Academies Press; 2012. Available at: www.iom.edu/reports/2012/acclerating-progress-in-obesity-prevention. aspx. Accessed July 16, 2013.
89. Bleich SN, Segal J, Wu Y, et al. Systematic review of community-based childhood obesity prevention studies. Pediatrics 2013;132(1):e201–10.
90. Khambalia AZ, Dickinson S, Hardy LL, et al. A synthesis of existing systematic reviews and meta-analyses of school-based behavioural interventions for controlling and preventing obesity. Obes Rev 2012;13(3):214–33.
91. Nixon CA, Moore HJ, Douthwaite W, et al. Identifying effective behavioural models and behaviour change strategies underpinning preschool- and school-based obesity prevention interventions aimed at 4–6-year-olds: a systematic review. Obes Rev 2012;13(Suppl 1):106–17.

92. Waters E, de Silva-Sanigorski A, Hall BJ, et al. Interventions for preventing obesity in children. Cochrane Database Syst Rev 2011;(12):CD001871.
93. McCrindle BW. Will childhood obesity lead to an epidemic of premature cardio-vascular disease? Evid Based Cardiovasc Med 2006;10(2):71–4.

Cardiomyopathies Encountered Commonly in the Teenage Years and Their Presentation

Michael D. Pettersen, MD

KEYWORDS

- Cardiomyopathy • Heart failure • Arrhythmia • Sudden death

KEY POINTS

- Cardiomyopathies represent an import cause of morbidity and mortality in the adolescent population as a result of the presence of systolic or diastolic dysfunction as well as the risk of cardiac dysrhythmia and sudden death.
- Dilated cardiomyopathy is the most common form of cardiomyopathy seen in patients younger than 18 years and is characterized by ventricular dilation and systolic dysfunction, resulting in signs and symptoms of congestive heart failure.
- Hypertrophic cardiomyopathy is a genetically inherited condition resulting in significant ventricular hypertrophy and fibrosis, and represents the most common cause of sudden, unexpected death in adolescents.
- Restrictive cardiomyopathy is a rare form of cardiomyopathy that results in ventricular diastolic dysfunction and carries a poor transplantation-free survival from the time of diagnosis.
- Knowledge of the typical clinical presentations of cardiomyopathy is important for physicians involved in the care of adolescent patients in order to facilitate early evaluation and intervention and to achieve the best clinical outcomes.

INTRODUCTION

Cardiomyopathy encompasses a genetically and clinically heterogeneous group of heart muscle disorders. They are defined by the presence of abnormal myocardial structure resulting in systolic or diastolic dysfunction, in the absence of ischemic heart disease or abnormal loading conditions. In affected children and adolescents, cardiomyopathy can have severe consequences, with up to 40% of individuals progressing to death or cardiac transplantation within 5 years of diagnosis.[1–4]

The classification of the cardiomyopathies is based on phenotype defined by clinical presentation and diagnostic evaluation of affected individuals, incorporating genetic diagnosis when possible. The most common cardiomyopathies encountered in adolescent patients include dilated cardiomyopathy (DCM), hypertrophic

Department of Pediatrics, Rocky Mountain Hospital for Children, 2055 High Street, Suite 255, Denver, CO 80205, USA
E-mail address: michael_pettersen@pediatrix.com

Pediatr Clin N Am 61 (2014) 173–186
http://dx.doi.org/10.1016/j.pcl.2013.09.017   **pediatric.theclinics.com**
0031-3955/14/$ – see front matter © 2014 Elsevier Inc. All rights reserved.

cardiomyopathy (HCM), and restrictive cardiomyopathy (RCM).[5] According to the US Pediatric Cardiomyopathy Registry, the annual incidence of cardiomyopathy is 1.13 per 100,000 children younger than 18 years, with DCM being the most common (56%), followed by HCM (30%).[6] Arrhythmogenic right ventricular cardiomyopathy is a rare, genetically inherited form of cardiomyopathy, which typically manifests as arrhythmia, syncope, or sudden death. Phenotypic manifestation does not usually occur until the third decade of life or beyond. Presentation in adolescents is rare, and this form of cardiomyopathy is not discussed further in this review.

The different types of cardiomyopathy can be associated with a wide range of symptoms ranging from none to severe. Most patients have pure forms of these disorders, which fulfill strict diagnostic criteria, although some have overlapping features with mixed forms of disease. Early recognition of these conditions by clinicians is important to allow prompt initiation of treatment, which is aimed at improving myocardial performance and hemodynamics, alleviating symptoms, and prolonging survival. For patients in whom medical management fails, heart transplantation is an option, with excellent intermediate-term success.

DCM
Background

DCM refers to congestive cardiac failure secondary to dilation and systolic dysfunction (with or without diastolic dysfunction) of the ventricles. Normal left ventricular ejection fraction is 50% to 65%. Anything less than 50% could indicate the presence of DCM. All 4 cardiac chambers are dilated and at times hypertrophied, with dilation more pronounced than hypertrophy. In the United States, the incidence of DCM is 0.57 cases per 100,000 children,[6] with genetic causes accounting for approximately 30% of DCM cases.

Cause

Multiple causes of myocardial damage have been identified, including infection (myocarditis), inborn errors of metabolism, neuromuscular disease, malformation syndromes, and toxins.[7] **Table 1** lists factors associated with myocardial damage and the development of DCM. However, in most cases, a specific cause is not identified and the cause remains idiopathic. An etiologic diagnosis could not be made in two-thirds of the cases of DCM in the North American Pediatric Cardiomyopathy Registry,[3] followed by myocarditis (16%), neuromuscular disorders (9%), familial DCM (5%), inborn errors of metabolism (4%), and malformation syndromes (1%). The genetics of DCM depend on the underlying cause. In children, 20% to 48% have a positive family history of the disease.[8] Inheritance is most commonly autosomal dominant, with X-linked, autosomal-recessive, and mitochondrial patterns of inheritance encountered less commonly. Multiple causative genes have been identified and predominantly encode 2 major subgroups of proteins, cytoskeletal, and sarcomeric proteins (**Table 2**).[7,9] Genetic testing is increasingly being performed by several commercial laboratories. In pure DCM, the yield of screening for many genes is low, with a causative gene abnormality identified in about 20% of cases.

History

Onset is usually insidious but may be acute in up to 25% of patients with DCM, especially if exacerbated by a complicating lower respiratory tract infection. Approximately 50% of patients with DCM have a history of a preceding viral illness. A detailed family history is important and is positive in 20% to 48% of cases.[8]

Common Presenting Symptoms	Less Common Presenting Symptoms
Fatigue	Chest pain
Shortness of breath	Orthopnea
Exercise intolerance	Hemoptysis
Syncope	Abdominal pain
Arrhythmia	Frothy sputum

Physical Examination

It is possible for a patient to have DCM and yet have a perfectly normal physical examination. With established disease, features of congestive heart failure may be prominent. Common physical examination findings include the following:

Systemic Findings	Cardiac Findings
Weak peripheral pulses	Tachycardia
Cool extremities	Displaced point of maximum impulse
Hepatomegaly	Active precordium
Low blood pressure, with decreased pulse pressure	Gallop rhythm
Shock	Accentuated P2 (with pulmonary hypertension)
Crackles or wheezing	Murmurs of mitral and tricuspid regurgitation
Peripheral edema	

Diagnostic Evaluation

Blood studies including a complete blood count, erythrocyte sedimentation rate, and C-reactive protein level may show evidence of acute inflammation in the setting of myocarditis. Similarly, antibody titers, viral culture, or polymerase chain reaction studies may suggest a viral cause. Serum carnitine levels may be low when the disease is caused by systemic carnitine deficiency. Biomarkers such as brain natriuretic peptide (BNP) and N-terminal prohormone BNP may be useful in the detection and risk stratification of patients with decompensated heart failure. A BNP level greater than 300 pg/mL was a strong predictor of death, transplantation, or heart failure hospitalization in a series of pediatric patients.[10]

Chest radiography shows cardiomegaly and may show evidence of pulmonary congestion or pulmonary venous hypertension. Increase of the left mainstem bronchus reflects dilation of the left atrium. In rare fulminant cases, cardiomegaly may not be prominent because the ventricle has not yet had time to dilate.

Changes on the electrocardiogram (ECG) are nonspecific and may include sinus tachycardia, abnormal frontal plane QRS axis, left atrial enlargement, left ventricular hypertrophy, deep Q waves with ST segment depression, and tall T waves in leads I, aVL, V_5, V_6 (reflecting left ventricular volume overload). It is important to identify evidence of myocardial ischemia, which might point to an anomalous coronary artery as the cause for heart failure. Cardiac arrhythmias such as supraventricular cardiomyopathy (SVT), or ventricular ectopy or tachycardia may be present in myocarditis. In some cases, sustained arrhythmias (eg, ectopic atrial tachycardia, atrial flutter, SVT) may be the cause of cardiomyopathy (ie, tachycardia-mediated cardiomyopathy).[11]

Table 1
Factors identified as causes of myocardial damage

Category of Factors	Specific Factors
Viral infections	Coxsackie virus, human immunodeficiency virus, echo virus, rubella, varicella, mumps, Epstein-Barr virus, cytomegalovirus, measles, polio
Bacterial infections	Diphtheria, *Mycoplasma*, tuberculosis, Lyme disease, septicemia
Neuromuscular disorders	Duchenne or Becker muscular dystrophy, Friedreich ataxia, Kearns-Sayre syndrome
Metabolic disorders	Glycogen storage diseases, carnitine deficiency, fatty acid oxidation defects
Endocrine disorders	Thyroid disease, pheochromocytoma, hypoglycemia
Hematologic disease	Sickle cell disease, thalassemia, iron deficiency anemia
Coronary artery disease	Anomalous left coronary artery from the pulmonary artery, Kawasaki disease
Drugs	Anthracycline, cyclophosphamide, chloroquine, iron overload, alcohol
Cardiac arrhythmia	SVT, atrial fibrillation/flutter, ventricular tachycardia

From Arola A, Jokinen E, Ruuskanen O, et al. Epidemiology of idiopathic cardiomyopathies in children and adolescents. A nationwide study in Finland. Am J Epidemiol 1997;146(5):385–93; with permission.

Echocardiography and Doppler studies form the basis for the diagnosis in most patients. Dilation of the left ventricle with global systolic dysfunction is the hallmark of the disease. The left ventricular shortening fraction is usually less than 25% (ejection fraction <50%). The presence of valvular regurgitation, parameters of diastolic function, and pulmonary artery pressures may be assessed. Pericardial effusion may be present. It is crucial to exclude anatomic abnormalities, which may be the cause of the cardiomyopathy, including anomalous left coronary artery arising from the pulmonary artery, mitral valve disease, and coarctation of the aorta.

Treatment

There have been tremendous improvements in the treatment of DCM over the last 20 years. Treatment is mainly directed at improving symptoms of heart failure and

Table 2
Genetic mutations associated with DCM

Mutation Associated With DCM		
Cardiac actin	Dystrophin	α-Myosin heavy chain
Desmin	Myosin-binding protein C	SUR2A
δ-Sarcoglycan	Muscle LIM protein	Lamin A/C
β-Myosin heavy chain	α-Actin-2	Metavinculin
Cardiac troponin T	Phospholamban	Cardiac troponin I
α-Tropomyosin	Cypher/LIM binding domain 3	Cardiac troponin type 2
Titin	Tafazzin	Myopalladin

From Jefferies JL, Towbin JA. Dilated cardiomyopathy. Lancet 2010;375:755, with permission; and Hsu DT, Canter CE. Dilated cardiomyopathy and heart failure in children. Heart Fail Clin 2010;6(4):418, with permission.

prevention of disease progression and related complication, such as end-organ dysfunction and stroke. Comprehensive guidelines for the treatment of pediatric heart failure have been published by the International Society for Heart and Lung Transplantation.[12] Many of the guidelines are based on small nonrandomized trials or are extrapolated from the adult literature. The mainstay of therapy includes afterload reduction using angiotensin-converting enzyme (ACE) inhibitors and β-blockade, with or without the use of diuretics to achieve euvolemia and minimize congestive symptoms. Digoxin continues to be widely used in the treatment of childhood DCM. Studies in adults failed to show a survival benefit from the use of digoxin but did report improvement of symptoms in some patients.[13] Treatment of decompensated heart failure is focused on diuresis with loop diuretics and afterload reduction with nitroglycerin, nitroprusside, or nesiritide. In patients with heart failure and clinical evidence of hypotension or hypoperfusion with increased filling pressures, treatment with intravenous inotropes or vasopressor therapy or both should be considered. Phosphodiesterase III inhibitors, such as milrinone, are useful in the treatment of cardiogenic shock because they increase contractility and reduce afterload by peripheral vasodilation without a consistent increase in myocardial oxygen consumption.[12]

In patients with severe symptomatic DCM refractory to medical management, mechanical assist devices have been increasingly used as device technology has improved. In adolescent patients, the use of a mechanical assist device results in successful bridging to transplantation in 80% of cases.[14] Heart transplantation remains the therapy of choice for end-stage DCM. Transplantation of children with DCM has the best survival of all the diagnostic groups. The Pediatric Heart Transplant Study Group recently analyzed 1098 patients with DCM listed for heart transplantation.[14] Mortality on the waiting list was 11%, and overall survival after listing for transplantation was 72% at 10 years.

Key message

- Most cases of DCM have no known cause (idiopathic)
- Family history may be positive in 20% to 48% of cases
- Echocardiography is diagnostic and helpful in ruling out other anatomic abnormalities that may present as heart failure
- Treatment includes management of heart failure symptoms and prevention of complications
- Heart transplantation is the therapy of choice for end-stage DCM

HCM
Background

HCM is defined by the presence of a hypertrophied, nondilated ventricle in the absence of an underlying hemodynamic cause (eg, systemic hypertension, aortic stenosis, coarctation of the aorta). Although once believed to be a rare disorder, HCM is believed to occur with an incidence of 1 in 500 in the general population and remains the most common cause of sudden death in adolescents and adults younger than 35 years.[15] HCM accounts for 30% of pediatric cardiomyopathy with an incidence of 0.47/100,000.[6] This condition can represent a complex mix of pathophysiologic mechanisms, including diastolic dysfunction, left (and in some cases, right) ventricular outflow tract obstruction, mitral regurgitation, myocardial ischemia, and cardiac arrhythmias. Treatment strategies are focused on alleviation of symptoms and prevention of sudden death.

Cause

The more common forms of HCM are inherited as an autosomal dominant trait and are caused by mutations in at least 10 identified genes. The most common are mutations on the genes that encode sarcomeric proteins and are listed in **Table 3**.[16] There are also rare familial forms of HCM caused by nonsarcomeric genes, including mitochondrial defects, potassium channel defects, and genes involved in calcium handling control mechanisms. A gene defect can be identified in 60% to 70% of patients. This finding suggests that novel HCM mutations are yet to be discovered. Earlier onset of the manifestations of HCM in childhood may represent a more heterogeneous group of disorders with a greater diversity than is seen in the adult population. **Table 4** provides a classification of HCM based on groupings of familial, syndromic, neuromuscular, and metabolic disorders.[17]

The HCM causative mutations result in myofibril disarray and fibrosis that progress and contribute to ventricular hypertrophy. The abnormal cellular architecture occurs even in areas of the myocardium that are not hypertrophied and may be the arrhythmogenic substrate for ventricular tachycardia and ventricular fibrillation. The ventricle becomes hypertrophied, but in most cases, it does not dilate, remaining normal in size or even small. Systolic function is generally normal or hyperdynamic; however, myocardial relaxation and filling are impaired. This situation may result in diastolic dysfunction and increased filling pressures. In late stages, a few patients may progress to heart failure with ventricular dilation and systolic dysfunction.[18]

A subset of patients with HCM present with left ventricular outflow tract obstruction, which is caused by asymmetrical septal hypertrophy and systolic motion of the anterior mitral leaflet. The obstruction is dynamic and dependent on the patient's volume status. Volume depletion increases the outflow gradient, whereas volume repletion decreases the obstruction. Some patients may have no outflow gradient at baseline but may develop obstruction with exertion.

History

Many adolescents with HCM are asymptomatic. They may come to medical attention in a variety of ways, including screening because of a positive family history, detection of a cardiac murmur, or presence of an abnormal ECG. They may also come to attention while being evaluated for syncope, chest pain, palpitations, angina, or out-of-hospital cardiac arrest.

Obtaining a detailed history is especially important in screening adolescents before sports participation. Sudden death, which is the most serious element of the natural history of this disease, is particularly common in teenagers and young adults. HCM

Table 3
Genetic mutations associated with HCM

Sarcomeric Mutations Associated With HCM	
β-Myosin heavy chain	Cardiac troponin I
α-Myosin heavy chain	α-Tropomyosin
Myosin essential light chain	Myosin-binding protein C
Myosin regulatory light chain	Titin
Cardiac troponin T	Actin

From Bos JM, Towbin JA, Ackerman MJ. Diagnostic, prognostic, and therapeutic implications of genetic testing for hypertrophic cardiomyopathy. J Am Coll Cardiol 2009;54(3):201–11; with permission.

Table 4
Phenotypically based classification of HCM

Category	Specific Conditions
Familial HCM	Sarcomeric HCM, maternally inherited HCM syndromes
Syndromic HCM	Noonan syndrome, Beckwith-Wiedemann syndrome, cardiofacial-cutaneous syndrome, Costello syndrome, lentiginosis (LEOPARD syndrome)
Neuromuscular disease	Friedreich ataxia
Metabolic disorders	Anabolic steroid therapy and abuse, carnitine deficiency, glycogenoses type 2, 3, and 9 (Pompe disease, Forbes disease, phosphorylase kinase deficiency), glycolipid lipidosis (Fabry disease), glycosylation disorders, I-cell disease, lipodystrophy, lysosomal disorders (Danon disease), mannosidosis, mitochondrial disorders, mucopolysaccharidoses type 1, 2, and 5 (Hurler syndrome, Hunter syndrome, Scheie syndrome), selenium deficiency

Adapted from Colan SD. Hypertrophic cardiomyopathy in childhood. Heart Fail Clin 2010;6(4):433–44; with permission.

is the most common cause of sudden cardiac death in young athletes and is usually caused by ventricular fibrillation.[19] The patient should be asked about previous episodes of syncope, especially if precipitated by physical exertion or the presence of palpitations or arrhythmia associated with exercise. Up to 50% to 60% of children with HCM have a positive family history.[8] A detailed review of the family history is therefore important. This review should include specific questions regarding the presence of known cardiomyopathy, sudden unexpected death at a young age, syncope, or the presence of a defibrillator or pacemaker in close relatives. All first-degree relatives of individuals who carry a diagnosis of HCM should receive additional cardiac and genetic screening. (Please refer to the article elsewhere in this issue for a detailed review on implications of positive family history.)

Among symptomatic patients, dyspnea is a common complaint. It is usually a consequence of diastolic dysfunction and increased left ventricular filling pressures. Symptoms are typically worse with exertion. The presence of left ventricular outflow tract obstruction may also contribute to the symptoms of dyspnea and may also cause a blunted increase in cardiac output with exercise, resulting in dizziness, presyncope, or syncope with exertion. Ventricular hypertrophy may increase myocardial oxygen demand, particularly during exertion, resulting in typical symptoms of angina. Symptoms of congestive heart failure may be present in patients with mitral regurgitation or severe diastolic dysfunction, and in rare patients who develop ventricular systolic dysfunction.

Physical Examination

Most adolescents with HCM do not have ventricular outflow obstruction and, therefore, may have a completely normal cardiac examination. Positive cardiac examination findings may include the following:

- Laterally displaced and forceful point of maximum impulse
- Double or triple apical impulse
- Bifid carotid pulse
- Murmur of dynamic left ventricular outflow obstruction

- Murmur of mitral insufficiency
- Fourth heart sound

Careful attention to auscultation for the presence of a cardiac murmur of ventricular outflow obstruction is particularly important when screening adolescents before sports participation. The murmur is typically a systolic ejection, crescendo-decrescendo–type murmur audible along the left sternal border, with radiation to the suprasternal notch and to the neck. With a mild degree of outflow tract obstruction, the murmur can be easily mistaken for an innocent flow murmur. With increasing degrees of left ventricular outflow tract obstruction, the murmur becomes louder, harsher, and higher in pitch. Maneuvers that decrease ventricular preload such as a Valsalva maneuver or having the patient stand increase the dynamic obstruction and increase the intensity of the murmur. This situation is in contrast to a murmur of aortic stenosis, in which these maneuvers decrease the intensity of the murmur. Because of this dynamic nature of the obstruction, it is important when performing screening adolescents to auscultate the patient in the supine, sitting, and standing positions or to have the patient perform a Valsalva maneuver in an attempt to provoke or intensify the murmur.

Diagnostic Evaluation

In contrast to the physical examination, which can be nonspecific, the ECG is abnormal in up to 95% of patients with HCM.[20,21] The classic ECG shows left ventricular hypertrophy (tall R wave in the left precordial leads and deep S waves in the right leads) and diffuse repolarization abnormalities (inverted T waves). Patients with restrictive ventricular filling may show atrial enlargement. Controversy exists regarding the role of routine ECG screening of athletes.

Echocardiography remains the gold standard for the diagnosis of HCM in children and adolescents. Left ventricular wall thickness of more than 2 standard deviations higher than the mean defines the presence of left ventricular hypertrophy. The pattern of hypertrophy is usually asymmetric, preferentially affecting the anterior mid to upper interventricular septum.[22] Left ventricular outflow obstruction is present at rest in 25% to 40% of children.[23] Echocardiographic findings of diastolic dysfunction and increased ventricular filling pressures are often present and may precede the onset of ventricular hypertrophy in children.[24] Early in childhood, echocardiographic manifestations of HCM may be absent but frequently develop during adolescence. Therefore, patients with an affected family member but without symptoms should be screened by echocardiography on a yearly basis during the adolescent years.[25]

Treatment

Treatment strategies are focused on alleviation of symptoms and prevention of sudden death. Physical activity restriction is an important component of the management of adolescents with HCM. Increased catecholamine levels associated with exercise may increase myocardial ischemia, leading to sudden death. American Heart Association recommendations advise that patients refrain from competitive athletics and intense isometric activities.[26]

The incidence of sudden death in HCM is less than 1% per year among adolescents. Patients considered to be at higher risk may benefit from placement of an implanted cardiac defibrillator (ICD). ICD implantation is generally recommended after an episode of aborted sudden death. It can also be considered for patients with specific factors placing them at higher risk, including spontaneously occurring ventricular tachycardia, family history of sudden cardiac death caused by HCM at a young age or in multiple relatives, identification of a high-risk gene mutation, abnormal blood pressure response to exercise, and possibly extreme ventricular hypertrophy (septal thickness >30 mm), although the last factor remains controversial.[18] Amiodarone can be considered for prevention of sudden death; however, an ICD seems to be superior in terms of efficacy.[27]

Pharmacologic treatment is reserved for patients who are symptomatic. β-Blockers are the primary treatment modality for symptomatic patients. This class of medication blocks the effect of catecholamines and slows the heart rate, reducing myocardial oxygen demand and enhancing diastolic filling. In patients whose symptoms are not controlled with a β-blocker, the addition of disopyramide can be considered, because its negative inotropic effects can further improve the outflow gradient and reduce symptoms.[15] In patients who are intolerant of β-blockers, a calcium channel blocker like verapamil can be considered.[28] Medical therapies, other than amiodarone, have not been shown to decrease the risk of sudden death.[18]

Surgical septal myomectomy is indicated in patients with significant symptoms in the presence of left ventricular outflow tract obstruction (>50 mm Hg) who are refractory to medical therapy. In experienced centers, operative mortality is 1% to 2%, with relief of symptoms in 70% of patients over intermediate-term follow-up.[18]

Key message

- The incidence of HCM in the general population is 1 in 500

- In the absence of left ventricular outflow tract obstruction, patients with HCM may be completely asymptomatic and have a normal cardiac examination

- Asymptomatic adolescents are frequently diagnosed during routine sports physical or because of a positive family history; a detailed family history is crucial, and genetic testing may be positive in 60% to 70% of patients with HCM

- Management strategies include activity restriction, alleviation of symptoms if present, and prevention of arrhythmia or sudden death

- Among adolescents, the incidence of sudden death is less than 1% per year

---

RCM
Background

RCM is a rare form of cardiomyopathy in childhood. It is characterized by restrictive filling and reduced diastolic function of either or both ventricles, usually with normal or near-normal systolic function and wall thicknesses.[5] The heart is structurally normal, but histologic abnormalities are often present. Although the incidence of RCM in children is unknown, it seems to be the least common cardiomyopathy, representing 2.5% to 5% of pediatric cardiomyopathies in the United States.[6,29] In certain tropical areas of Africa, Asia, and South America, it is endemic and secondary to endomyocardial fibrosis. In these regions, RCM may account for up to 20% of cases of cardiomyopathy.[30] Prognosis for children with RCM is poor, with a median survival time to death or transplantation of 2.2 years.[29] Cardiac transplantation is generally considered early in the course of this disease.

Cause

This condition may represent a primary abnormality or may be secondary to another disease (such as amyloidosis, which is the most common cause of RCM in adults in the United States). **Table 5** lists the causes of RCM.[31] Infiltrative and storage disorders, such as amyloidosis and sarcoidosis, are rare in children, and these diagnoses are almost never made outside the adult population. Increasingly, disease-causing mutations involving sarcomeric and nonsarcomeric genes are being discovered as a causative factor in RCM. Some of these mutations can have overlapping phenotypes with dilated and HCM. The prevalence of sporadic versus familial RCM is not known. Endomyocardial biopsy findings are usually nonspecific, including interstitial fibrosis and myocyte hypertrophy.

History

Clinical signs and symptoms in RCM are dependent on the severity of diastolic dysfunction, the degree of systemic and pulmonary venous congestion, and the resultant amount of reduced cardiac output. Common historical findings and indications for referral to cardiology include the following:

- Respiratory symptoms: dyspnea at rest or with exertion, paroxysmal nocturnal dyspnea, orthopnea
- Typical history of congestive heart failure
- Generalized fatigue or weakness
- Ascites or peripheral edema
- Palpitations or syncope
- Positive family history

Physical Examination

Abnormal physical examination findings are common in RCM, reflecting increased right and left ventricular filling pressures, diminished cardiac output, and the presence of pulmonary hypertension. Mildly affected individuals may have a normal physical examination. Common physical examination findings may include the following:

Systemic Findings	Cardiac Findings
Tachypnea	Tachycardia
Weak peripheral pulses	Murmurs of mitral and tricuspid regurgitation
Cool extremities	Gallop rhythm
Hepatomegaly	Accentuated P2 (with pulmonary hypertension)
Jugular venous distension	
Low blood pressure, with decreased pulse pressure	
Crackles or wheezing	
Peripheral edema or ascites	

Diagnostic Evaluation

ECG abnormalities are present in 98% of patients with RCM at presentation.[32] The most common abnormalities include right or left atrial enlargement, ST segment depression, and T wave abnormalities. Right or left ventricular hypertrophy and cardiac conduction abnormalities may be seen. Holter monitoring is useful to identify rhythm abnormalities, including atrial flutter, atrial fibrillation, and second-degree or third-degree heart block. Cardiac arrhythmias have been reported in 15% of pediatric patients with RCM.[33]

Echocardiography is usually diagnostic in RCM. Classic echocardiographic findings included marked atrial enlargement in the absence of significant atrioventricular valve

Table 5	
Causes of RCM	
Category	**Specific Conditions**
Genetic	Sarcomeric mutations: troponin I, troponin T, α cardiac actin, myosin-binding protein C, β myosin heavy chain, myosin light chain Nonsarcomeric mutations: desmin, RSK2 (Coffin-Lowry), lamin A/C (Emery Dreifuss), transthyretin (amyloidosis)
Mixed	Amyloidosis, endocardial fibroelastosis
Acquired	Endomyocardial fibroelastosis, myocarditis, cardiac transplant, pseudoxanthoma elasticum, diabetic cardiomyopathy, sarcoidosis, hemochromatosis, Fabry disease, Gaucher disease, glycogen storage disease, Löffler syndrome, scleroderma, carcinoid, metastatic cancers, radiation, drugs, fatty infiltration

Adapted from Denfield SW, Webber SA. Restrictive cardiomyopathy in childhood. Heart Failure Clin 2010;6:445–52; with permission.

regurgitation, with normal end-diastolic ventricular volumes.[34] Atrial thrombi may be detected. Doppler evaluation can be useful in assessing diastolic abnormalities and distinguishing RCM from constrictive pericarditis.[35]

Cardiac catheterization plays an important role in the evaluation of patients with RCM and should be performed at the time of diagnosis. Ventricular filling pressures are increased, with the end-diastolic pressure in the left ventricle usually being significantly higher than the right ventricle. Pulmonary hypertension is common, and pulmonary vasoreactivity can be tested with agents such as inhaled nitric oxide.[36] Patients with increased and fixed pulmonary vascular resistance may be precluded from isolated heart transplantation. Endomyocardial biopsy can be considered; however, biopsy specimens are usually nondiagnostic in children, and the procedure is not without risk in these potentially fragile patients.[37]

Treatment

None of the medical therapies has been clearly shown to improve clinical outcomes in children with RCM. Pharmacologic therapy is directed predominantly at improving symptoms. Diuretic therapy can be used to improve symptoms related to systemic and pulmonary venous congestion. However, excessive diuresis should be avoided, because these patients may be preload dependent to maintain cardiac output. Patients with RCM have been shown to have a significant risk of thromboembolic complication.[38] Anticoagulation should be considered, in the absence of any specific contraindication, with appropriate monitoring of coagulation parameters. Previous pediatric studies have suggested that ACE inhibitors may decrease systemic blood pressure without increasing cardiac output; therefore, these medications should probably be avoided for this condition.[39]

Because of the poor long-term survival of children with RCM, orthotopic cardiac transplantation should be considered early in the course of the disease, particularly if the patient is symptomatic or has evidence of pulmonary hypertension. Most experts agree that progressive increase in pulmonary vascular resistance should lead to early referral for transplantation. Fixed, irreversible pulmonary vascular disease may necessitate combined heart-lung transplantation.[38,40] Rare patients have shown prolonged survival without transplantation, but there are no well-defined predictors for determining which patients may be conservatively followed.

Key message

- RCM is rare in children and adolescents

- Echocardiography along with cardiac catheterization plays an important role in the diagnosis of restricted ventricular filling with significantly increased ventricular end-diastolic pressures (left ventricle more than right ventricle)

- Management centers around symptom control, prevention of thromboembolic complication, and heart transplantation

- These patients are preload dependent, and excessive diuresis may be harmful

---

SUMMARY

Cardiomyopathy is rare during adolescence but represents an important cause of morbidity and mortality in this patient population. It is important for the primary care physician to have a thorough understanding of the pathophysiology and typical clinical presentation of these disorders, allowing prompt referral to pediatric cardiology. Treatment is directed at alleviation of symptoms and prevention of sudden death. For patients in whom medical management fails, cardiac transplantation provides an option with excellent intermediate-term success. Early recognition of these disorders and prompt referral help achieve optimal clinical results.

REFERENCES

1. Arola A, Jokinen E, Ruuskanen O, et al. Epidemiology of idiopathic cardiomyopathies in children and adolescents. A nationwide study in Finland. Am J Epidemiol 1997;146(5):385–93.
2. Daubeney PE, Nugent AW, Chondros P, et al. Clinical features and outcomes of childhood cardiomyopathy: results from a population based study. Circulation 2006;114(24):2671–8.
3. Towbin JA, Lowe AM, Colan SD, et al. Incidence, causes, and outcomes of dilated cardiomyopathy in children. JAMA 2006;296(15):1867–76.
4. Colan SD, Lipshultz SE, Lowe AM, et al. Epidemiology and cause-specific outcome of hypertrophic cardiomyopathy in children: findings form the Pediatric Cardiomyopathy Registry. Circulation 2007;115(6):773–81.
5. Richardson P, McKenna W, Bristow M, et al. Report of the 1995 World Health Organization/International Society and Federation of Cardiology Task Force on the definition and classification of cardiomyopathies. Circulation 1996;93: 841–2.
6. Lipshultz SE, Sleeper LA, Towbin JA, et al. The incidence of pediatric cardiomyopathy in two regions of the United States. N Engl J Med 2003;348:1647–55.
7. Jefferies JL, Towbin JA. Dilated cardiomyopathy. Lancet 2010;375:752–62.
8. Towbin JA, Bowles NE. The failing heart. Nature 2002;415:83–97.
9. Hsu DT, Canter CE. Dilated cardiomyopathy and heart failure in children. Heart Fail Clin 2010;6(4):415–32.
10. Price JF, Thomas AK, Grenier M, et al. B-type natriuretic peptide predicts adverse cardiovascular events in pediatric outpatients with chronic left ventricular systolic dysfunction. Circulation 2006;114(10):1063–9.
11. Medi C, Kalman JM, Haqqani H, et al. Tachycardia-mediated cardiomyopathy secondary to focal atrial tachycardia: long-term outcome after catheter ablation. J Am Coll Cardiol 2009;53(19):1791–7.

12. Rosenthal D, Chrisant MR, Edens E, et al. International Society for Heart and Lung Transplantation: practice guidelines for management of heart failure in children. J Heart Lung Transplant 2004;23(12):1313–33.

13. Jessup M, Abraham WT, Casey DE, et al. 2009 focused update: ACCF/AHA Guidelines for the diagnosis and management of heart failure in adults: a report of the American College of Cardiology Foundation/American Heart Association Task Force on Practice Guidelines. Circulation 2009;119(14):1977–2016.

14. Kirk R, Naftel D, Hoffman TM, et al. Outcome of patients with dilated cardiomyopathy listed for transplant: a multi-institutional study. J Heart Lung Transplant 2009; 28(12):1322–8.

15. Nishimura RA, Homes DR. Hypertrophic obstructive cardiomyopathy. N Engl J Med 2004;350:1320–7.

16. Bos JM, Towbin JA, Ackerman MJ. Diagnostic, prognostic, and therapeutic implications of genetic testing for hypertrophic cardiomyopathy. J Am Coll Cardiol 2009;54(3):201–11.

17. Colan SD. Hypertrophic cardiomyopathy in childhood. Heart Fail Clin 2010;6(4): 433–44.

18. Maron BJ, McKenna WJ. American College of Cardiology/European Society of Cardiology clinical expert consensus document of hypertrophic cardiomyopathy. J Am Coll Cardiol 2003;42:1687–713.

19. Maron BJ. Sudden death in young athletes. N Engl J Med 2003;349:1065–75.

20. Corrado D, Basso C, Schiavon M, et al. Screening for hypertrophic cardiomyopathy in young athletes. N Engl J Med 1998;339:364–9.

21. Montgomery JV, Harris KM, Casey SA, et al. Relation of electrocardiographic patterns to phenotypic expression and clinical outcome in hypertrophic cardiomyopathy. Am J Cardiol 2005;96:270–5.

22. Klues HG, Schiffers A, Maron BJ. Phenotypic spectrum and patterns of left ventricular hypertrophy in hypertrophic cardiomyopathy: morphologic observations and significance as assessed by two-dimensional echocardiography in 600 patients. J Am Coll Cardiol 1995;26:1699–708.

23. Nugent AW, Daubeney PE, Chondros P, et al. Clinical features and outcomes of childhood hypertrophic cardiomyopathy: results from a national population-based study. Circulation 2005;112:1332–8.

24. McMahon CJ, Nagueh SF, Pignatelli RH, et al. Characterization of left ventricular diastolic function by tissue Doppler imaging and clinical status in children with hypertrophic cardiomyopathy. Circulation 2004;109:1756–62.

25. Moak JP, Kaski JP. Hypertrophic cardiomyopathy in children. Heart 2012;98: 1044–54.

26. Maron BJ. AHA scientific statement. Recommendations for physical activity and recreational sports participation for young patients with genetic cardiovascular diseases. Circulation 2004;109:2807–16.

27. Maron BJ, Estes N III, Maron MS, et al. Primary prevention of sudden death as a novel treatment strategy in hypertrophic cardiomyopathy. Circulation 2003;10: 2872–5.

28. Bonow RO, Dilsizian V, Rosing DR, et al. Verapamil-induced improvement in left ventricular diastolic filling and increased exercise tolerance in patients with hypertrophic cardiomyopathy: short- and long-term effect. Circulation 1985;72:853–64.

29. Russo LM, Webber SA. Idiopathic restrictive cardiomyopathy in children. Heart 2005;91(9):1199–202.

30. Kushwaha SS, Fallon JT, Fuster V. Restrictive cardiomyopathy. N Engl J Med 1997;336(4):267–76.

31. Denfield SW, Webber SA. Restrictive cardiomyopathy in childhood. Heart Failure Clin 2010;6:445–52.

32. Denfield SW. Sudden death in children with restrictive cardiomyopathy. Card Electrophysiol Rev 2002;6:163–7.

33. Rivenes SM, Kearney DL, Smith EO, et al. Sudden death and cardiovascular collapse in children with restrictive cardiomyopathy. Circulation 2000;102: 876–82.

34. Ceta F, O'Leary PW, Seward JB, et al. Idiopathic restrictive cardiomyopathy in childhood: diagnostic features and clinical outcome. Mayo Clin Proc 1995;70: 634–40.

35. Gewillig M, Mertens L, Moerman P, et al. Idiopathic restrictive cardiomyopathy in childhood. A diastolic disorder characterized by delayed relaxation. Eur Heart J 1996;17:1413–20.

36. Hughes ML, Kleinert S, Keogh A, et al. Pulmonary vascular resistance and reactivity in children with end-stage cardiomyopathy. J Heart Lung Transplant 2000; 19:701–94.

37. Yoshizato T, Edwards WT, Alboliras ET, et al. Safety and utility of endomyocardial biopsy in infants, children and adolescents: a review of 66 procedures in 53 patients. J Am Coll Cardiol 1990;15(2):436–42.

38. Weller RJ, Weintraub R, Addonizo LJ, et al. Outcome of idiopathic restrictive cardiomyopathy in children. Am J Cardiol 2002;90:501–6.

39. Bengur AR, Beekman RH, Rocchini AP. Acute hemodynamic effects of captopril in children with a congestive or restrictive cardiomyopathy. Circulation 1991; 83(2):523–7.

40. Fenton MJ, Chubb H, McMahon AM, et al. Heart and heart-lung transplantation for idiopathic restrictive cardiomyopathy in children. Heart 2006;92:85–9.

A Pediatric Approach to Family History of Cardiovascular Disease
Diagnosis, Risk Assessment, and Management

Erin M. Miller, MS, CGC*, Robert B. Hinton, MD

KEYWORDS

- Family history • Counseling • Risk assessment • Congenital heart disease
- Sudden death • Genetic syndromes • Pediatrics • Cardiovascular malformation
- Cardiomyopathy

KEY POINTS

- Complete detailed family histories are critical for the optimal management of children and families.
- Awareness of family history is important for individual health.
- Evaluation of family history may provide reassurance regarding disease risk and allow patients to avoid unnecessary testing.
- Family history evaluation may allow early diagnosis and improved outcomes.

INTRODUCTION

The medical family history is a record of illnesses and other pertinent health information among family members.[1] Applications of the family history include confirming medical diagnoses, identifying family members at risk for various conditions, and calculating risk for developing a particular disease.[2,3] A detailed family history provides the first genetic screen for an individual and contains substantial medical information. As genetic testing becomes more available, and clinicians embrace primary prevention and early intervention, the family history will become increasingly important in clinical decision making, especially in pediatrics, where universal screening approaches are already engrained in the culture. Further, because clinicians are learning that many of the supposedly acquired diseases of adulthood have developmental causes, the genetic basis of these conditions need to be understood and proactively acted on even though the clinical conditions may not typically manifest in the pediatric age range. At present, many efforts are being directed toward increasing awareness of

Disclosures: The authors have no disclosures to make.
Division of Cardiology, The Heart Institute, Cincinnati Children's Hospital Medical Center, 3333 Burnet Avenue, Cincinnati, OH 45229, USA
* Corresponding author. 3333 Burnet Avenue, MLC 7020, Cincinnati, OH 45229.
E-mail address: erin.miller@cchmc.org

the value of the family history and identifying efficient and practical ways to use the family history information.[4,5] In summary, family history has a central usefulness for all health care providers and a significant impact on clinical management in the emerging genetic era.

A pedigree, also known as a family tree, is a graphic representation of a family history using symbols. The pedigree is used for many clinical and research purposes including: making a diagnosis, establishing a pattern of inheritance, identifying family members at risk, calculating risk, making decisions regarding tests and surveillance strategies, and patient education.[1,6–8] Given the universal use of this tool, the National Society of Genetic Counselors (NSGC) formed a Pedigree Standardization Task Force and developed standard nomenclature for pedigrees.[9,10] Because the family history affects all areas of medicine, it is important that all health care professionals have a working knowledge of pedigree structure. Practical suggestions for recording a medical pedigree are included in **Box 1**. The family history is dynamic and needs to be revisited and updated periodically. Once the detailed family history is obtained, time and effort needs to be invested to maintain the accuracy and value of the information.[11] There are significant barriers to the optimal use of family history information, primarily a lack of awareness on the family's part and considerable time restrictions on the health care professional's part. In an effort to increase family history awareness, tools have been developed and are available to the general public to generate and maintain a detailed family history (**Table 1**). For example, the Health and Human Services Family History Initiative has designed a publicly available, Web-based program providing a means to generate and maintain a detailed family history, as well as keeping track of prenatal genetic and environmental risk factors.[2,12] Further, as electronic

---

Box 1
Tips for pedigree documentation

Start with the patient or proband and work backwards

Indicate the proband with an arrow

Confirm whether the proband has siblings and clarify whether they share 1 (half siblings) or both parents (full siblings)

Ask about the mother, followed by her siblings and their children, and maternal grandparents

Repeat with father's side of the family

Ask specifically about each individual:

- For affected individuals, document the age at diagnosis and the diagnosis

- For unaffected individuals, document specific cardiovascular symptoms and any completed cardiac screening

- For all individuals, document current age or age and cause of death

Be consistent when documenting:

- Include the father/male partner on the left hand side and the mother/female partner on the right hand side

- Keep generations (ie, proband, siblings, maternal and paternal first cousins) on the same horizontal level

- Place siblings in birth order (oldest on left, youngest on right)

Refer the most severely affected individual for genetic counseling, evaluation, and testing when possible

Table 1	
Resources for family history ascertainment and awareness	
Health and Human Services Family History Initiative	www.hhs.gov/familyhistory
Online Mendelian Inheritance of Man	www.ncbi.nlm.nih.sov/Omim
US Centers for Disease Control and Prevention	www.cdc.gov/genomics
March of Dimes	www.marchofdimes.com
National Coalition for Health Professional Education in Genetics	www.nchpeg.org
NSGC	www.nscg.org
American Academy of Pediatrics	www.aap.org
American Medical Association	www.ama-assn.ore
American Society of Human Genetics	www.ashg.ore
Gene Tests	www.genetests.org

medical records become increasingly sophisticated and personalized medicine initiatives are implemented, there will be a need to combine this information in a way that the patient can access and use.[13,14]

The family history is widely used in pediatrics, and this article describes specific approaches to family history in the context of pediatric cardiovascular disease. The various approaches to family history in cardiovascular malformation (CVM) are reviewed, along with known cardiovascular diseases with a genetic basis, including cardiomyopathy, arrhythmia, thoracic aortic aneurysm, and sudden cardiac death, and the practical applications of family history information, including diagnosis, risk stratification, and management, are also discussed.

FAMILY HISTORY OF CVM

Pediatric heart disease includes CVM, also known as congenital heart disease (CHD), cardiomyopathy, channelopathy, and aortopathy. CVM refers to malformation of the cardiovascular system that is present at birth. These cardiovascular anomalies are the most common birth defects and a leading cause of infant mortality. Despite advances in the diagnosis and treatment of CVM, there continues to be significant associated mortality, morbidity, and economic burden.[15,16] The incidence of CVM is classically cited as 8 per 1000 live births, or approximately 1%, but the true incidence of all CVM is estimated to be 5 per 100, or 5% of live births.[17] A substantial number of spontaneous abortuses have CVM, with an estimated incidence of 20 per 100, suggesting that the true incidence of CVM is even higher.[18]

Because the detection of cardiovascular disease, especially CVM, is increasingly occurring during gestation, the role of prenatal counseling is rapidly evolving and is necessary for optimal care. The primary goals of genetic counseling for CVM in the prenatal period are to determine whether the specific CVM suggests an underlying genetic syndrome and whether genetic testing is indicated. Parents receive comprehensive information about the diagnosis for anticipatory care. A prenatal confirmation of the cause prepares both the family and health care providers before delivery and often affects medical management and family decision making. With the advent of noninvasive prenatal diagnosis, certain chromosomal abnormalities can be identified without the risk of miscarriage associated with amniocentesis and chorionic villus sampling. Genetic counselors are positioned to help the family understand the diagnosis and possible associated genetic conditions, to discuss the risks and benefits of genetic testing if indicated, and to provide psychosocial support to the family. Genetic counseling during the preconception or prenatal period may also be indicated for individuals affected with CVM. The goals of prenatal genetic counseling may include discussion of recurrence risks for CVM and recommendations for fetal echocardiography.

The Baltimore-Washington Infant Study, the largest and most comprehensive epidemiologic study of CVM, recognized diabetes and environmental teratogens such as retinoic acid as risk factors for CVM, but more importantly identified a positive family history as the most common risk factor for CVM.[19] Classification schemes have evolved substantially since Maude Abbott generated *The Atlas of Congenital Cardiac Disease* more than 100 years ago, which is widely regarded as the first classification system for CVM. An exquisite clinical taxonomy was established based on anatomy and physiology, but classification paradigms have been developed recently that attempt to account for the underlying causes of CVM by using the developmental relationships of lesions.[20–22] For example, the National Birth Defects Prevention Study developed a comprehensive taxonomy that organizes CVM in several ways, including the most specific definition of a single defect, such as hypoplastic left heart syndrome (the splitting approach), the most broad groupings, such as left-sided outflow tract obstruction lesions (the clumping approach), and an intermediate level that allows flexibility with the analysis of common associations, such as aortic stenosis and coarctation of the aorta. Overall, a classification system that incorporates causal factors as well as deep phenotyping is necessary for informed counseling and optimal risk assessment.

Given the high incidence of CVM, a positive family history is likely to be encountered by any health care provider obtaining family histories routinely. As with any reported family history, confirming the specific defect is necessary to guide appropriate counseling and recommendations. In addition, it is important to consider possible causes, which are broad and include chromosomal imbalances and single-gene sequence variants, with most arising through various combinations of genetic and environmental factors. This information should be used to determine whether genetic evaluation and/or cardiac screening may be indicated for the patient. Understanding the family history of CVM may allow the identification of important genetic reproductive risks for the patient and family.

Approximately 7% to 12% of individuals with CVM have an underlying chromosome abnormality including trisomy 21, trisomy 18, 22q11 deletion, and trisomy 13.[23,24] Of these diagnoses, 22q11 deletion syndrome is most frequently transmitted from parent to child. In addition, features of 22q11.2 deletion syndrome are variable and, in some families, diagnosis may be missed or delayed. CVMs that should prompt further questioning and consideration of 22q11.2 deletion syndrome include interrupted aortic arch, truncus arteriosus, tetralogy of Fallot, ventricular septal defect (VSD) with aortic arch anomaly, and isolated aortic arch anomalies, including a right-sided aortic arch that can be associated with vascular rings.[15] There are also well-described genetic syndromes caused by DNA sequence variants in known genes including Noonan syndrome, Holt Oram syndrome, and Alagille syndrome. A summary of CVMs with commonly associated genetic syndromes is given in **Table 2**. If the CVM is associated with a known underlying genetic syndrome, caused by either a chromosomal or single-gene abnormality, the inheritance pattern is readily known and the presence or absence of extracardiac features in the patient and relatives is often easy to assess, thus allowing the provision of risk assessment.

Most CVM is not associated with a well-described chromosome abnormality or genetic syndrome. The emergence of chromosome microarray technology has identified

Table 2 CVM and associated genetic syndrome		
CVM	**Genetic Syndrome**	**Frequency (%)**
Supravalvar aortic stenosis	Williams syndrome	75
Pulmonary stenosis (peripheral and branch)	Alagille syndrome	67
Conotruncal defects (IAA, VSD with AA, TA, TOF, AAA)	Deletion 22q syndrome	>50
Pulmonary valve stenosis	Noonan syndrome	20–50

Abbreviations: AAA, aortic arch anomaly; IAA, interrupted aortic arch; TA, truncus arteriosus; TOF, tetralogy of Fallot.

chromosomal imbalances not previously detected by traditional karyotype in approximately 18% to 20% of cases of CVM when additional features, such as other congenital anomalies or intellectual impairment, are present.[25–27] The yield of chromosome microarray testing in isolated CVM is not known and likely depends on the age of the affected individual, with a potentially higher yield in infants, given the inability to evaluate for developmental delay and other late-onset features.[27,28] If a family history of CVM is reported and the affected individual has additional congenital anomalies or intellectual impairment, genetic evaluation is typically indicated. For example, a patient with pulmonary valve stenosis and short stature should be referred for genetic evaluation with specific consideration of Noonan syndrome. In addition, a patient with tetralogy of Fallot and mental illness should be referred for consideration of 22q11.2 deletion syndrome. Even if the cardiac and noncardiac features do not suggest a specific syndrome, the presence of CVM in the context of other medical or developmental concerns warrants genetic evaluation.

More than 30 genes have been associated with nonsyndromic forms of CVM.[29,30] The contribution both in terms of risk for malformation and number of cases remains uncertain but has been reported to be between 3% and 5%.[15] Studies regarding heritability of isolated CVM suggest that genetic factors play an important role and the contribution of single genes may be greater than currently reported.[31,32] Single-gene testing is not typically indicated in cases of isolated CVM unless there are multiple affected individuals in the family. One example of this is the association of mutations in the NKX2.5 gene with familial CVM, specifically atrial septal defects and atrioventricular block.[33,34] Mutations in this gene are inherited in an autosomal dominant manner with reduced penetrance and variable expressivity, underscoring the common observation that what seems to be mendelian inheritance is complex inheritance (ie, a single gene does not fully explain inheritance). The findings of genetic heterogeneity, reduced penetrance, and variable expressivity are typical in nonsyndromic CVM and suggest that most of these defects are polygenic.

Despite the well-known genetic basis of CVM, less than 20% have a known genetic cause.[12,35] Environmental factors have been shown to be associated with increased risk for CVM, including maternal health, maternal exposures, and pregnancy complications.[12] Diabetes is known to be associated with an increased risk for CVM in addition to other congenital anomalies.[36] Fertility medications and maternal smoking during pregnancy were recently associated with an increased risk of CVM. Although these risk factors are considered nongenetic, they may still be shared within the family and result in an increased risk of CVM for future pregnances or other relatives. Given what is known regarding genetic and environmental risk factors for CVM, it is likely that most defects are the result of multifactorial inheritance. In light of the currently limited knowledge and understanding about the multifactorial traits, the family history tool remains the most reliable in establishing risk.[4,7,12]

The overall recurrence risk of nonsyndromic CVM generally ranges from 2% to 10%.[23,37] The risk of recurrence is based on the specific CVM, the relationship to the affected individual, and the gender of the affected individual. For example, the likelihood of a couple having a child with a CVM is higher if the mother has a personal history of CVM as opposed to the father, and the risk is greater if the affected first-degree relative is a parent as opposed to a sibling. A severe left ventricular outflow tract obstruction lesion (LVOTO), hypoplastic left heart syndrome (HLHS), has been shown to have a high degree of heritability with an empiric recurrence risk for CVM being approximately 20%.[12,38] In addition, HLHS and bicuspid aortic valve (BAV) are genetically related, with an increased risk of BAV among relatives. Thus, cardiac screening may be indicated for individuals with a family history of an LVOTO lesion.[39] This finding again shows the importance of confirming the family history and specific lesion in order to provide the most accurate risk assessment and cardiac screening recommendations.

Key message

- Positive family history is a common risk factor for CVM
- Confirmation of a specific CVM may help guide appropriate counseling, risk assessment, and testing
- Individuals with CVM and an additional congenital anomaly or intellectual impairment may benefit from genetic evaluation
- Single-gene mutations are not known to be a common cause of isolated familial CVM; however, they may be underreported
- Most CVMs are attributed to multifactorial inheritance

FAMILY HISTORY OF KNOWN GENETIC DISEASE

As discussed in detail earlier, virtually any disease can be attributed to the result of the combined action of genes and environment, with the relative role of the genetic component varying depending on the disease. The role of genetics in syndromic and isolated CVM was discussed earlier. Other inherited cardiac diseases that may manifest in the pediatric age range include cardiomyopathy, channelopathy, and thoracic aortic aneurysm. Rather than chromosome abnormalities, most of these conditions result from variation in DNA sequence that alters protein structure or function.

Hypertrophic Cardiomyopathy

As a group, the cardiomyopathies are chronic and often progressive diseases that can affect infants, children, and adults. The World Health Organization recognizes 4 clinical phenotypes: hypertrophic cardiomyopathy (HCM), dilated cardiomyopathy (DCM), restrictive cardiomyopathy (RCM), and arrhythmogenic right ventricular cardiomyopathy (ARVC).[40] Among heart disease caused wholly or partly by genetic factors, HCM is one of the most common (1 in 500 adults) and is clinically characterized by unexplained left ventricular hypertrophy with hyperdynamic function.[41–43] Potential causes are broad and include both environmental and heritable causes; however, most cases are caused by mutations in genes that encode elements of the sarcomere and cytoskeleton in cardiomyocytes.[44,45] The yield of genetic testing in HCM is approximately 40% to 70%.[44,46,47] One of the primary indications for genetic testing in HCM is the ability to offer known variant testing to at-risk relatives. Previous literature suggests that genetic testing is being used in this way.[48] Although HCM most often occurs without extracardiac features, it is also known to be associated with genetic syndromes including Noonan syndrome and Pompe disease.[15,49] If there is a reported family history of HCM in a first-degree relative, referral for cardiac screening is indicated.[46,50,51] **Fig. 1** shows the use of family history and cardiac screening following a diagnosis of HCM.

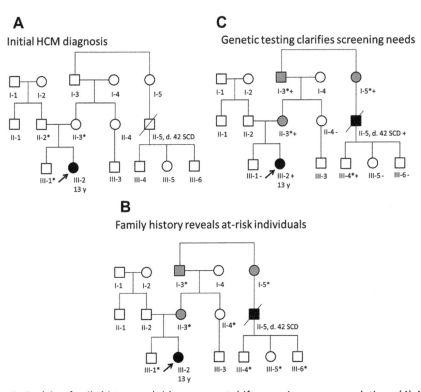

Fig. 1. Evolving family history and risk assessment shift screening recommendations. (A) At-risk relatives for whom cardiac screening is indicated based on the diagnosis of HCM in this 13-year-old. First-degree relatives (III-1, II-2, and II-3; *asterisks*) are at 50% risk. (B) Additional at-risk relatives identified when a second HCM diagnosis (II-5) is revealed in a maternal relative on review of the final autopsy report. Cardiac screening is also indicated for this individual's first-degree relatives (III-4, III-5, III-6, I-5). Three relatives are considered obligate carriers of the autosomal dominant genetic variant (I-5, I-3, and II-3; *light shading*). These individuals are at known risk for disease. First-degree relatives of an obligate carrier are at 50% risk and should also have cardiac screening. The patient's father (II-2) is no longer considered to be at risk. (C) Genetic testing allows definitive risk stratification. Several family members at 50% risk (III-5, III-6, II-4, III-1) did not inherit the disease-causing variant; these individuals and their children do not require cardiac screening. arrow, proband (affected individual that brought the family to medical attention). +, genetic variant present; −, genetic variant absent; circles, women; slash mark, deceased individual; squares, men.

Long QT Syndrome

There are several inherited conditions associated with increased risk for ventricular arrhythmia and sudden cardiac death (SCD), including long QT syndrome (LQTS), Brugada syndrome, and catecholaminergic ventricular tachycardia (CPVT). LQTS is the most common inherited arrhythmia, with an estimated prevalence of 1 in 3000.[52] LQTS is characterized by prolongation of the corrected QT interval (QTc) and T wave abnormalities by electrocardiogram (ECG).[53,54] There are several drugs associated with prolongation of QT interval (www.sads.org/living-with-sads/Drugs-to-Avoid), but most cases are caused by mutations in genes that encode for potassium or sodium cardiac ion channels or interacting proteins.[55] Individuals taking a drug known to prolong the QT interval may have the genetic basis for LQTS. Individuals with LQTS have a predisposition for syncope and the characteristic arrhythmia is referred to as torsades de pointes.[56] As with other genetic cardiac diseases, LQTS shows variable expressivity and decreased penetrance of both the ECG findings and clinical symptoms. Overall, approximately 31% of individuals with a disease-causing mutation have a normal QTc interval and more than 30% of individuals with LQTS remain asymptomatic with no reported history of syncope.[57,58]

LQTS is inherited in an autosomal dominant manner, but there is a recessive condition associated with a prolonged QT interval, known as Jervell and Lange-Neilson syndrome (JLNS). Homozygous or compound heterozygous disease-causing variants in 2 of the same genes that cause LQTS (KCNQ1 and KCNE1) result in JLNS. In general, the inherited channelopathies show autosomal dominant inheritance and variable expressivity. If a patient reports a family history that suggests an inherited channelopathy, confirmation of the diagnosis is important and guides cardiac screening and genetic testing recommendations necessary to identify at-risk relatives. If a patient reports a family history suggesting an inherited channelopathy, at-risk (first-degree) relatives should be referred for a baseline ECG and, if possible, an affected relative should be referred for further evaluation of a genetic cause.

Thoracic Aortic Aneurysm and Dissection

Thoracic aortic aneurysm (TAA) is a subclinical disease state that is typically recognized late in life but can be associated with dissection and sudden death.[59–61] TAA has been recognized as a structural defect with increasing interest in genetic and developmental contributions to malformation of the aortic wall.[62–64] Based on this new information, aortic malformation is a CVM that is present at birth (even if the aorta dimensions are normal) and predisposes the individual to progressive aortic dilation (TAA). Association of TAA with known connective tissue disorders, such as Marfan syndrome and Loeys-Dietz syndrome, and genetic causes of nonsyndromic (familial or isolated) cases of TAA, including mutations in the genes ACTA2, MYH11, and TGFBR2, have been established.[65–67] In the future, genetic testing will play an increasing role in the clinical management of patients with TAA. Screening guidelines for TAA now incorporate genetic information, as do the new Ghent criteria for Marfan syndrome. As more is learned about the genetic basis of nonsyndromic TAA, the yield of clinical genetic testing and the usefulness of genotype information will improve.[61,68] Genotype definition and phenotype stratification will significantly affect counseling (prognosis, recurrence risk), timing and choice of medication, and surgical disposition (timing and approach). Genotype definition may eventually be able to identify those patients with TAA who are at risk (or not at risk) of developing dissection or the need for surgery, affecting clinical management decisions.

If a family history of cardiomyopathy, channelopathy, or aortopathy is reported, the first step is to confirm the diagnosis and degree of relation to the affected individual. It is important to clarify the etiology as there are acquired causes of disease that result in different recommendations. For example, ischemic cardiomyopathy is the most common type of DCM and is characterized by dilatation and dysfunction of the left ventricle. These findings are secondary to ischemia caused by coronary artery disease (CAD) and myocardial infarctions. Most often, cardiac screening or evaluation is indicated for first-degree relatives (parent, sibling, and child); however, screening in second-degree relatives (grandparent, aunt/uncle, and half-sibling) may be indicated. Cardiac screening for second-degree relatives should be considered if there is a history of cardiovascular symptoms or if that relative participates in activities that may be considered high risk for a sudden cardiac arrest (SCA), such as competitive sports.[69] These diseases are typically inherited in an autosomal dominant manner and are observed with significant clinical variability and decreased penetrance. There have been reports of de novo mutations with HCM, LQTS, and TAA in which case the mutation was not inherited, but affected individuals can pass the mutation on to their children. Identification of a disease-causing mutation allows for optimal care of the patient, as well as risk stratification of relatives through known mutation testing. Genetic testing should be initiated in the most severely affected individual in the family when possible. A living affected relative is typically the best candidate for genetic testing; however, in the case of SCD, postmortem genetic testing may be most informative (discussed later). At-risk individuals may be identified before development of cardiac disease and or cardiovascular symptoms, allowing early diagnosis or the ability to reassure families and avoid time-consuming and costly cardiac screening. Identification of at-risk individuals is particularly important because many of these conditions may present with SCD as the initial symptom secondary to arrhythmia or aortic dissection.

Primary care physicians are perfectly positioned to identify potential health risks in the patients and families they care for, including an increased risk for cardiovascular disease and SCD. Most inherited cardiovascular diseases show genetic and phenotypic heterogeneity and require tertiary care for complete genetics evaluation and potential testing. Consensus statements endorsed by numerous organizations recommend genetic testing and genetic counseling for inherited cardiovascular disease as part of standard clinical care.[51,61,70] With the increasing understanding of the genetic contribution to heart disease, cardiovascular genetic counseling has emerged as a specialty critical to the care of patients with heritable cardiovascular disease. These genetic counselors are masters-trained health care professionals in medical genetics and psychosocial counseling with specialization in cardiovascular genetics. Genetic counselors have expertise in obtaining and assessing medical and family history, facilitating genetic testing, providing emotional support and or resources, and liaising with other health care professionals. The NSGC Web site has up-to-date member contact information to help locate a cardiac genetic counselor (www.nsgc.org) based on geographic areas.

Key message

- Hypertrophic cardiomyopathy is the most common heart disease with a genetic basis, and the yield of genetic testing is up to 70% in familial cases

- Hypertrophic cardiomyopathy may be associated with genetic syndromes, including Noonan syndrome and Pompe disease

(continued on next page)

Key message (*continued*)

- Inherited arrhythmic disorders include LQTS, Brugada syndrome, and catecholaminergic ventricular tachycardia

- In patients with a positive family history of heritable arrhythmic disorders, a specific diagnosis and genetic testing results guide screening recommendations

- In patients with a family history of cardiomyopathy, channelopathy, or aortopathy, confirmation of the specific diagnosis is important and should guide referral for cardiac screening and or genetic testing

- Cardiac screening for second-degree relatives may be considered in the presence of a cardiovascular symptom or if that relative participates in activities considered high risk for an SCA, such as competitive sports

---

FAMILY HISTORY OF SCD

SCD is the abrupt loss of heart function in a person who may or may not have diagnosed cardiovascular disease. The time and mode of death are unexpected and death occurs instantly or shortly after symptoms appear. If the death remains unexplained despite postmortem examination, the term sudden arrhythmic death syndromes may be used.[71] This term is comparable with sudden infant death syndrome as a diagnosis of exclusion after other causes of death are ruled out. The American Heart Association (AHA) reports that nearly 360,000 out-of-hospital cardiac arrests occur in the United States each year, with an overall survival rate of approximately 9.5%,[72] but this represents only those cases reported by emergency medical services and therefore may be artificially low, underscoring the importance of early screening and diagnosis for family members.

The evaluation of family members, when a SCD occurs, should proceed outward from the index case in a logical and stepwise fashion. A detailed family history, as outlined earlier, must be obtained and information must be gathered from available medical records or postmortem examinations to determine the cause of death and potential for a genetic cause. In some cases, the cause of death remains unknown despite request and review of available records. In this case, a more complete cardiac evaluation with echocardiogram, ECG, and lipid screening may be indicated. However, if the autopsy confirms extensive CAD resulting in a myocardial infarction, relatives do not need to undergo cardiac imaging but should be evaluated and assertively counseled regarding traditional risk factors for CAD (eg, dyslipidemia, tobacco use, hypertension) with the primary goal being behavior modification. In addition to confirming the cause of sudden death in the family, the degree of relation to the deceased individual is important. As discussed previously, further evaluation is most often indicated for first-degree relatives only. Although parents and families are often anxious and worried, recommending cardiac testing and receiving normal results may provide false reassurance if the cause of death is not known. If a heritable cause for SCD is suspected then it may be wise to involve genetic counseling as a prudent first step in risk assessment and developing a coordinated approach to evaluation in the family.

SCD accounts for approximately 7% of all deaths in the young; however, the incidence rate has been difficult to determine, with reported incidences ranging from 1.3 to 8.5 per 100,000 individuals.[73,74] SCD is not common, but it has a severe impact on families, care providers, and the community and attracts significant public and media attention. Preexisting CAD remains the most common cardiac cause of sudden unexplained deaths in the young. However, incidence figures collected by departments of community health frequently include young adults in their third or fourth decade of life when reporting this incidence. Diagnoses that predispose teens to SCD include HCM, coronary artery anomalies, ARVC and channelopathies.[73,74] SCD related to these diagnoses has been documented in infancy and during competitive athletics. These diseases are typically undetected before the SCD event. An autopsy is essential in cases of SCD; however, no identifiable cause is found at autopsy in up to one-third of young people.[73,75] Lack of knowledge about the cause of SCD poses the greatest challenge in understanding the potential heritability of the underlying disease and risk of sudden death for surviving relatives.

Assessing a young person's risk of SCD can be challenging and requires consideration of both personal and family history. Pediatric patients are frequently referred for cardiac evaluation based on personal risk factors for SCD such as a history of syncope or seizure with exertion, excitement, or startle, as well as other cardiovascular symptoms such as chest pain with exertion. Factors that contribute to risk of CAD, including tobacco use, hypertension, high cholesterol, obesity, diabetes mellitus, sedentary lifestyle, and excessive alcohol use, are important in assessing risk for SCD among individuals of all ages. Patients may also be referred for cardiac evaluation based on a significant family history such as early sudden death, known heart disease, or knowledge of a specific cardiac diagnosis such as HCM, DCM, or LQTS in one or more relatives. A retrospective study investigating warning symptoms and family history of cardiovascular disease following SCA in a young person identified that most victims (72%) experienced at least one cardiovascular symptom before SCA and a significant family history was present in 40% of cases, with 27% reporting a family history of sudden death before the age of 50 years.[76] Routine well-child visits are standard of care in the United States. However, current recommendations lack emphasis on defining family history that may predispose a patient to SCD. A more specific cardiovascular personal and family history focused on identifying risk factors that lead to SCD has been emphasized in the context of athletic participation.[77]

Sports activity in adolescents and young adults has been associated with an increased risk of SCD in susceptible athletes.[78] Initial recommendations for screening among athletes were published in 1996 and have been reviewed and updated.[79] The 12-element AHA recommendations for screening include the presence of premature death before the age 50 years of age caused by heart disease in one or more relatives, disability from heart disease in a close relative less than 50 years of age, or specific knowledge of a certain cardiac condition in a relative (eg, HCM, DCM, LQTS, or other arrhythmia; Marfan syndrome). In addition, a family history of drowning or near drowning or a single-motor-vehicle accident of unknown cause may mask the presence of an inherited cardiac disease in a relative, showing the need for an understanding of both the underlying cause of death (ie, several causes of SCD may occur in the context of drowning) and specific risk factors (eg, swimming and some forms of LQTS). The degree of relation to the affected individual is important. The more closely related the patient is to the affected individual, the greater the chances that the patient may be at increased risk. In addition, the more closely related the affected individual, the more easily the necessary medical records and information regarding diagnosis and cause of death may be obtained. The most common cause of SCD in young athletes is HCM, which accounts for approximately 36% of cases.[80] CVM accounts for approximately 14% of cases and includes aortic stenosis, aortic dissection, and mitral valve prolapse. These diagnoses can be confirmed on postmortem examination.

Postmortem genetic testing may identify or confirm the cause of death and allow risk stratification of surviving relatives (**Fig. 2**). Identifying the cause of SCD is a high priority and necessary in order to provide accurate risk assessment for family members. If the sudden death is recent, ensuring that the medical examiner obtains and

stores a sample viable for genetic testing is important. One barrier to postmortem genetic testing has been a lack of uniform standards for the retention of blood and tissue
samples following sudden death. The National Association of Medical Examiners
recently published a position paper on sample retention and the NSGC has a dedi-
cated Web page for postmortem genetic testing (nsgc.org). Additional barriers to
postmortem testing beyond sample collection include lack of reimbursement among
third-party payers.

Known Cause of SCD

When the cause of SCD is confirmed, either because of a prior cardiac or postmortem
diagnosis, genetic testing should be performed based on the specific diagnosis. If a
disease-causing mutation is found, testing for known mutation should be used for
risk stratification of relatives.[46] Clinical genetic testing is available for several cardiac
diseases associated with an increased risk for SCD. The yield of genetic testing varies
by disease and is summarized in **Table 3**. If a diagnosis is confirmed on autopsy and a
postmortem sample is not available for further genetic testing, cardiac screening in at-
risk relatives should be based on the specific diagnosis. Screening guidelines for many
of the diseases associated with increased risk of SCD[81] have previously been published.[46,51,82] If the patient or other relative is subsequently diagnosed with cardiac
disease, genetic testing should be initiated in the affected individual. Initiating genetic

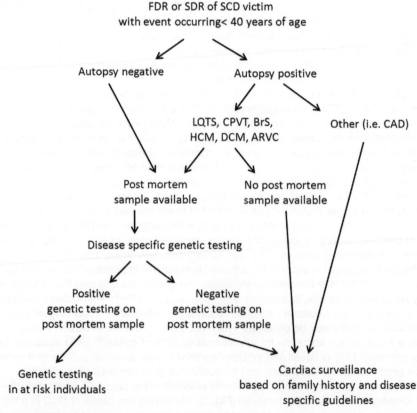

Fig. 2. Cardiac screening and genetic testing approach to a family history of SCD. BrS,
Brugada syndrome; FDR, first-degree relative; SDR, second-degree relative.

Table 3
Summary of genetic testing yield for diseases with increased risk of SCD

Cardiac Disease	Yield of Genetic Testing (%)
LQTS	75
Catecholaminergic polymorphic ventricular tachycardia	60
Brugada syndrome	20
Hypertrophic cardiomyopathy	60
Dilated cardiomyopathy	30
ARVC	40–60
Sudden unexplained death syndromes	26[78]

Yield of genetic testing is derived from laboratory Web sites performing clinically available genetic testing and represents the likelihood of identifying a disease-causing mutation in an individual with an unequivocal disease phenotype. Information available at: www.genetests.org.

testing in an unaffected individual is typically not recommended because the result interpretation is difficult and results are unlikely to be helpful in diagnosis, risk assessment, and management.

Unknown Cause of SCD

Postmortem genetic testing can be helpful in cases of negative autopsy with sudden unexplained death and genetic testing for channelopathies should be considered.[81] In cases of sudden unexplained death, postmortem genetic testing may reveal a cause of death in approximately 26% of cases.[81] LQTS-associated gene mutations were identified in 14.5% of cases and a mutation in the *RYR2* gene associated with CPVT was identified in 12.1%. Both LQTS and CPVT show autosomal dominant inheritance with decreased penetrance and variable expressivity, thus 50% of the relatives may have inherited the identified gene mutation but may have normal cardiac testing. Another major function of such testing is reassurance of relatives who did not inherit the disease-causing mutation and avoidance of unnecessary screening and treatment. Even though postmortem genetic testing confirms a diagnosis in only a minority of sudden unexplained death cases, the potential health benefits warrant testing.

Key message

- SCD is a rare but serious event among adolescents and young adults.
- Sports activity in adolescents has been associated with an increased risk of SCD.
- The 12-element AHA recommendations for screening young athletes include 8 items for personal and family history and 4 items for physical examination.
- Routine visits for athletic participation that emphasize family history may play an important role in prevention of SCD.
- For patients referred to a subspecialist for a positive family history of SCD, a specific diagnosis is crucial for counseling and further management.
- Evaluation of family members with family history of SCD should proceed outward from the index case in a logical and stepwise fashion.
- Lack of knowledge of the specific cause for SCD in a family member is common.
- Postmortem genetic testing can be helpful in SCD cases associated with either a negative autopsy or a heritable heart disease.
- If the autopsy confirms CAD and myocardial infarction, no cardiac imaging is indicated. Family members should be evaluated and assertively counseled regarding traditional risk factors for CAD (eg, dyslipidemia, tobacco use, hypertension) with the primary goal of behavior modification.

Box 2
Summary: conclusions

A detailed family history is necessary for optimal clinical care

The family history should be confirmed with medical records and updated on a routine basis

The pedigree is a useful tool for consolidating medical information

Regular collection of family history information is an opportunity for family education

The family history may indicate the need for genetic counseling and testing

Evaluation of family history may provide reassurance regarding disease risk and may allow patients to avoid unnecessary testing

The family history may allow early diagnosis and improved outcomes

Health care providers can locate local genetic counselors via the NSGC Web site (www.nsgc.org)

Family history is the most reliable tool for establishing risk of disease

Box 3
Summary: future directions

A dynamic family history and pedigree becomes part of an interactive electronic medical record

Transferrable electronic medical records may integrate family history with genetic testing results

Family history may empower patients by improving knowledge and linking them to guidelines and clinical trials

The family history is critical to the continued success of biobanks and human genetics research

Increased access to genetic counselors will play an important role in evaluation of family history and integration into clinical care

SUMMARY

Taken together, the family history facilitates diagnosis, risk stratification, and disease management. The application of family history is vital to delivering optimal care, and, as more is learned about the genetic basis of pediatric cardiovascular disease, the family history will play an increasingly central role in management (**Box 2**). Family history will be a necessary part of the transformative changes that are taking place as progress in genetics is applied to the care of patients (**Box 3**). A working knowledge of the family history and counseling and genetics services will be necessary to fulfill the promise of comprehensive care.

REFERENCES

1. Bennett RL. The practical guide to the genetic family history. New York: John Wiley; 1999.
2. Guttmacher AE, Collins FS, Carmona RH. The family history—more important than ever. N Engl J Med 2004;351(22):2333–6.
3. Yoon PW, Scheuner MT, Peterson-Oehlke KL, et al. Can family history be used as a tool for public health and preventive medicine? Genet Med 2002;4(4): 304–10.

4. Romitti PA. Utility of family history reports of major birth defects as a public health strategy. Pediatrics 2007;120(Suppl 2):S71–7.
5. Robin NH, Tabereaux PB, Benza R, et al. Genetic testing in cardiovascular disease. J Am Coll Cardiol 2007;50(8):727–37.
6. Scheuner MT, Wang SJ, Raffel LJ, et al. Family history: a comprehensive genetic risk assessment method for the chronic conditions of adulthood. Am J Med Genet 1997;71(3):315–24.
7. Williams RR, Hunt SC, Heiss G, et al. Usefulness of cardiovascular family history data for population-based preventive medicine and medical research (the Health Family Tree Study and the NHLBI Family Heart Study). Am J Cardiol 2001;87(2):129–35.
8. Trotter TL, Martin HM. Family history in pediatric primary care. Pediatrics 2007; 120(Suppl 2):S60–5.
9. Bennett RL, Steinhaus KA, Uhrich SB, et al. Recommendations for standardized human pedigree nomenclature. Pedigree Standardization Task Force of the National Society of Genetic Counselors. Am J Hum Genet 1995;56(3):745–52.
10. Bennett RL, French KS, Resta RG, et al. Standardized human pedigree nomenclature: update and assessment of the recommendations of the National Society of Genetic Counselors. J Genet Couns 2008;17(5):424–33.
11. Ciarleglio LJ, Bennett RL, Williamson J, et al. Genetic counseling throughout the life cycle. J Clin Invest 2003;112(9):1280–6.
12. Fung A, Manlhiot C, Naik S, et al. Impact of prenatal risk factors on congenital heart disease in the current era. J Am Heart Assoc 2013;2(3):e000064.
13. Green RF. Summary of workgroup meeting on use of family history information in pediatric primary care and public health. Pediatrics 2007;120(Suppl 2):S87–100.
14. Pulley JM, Denny JC, Peterson JF, et al. Operational implementation of prospective genotyping for personalized medicine: the design of the Vanderbilt PREDICT project. Clin Pharmacol Ther 2012;92(1):87–95.
15. Pierpont ME, Basson CT, Benson DW Jr, et al. Genetic basis for congenital heart defects: current knowledge: a scientific statement from the American Heart Association Congenital Cardiac Defects Committee, Council on Cardiovascular Disease in the Young: endorsed by the American Academy of Pediatrics. Circulation 2007;115(23):3015–38.
16. Hospital stays, hospital charges, and in-hospital deaths among infants with selected birth defects–United States, 2003. MMWR Morb Mortal Wkly Rep 2007;56(2):25–9.
17. Hoffman JI, Kaplan S. The incidence of congenital heart disease. J Am Coll Cardiol 2002;39(12):1890–900.
18. Hoffman JI. Incidence of congenital heart disease: I. Postnatal incidence. Pediatr Cardiol 1995;16(3):103–13.
19. Ferencz C, Rubin JD, McCarter RJ, et al. Congenital heart disease: prevalence at livebirth. The Baltimore-Washington Infant Study. Am J Epidemiol 1985; 121(1):31–6.
20. Fyler DC, Rudolph AM, Wittenborg MH, et al. Ventricular septal defect in infants and children; a correlation of clinical, physiologic, and autopsy data. Circulation 1958;18(5):833–51.
21. Clark EB. Pathogenetic mechanisms of congenital cardiovascular malformations revisited. Semin Perinatol 1996;20(6):465–72.
22. Botto LD, Lin AE, Riehle-Colarusso T, et al. Seeking causes: classifying and evaluating congenital heart defects in etiologic studies. Birth Defects Res A Clin Mol Teratol 2007;79(10):714–27.

23. Oyen N, Poulsen G, Boyd HA, et al. Recurrence of congenital heart defects in families. Circulation 2009;120(4):295–301.

24. Hartman RJ, Rasmussen SA, Botto LD, et al. The contribution of chromosomal abnormalities to congenital heart defects: a population-based study. Pediatr Cardiol 2011;32(8):1147–57.

25. Breckpot J, Thienpont B, Peeters H, et al. Array comparative genomic hybridization as a diagnostic tool for syndromic heart defects. J Pediatr 2010;156(5): 810–7, 817.e1–e4.

26. Lu XY, Phung MT, Shaw CA, et al. Genomic imbalances in neonates with birth defects: high detection rates by using chromosomal microarray analysis. Pediatrics 2008;122(6):1310–8.

27. Connor JA, Hinton RB, Miller EM, et al. Genetic testing practices in infants with congenital heart disease. Congenit Heart Dis 2013. [Epub ahead of print].

28. Soemedi R, Wilson IJ, Bentham J, et al. Contribution of global rare copy-number variants to the risk of sporadic congenital heart disease. Am J Hum Genet 2012; 91(3):489–501.

29. Wessels MW, Willems PJ. Genetic factors in non-syndromic congenital heart malformations. Clin Genet 2010;78(2):103–23.

30. Blue GM, Kirk EP, Sholler GF, et al. Congenital heart disease: current knowledge about causes and inheritance. Med J Aust 2012;197(3):155–9.

31. Fahed AC, Gelb BD, Seidman JG, et al. Genetics of congenital heart disease: the glass half empty. Circ Res 2013;112(4):707–20.

32. Wang X, Wang J, Zhao P, et al. Familial congenital heart disease: data collection and preliminary analysis. Cardiol Young 2013;23(3):394–9.

33. Schott JJ, Benson DW, Basson CT, et al. Congenital heart disease caused by mutations in the transcription factor NKX2-5. Science 1998;281(5373):108–11.

34. McElhinney DB, Geiger E, Blinder J, et al. NKX2.5 mutations in patients with congenital heart disease. J Am Coll Cardiol 2003;42(9):1650–5.

35. Richards AA, Santos LJ, Nichols HA, et al. Cryptic chromosomal abnormalities identified in children with congenital heart disease. Pediatr Res 2008;64(4): 358–63.

36. Jenkins KJ, Correa A, Feinstein JA, et al. Noninherited risk factors and congenital cardiovascular defects: current knowledge: a scientific statement from the American Heart Association Council on Cardiovascular Disease in the Young: endorsed by the American Academy of Pediatrics. Circulation 2007;115(23): 2995–3014.

37. Fesslova V, Brankovic J, Lalatta F, et al. Recurrence of congenital heart disease in cases with familial risk screened prenatally by echocardiography. J Pregnancy 2011;2011:368067.

38. Hinton RB Jr, Martin LJ, Tabangin ME, et al. Hypoplastic left heart syndrome is heritable. J Am Coll Cardiol 2007;50(16):1590–5.

39. Hinton RB, Martin LJ, Rame-Gowda S, et al. Hypoplastic left heart syndrome links to chromosomes 10q and 6q and is genetically related to bicuspid aortic valve. J Am Coll Cardiol 2009;53(12):1065–71.

40. Richardson P, McKenna W, Bristow M, et al. Report of the 1995 World Health Organization/International Society and Federation of Cardiology Task Force on the definition and classification of cardiomyopathies. Circulation 1996;93(5):841–2.

41. Maron BJ, Towbin JA, Thiene G, et al. Contemporary definitions and classification of the cardiomyopathies: an American Heart Association Scientific Statement from the Council on Clinical Cardiology, Heart Failure and Transplantation Committee; Quality of Care and Outcomes Research and Functional

Genomics and Translational Biology Interdisciplinary Working Groups; and Council on Epidemiology and Prevention. Circulation 2006;113(14):1807–16.

42. Morita H, Larson MG, Barr SC, et al. Single-gene mutations and increased left ventricular wall thickness in the community: the Framingham Heart Study. Circulation 2006;113(23):2697–705.

43. Zou Y, Song L, Wang Z, et al. Prevalence of idiopathic hypertrophic cardiomyopathy in China: a population-based echocardiographic analysis of 8080 adults. Am J Med 2004;116(1):14–8.

44. Morimoto S. Sarcomeric proteins and inherited cardiomyopathies. Cardiovasc Res 2008;77(4):659–66.

45. Watkins H, Ashrafian H, Redwood C. Inherited cardiomyopathies. N Engl J Med 2011;364(17):1643–56.

46. Ackerman MJ, Priori SG, Willems S, et al. HRS/EHRA expert consensus statement on the state of genetic testing for the channelopathies and cardiomyopathies this document was developed as a partnership between the Heart Rhythm Society (HRS) and the European Heart Rhythm Association (EHRA). Heart Rhythm 2011;8(8):1308–39.

47. Kindel SJ, Miller EM, Gupta R, et al. Pediatric cardiomyopathy: importance of genetic and metabolic evaluation. J Card Fail 2012;18(5):396–403.

48. Miller EM, Wang Y, Ware SM. Uptake of cardiac screening and genetic testing among hypertrophic and dilated cardiomyopathy families. J Genet Couns 2013; 22(2):258–67.

49. Leslie N, Tinkle BT. Glycogen storage disease type II (Pompe disease). In: Pagon RA, Adam MP, Bird TD, et al, editors. Seattle (WA): GeneReviews; 1993.

50. Charron P, Arad M, Arbustini E, et al. Genetic counselling and testing in cardiomyopathies: a position statement of the European Society of Cardiology Working Group on Myocardial and Pericardial Diseases. Eur Heart J 2010;31(22): 2715–26.

51. Hershberger RE, Lindenfeld J, Mestroni L, et al. Genetic evaluation of cardiomyopathy–a Heart Failure Society of America practice guideline. J Card Fail 2009; 15(2):83–97.

52. Alders M, Mannens M. Romano-Ward syndrome. In: Pagon RA, Adam MP, Bird TD, et al, editors. Seattle (WA): GeneReviews; 1993.

53. Schwartz PJ, Crotti L. QTc behavior during exercise and genetic testing for the long-QT syndrome. Circulation 2011;124(20):2181–4.

54. Vincent GM. Long QT syndrome. Cardiol Clin 2000;18(2):309–25.

55. Splawski I, Shen J, Timothy KW, et al. Spectrum of mutations in long-QT syndrome genes. KVLQT1, HERG, SCN5A, KCNE1, and KCNE2. Circulation 2000;102(10):1178–85.

56. Zhang L, Timothy KW, Vincent GM, et al. Spectrum of ST-T-wave patterns and repolarization parameters in congenital long-QT syndrome: ECG findings identify genotypes. Circulation 2000;102(23):2849–55.

57. Vincent GM, Timothy KW, Leppert M, et al. The spectrum of symptoms and QT intervals in carriers of the gene for the long-QT syndrome. N Engl J Med 1992; 327(12):846–52.

58. Zareba W, Moss AJ, Schwartz PJ, et al. Influence of genotype on the clinical course of the long-QT syndrome. International Long-QT Syndrome Registry Research Group. N Engl J Med 1998;339(14):960–5.

59. Ince H, Nienaber CA. Etiology, pathogenesis and management of thoracic aortic aneurysm. Nat Clin Pract Cardiovasc Med 2007;4(8):418–27.

60. Januzzi JL, Isselbacher EM, Fattori R, et al. Characterizing the young patient with aortic dissection: results from the International Registry of Aortic Dissection (IRAD). J Am Coll Cardiol 2004;43(4):665–9.

61. Hiratzka LF, Bakris GL, Beckman JA, et al. 2010 ACCF/AHA/AATS/ACR/ASA/ SCA/SCAI/SIR/STS/SVM guidelines for the diagnosis and management of patients with thoracic aortic disease: a report of the American College of Cardiology Foundation/American Heart Association Task Force on Practice Guidelines, American Association for Thoracic Surgery, American College of Radiology, American Stroke Association, Society of Cardiovascular Anesthesiologists, Society for Cardiovascular Angiography and Interventions, Society of Interventional Radiology, Society of Thoracic Surgeons, and Society for Vascular Medicine. Circulation 2010;121(13):e266–369.

62. Milewicz DM, Guo DC, Tran-Fadulu V, et al. Genetic basis of thoracic aortic aneurysms and dissections: focus on smooth muscle cell contractile dysfunction. Annu Rev Genomics Hum Genet 2008;9:283–302.

63. Lindsay ME, Dietz HC. Lessons on the pathogenesis of aneurysm from heritable conditions. Nature 2011;473(7347):308–16.

64. Eagle KA. Rationale and design of the National Registry of Genetically Triggered Thoracic Aortic Aneurysms and Cardiovascular Conditions (GenTAC). Am Heart J 2009;157(2):319–26.

65. Guo DC, Pannu H, Tran-Fadulu V, et al. Mutations in smooth muscle alpha-actin (ACTA2) lead to thoracic aortic aneurysms and dissections. Nat Genet 2007; 39(12):1488–93.

66. Zhu L, Vranckx R, Khau Van Kien P, et al. Mutations in myosin heavy chain 11 cause a syndrome associating thoracic aortic aneurysm/aortic dissection and patent ductus arteriosus. Nat Genet 2006;38(3):343–9.

67. Tran-Fadulu V, Pannu H, Kim DH, et al. Analysis of multigenerational families with thoracic aortic aneurysms and dissections due to TGFBR1 or TGFBR2 mutations. J Med Genet 2009;46(9):607–13.

68. Loeys BL, Dietz HC, Braverman AC, et al. The revised Ghent nosology for the Marfan syndrome. J Med Genet 2010;47(7):476–85.

69. Maron BJ, Chaitman BR, Ackerman MJ, et al. Recommendations for physical activity and recreational sports participation for young patients with genetic cardiovascular diseases. Circulation 2004;109(22):2807–16.

70. Ashley EA, Hershberger RE, Caleshu C, et al. Genetics and cardiovascular disease: a policy statement from the American Heart Association. Circulation 2012;126(1):142–57.

71. Behr E, Wood DA, Wright M, et al. Cardiological assessment of first-degree relatives in sudden arrhythmic death syndrome. Lancet 2003;362(9394):1457–9.

72. Roger VL, Go AS, Lloyd-Jones DM, et al. Heart disease and stroke statistics– 2012 update: a report from the American Heart Association. Circulation 2012; 125(1):e2–220.

73. Winkel BG, Holst AG, Theilade J, et al. Nationwide study of sudden cardiac death in persons aged 1-35 years. Eur Heart J 2011;32(8):983–90.

74. Liberthson RR. Sudden death from cardiac causes in children and young adults. N Engl J Med 1996;334(16):1039–44.

75. Doolan A, Langlois N, Semsarian C. Causes of sudden cardiac death in young Australians. Med J Aust 2004;180(3):110–2.

76. Drezner JA, Fudge J, Harmon KG, et al. Warning symptoms and family history in children and young adults with sudden cardiac arrest. J Am Board Fam Med 2012;25(4):408–15.

77. Maron BJ, Douglas PS, Graham TP, et al. Task force 1: preparticipation screening and diagnosis of cardiovascular disease in athletes. J Am Coll Cardiol 2005;45(8):1322–6.
78. Corrado D, Basso C, Rizzoli G, et al. Does sports activity enhance the risk of sudden death in adolescents and young adults? J Am Coll Cardiol 2003; 42(11):1959–63.
79. Maron BJ, Thompson PD, Puffer JC, et al. Cardiovascular preparticipation screening of competitive athletes. A statement for health professionals from the Sudden Death Committee (clinical cardiology) and Congenital Cardiac Defects Committee (cardiovascular disease in the young), American Heart Association. Circulation 1996;94(4):850–6.
80. Maron BJ, Thompson PD, Ackerman MJ, et al. Recommendations and considerations related to preparticipation screening for cardiovascular abnormalities in competitive athletes: 2007 update: a scientific statement from the American Heart Association Council on Nutrition, Physical Activity, and Metabolism: endorsed by the American College of Cardiology Foundation. Circulation 2007;115(12):1643–55.
81. Tester DJ, Medeiros-Domingo A, Will ML, et al. Cardiac channel molecular autopsy: insights from 173 consecutive cases of autopsy-negative sudden unexplained death referred for postmortem genetic testing. Mayo Clin Proc 2012;87(6):524–39.
82. van Langen IM, Hofman N, Tan HL, et al. Family and population strategies for screening and counselling of inherited cardiac arrhythmias. Ann Med 2004; 36(Suppl 1):116–24.

Caring for a Teen with Congenital Heart Disease

Pooja Gupta, MD

KEYWORDS

- Congenital heart disease • Adolescents • Transition • Primary care provider
- Psychosocial

KEY POINTS

- Adolescents with CHD are a rapidly growing population.
- They require lifelong cardiac and noncardiac care.
- Identity formation is a core developmental task during the teenage years.
- Special attention to psychosocial issues is required to prevent maladaptive outcomes during this vulnerable period.
- A seamless successful transition process is central to prevention of patients lost to follow-up and to foster self-care behaviors.

INTRODUCTION

Rapid advancements in medical and surgical sciences have resulted in an increased number of patients with congenital heart disease (CHD) entering teenage and adulthood. CHD is the most common birth defect in United States and the incidence of CHD is approximately 9 per 100,000 live births.[1,2] Each year, 40,000 babies are born with CHD in the United States and 85% to 90% of these patients are surviving into adulthood; the total number of adults with CHD in the United States has exceeded 1,000,000.[3] For the first time in the history of medicine, adults with CHD outnumber pediatric patients with CHD. A 400% increase in adult CHD outpatient workload was reported in Canada.[4]

With these statistics in mind, it is inevitable that pediatricians will provide care to this special and complex group of patients during their teenage years. Because teenagers may be vulnerable in many different ways, even in the absence of a disease, the presence of a chronic disease such as CHD poses an extreme challenge for health care providers. The goal of care for patients with CHD during their adolescence is to best prepare them to deal with the issues that may arise now or in the future. Critical to this process is a successful transition from a pediatric to an adult health care

Disclosures: None.
Division of Cardiology, The Carman and Ann Adams Department of Pediatrics, Wayne State University School of Medicine, 3901 Beaubien Boulevard, Detroit, MI 48201-2119, USA
E-mail address: pgupta2@dmc.org

Pediatr Clin N Am 61 (2014) 207–228
http://dx.doi.org/10.1016/j.pcl.2013.09.019
0031-3955/14/$ – see front matter © 2014 Elsevier Inc. All rights reserved.
pediatric.theclinics.com

setting, both in terms of primary care and specialized care. As stated by the American Academy of Pediatrics, "The goal of transition in health care for young adults with special health care needs is to maximize lifelong functioning and potential through the provision of high-quality, developmentally appropriate health care services that continue uninterrupted as the individual moves from adolescence to adulthood."[5]

This article reviews the unique issues pertaining to teens with CHD that a pediatric health care provider should be familiar with when taking care of these patients to ensure a smooth transition into adulthood. Details of individual cardiac lesions are not discussed in this article. To understand how chronic illness such as CHD can affect developmental milestones, awareness of normal developmental milestones is necessary.[6–8] All teenagers with CHD require primary care and ongoing specialized cardiac care.[9] As defined by the American Academy of Pediatrics' medical home policy statement, patients with chronic lifelong health care needs should have easy access to a "medical home" where they receive primary, family-centered care.[10–13] This role can be played by pediatricians, family practitioners, or internal medicine-pediatric experts. When these patients are cared for by family practitioners or internal medicine-pediatric experts, it reduces the total number of physician transfers that they have to go through in their lifetime. Expertise in adolescent medicine might be beneficial in dealing with general teenage issues in addition to issues specific to CHD and allow for a smooth transition into adulthood.

APPROACH TO A TEEN WITH CHD: ROLE OF A PRIMARY PROVIDER

Teenagers with CHD may have various cardiac, noncardiac medical and surgical needs because of coexisting diseases or anomalies. Good record keeping and coordination of care with the various subspecialists is central to optimal primary care. It is crucial that there be a strong mechanism of communication between the cardiologist, the primary care provider (PCP), and any other specialists involved. The PCP should take charge of their patients' care, prevent fractionated care, and involve the family members and the patient in medical decision making with ongoing education. Updated, accurate personal health information documented in the format of a passport[8] is not only beneficial for the health care providers in various settings but may also improve patient knowledge and understanding about their heart disease.[14] Providers should be aware of the patient's diagnosis, anticipated and ongoing issues, current medications, baseline functional status, and current recommendations regarding exercise and endocarditis prophylaxis, which are discussed later in this article. This knowledge enables them to take care of their patients appropriately when they report any new symptoms or concerns. Information about current medications help to guard against potential drug interactions if they are on multiple medications or if a new drug is prescribed. The American Heart Association (AHA) Scientific Statement regarding "Best practices in managing transition to adulthood for adolescents with CHD" lists all of the health maintenance needs of a patient with CHD that a PCP may handle including vaccinations, cholesterol screening, hypertension screening, cancer screening at appropriate ages, assessment of tobacco, alcohol and or drug use, nutritional counseling, contraception, and sexuality issues.[15] It is important that all primary care givers spend some time alone with adolescent patients discussing various issues unique to this age group. Lapse in cardiac care is likely to occur during the transition from adolescence to adulthood[16] and may occur despite being in contact with health care.[17] For compliant teenagers, the rate of retention by a pediatric cardiologist is surprisingly high.[18] A primary provider can play an active role in transitioning this group of patients from the pediatric to adult care setting in a seamless manner as opposed to an abrupt transfer.[19] During transition, it is important that there is a period of overlap of care between the 2 kinds of services (pediatric and adult). Ideally, the transition of primary care and subspecialty care should not occur at the same time.[15]

Compliance Issues: Lost to Follow-Up

Most adults with complex CHD are either lost from specialized cardiac care or are taken care of by cardiologists with no CHD expertise and training.[20,21] Less than 30% of adults with CHD are seen by specialized providers.[22] In 2004, Reid and colleagues[23] reported that 48% of adolescents with CHD underwent successful transition. Their data suggested that ongoing care during adolescence with continued discussion of the importance of transition was important for successful transition. Unfortunately, this component of discussion and patient education is often missing.[24] The other likely reasons for lost to follow-up may be the false perception that the heart has been fixed. which is supported by a lack of symptoms or a lack of knowledge about the need for follow-up. This issue can be further aggravated by insurance barriers. Wacker and colleagues,[21] in their study of 10,500 German patients, reported lack of follow-up at a specialized adult CHD center in a 5-year period in 76% of their patients. Yeung and colleagues[25] cited the most common reason for lack of follow-up was the message "no need to follow up." They also report an association between lapse of medical care and adverse outcome. The American College of Cardiology (ACC)/AHA 2008 Guidelines on the "Management of Adults with Congenital Heart Disease" recommends that the transition process for patients with CHD begin at 12 years of age to prepare the patient for transfer to adult care.[9] The lost to follow-up concept is not only seen with cardiac care but also for primary care. As the need for immunizations and other health-related issues decline in this age group, it is easier for patients to fall out of the system. Some patients and families may perceive their cardiologist as the primary care giver potentiating noncompliance with PCP visits.

Key message

- All patients with significant CHD (repaired or unrepaired) need lifelong care and follow-up with a CHD specialist and primary provider

- Good record keeping and coordination of care with all the specialists involved is central to optimal care

- Adolescent patients are likely to fall out of the medical system at some time during the teenage years for several reasons

- Lack of symptoms, lack of knowledge about the need for follow-up, and lack of insurance results in high rates of lost to follow-up

- Ongoing patient education and discussion regarding the importance of follow-up might improve lost to follow-up rates

- Both the primary provider and cardiologist can be instrumental in improving compliance

- The ACC/AHA recommend that the transition process whereby patients are handed over from the pediatric to adult care setting should start at 12 years of age

---

Interventions

Cardiac interventions and reinterventions

The number of unrepaired adolescent patients with significant CHD is steadily declining particularly in developed countries. Late diagnosis may be encountered in some cases. However, most adolescents with moderate to severe CHD have already gone through a surgical intervention.[26,27] Therefore, reoperations are more common than primary repair in this age group. Monro and colleagues[27] report a 15% incidence of reintervention up to 26 years after the first operation with a 20-year survival rate of 86%. However, the incidence of reoperation varies based on the specific cardiac lesion, type, and age at repair. The perioperative issues encountered in adolescents and young adults during cardiac and noncardiac surgeries are discussed by Mott and colleagues.[28] Optimal management of other coexisting conditions and patient education is central to prompt recovery. In those patients diagnosed with CHD for the first time, referral should be made to a tertiary care center after careful consideration of the expertise of the cardiac surgeon for that particular CHD and the adequacy of postoperative care at that particular institution.

Key message

- Reinterventions are more common during adolescence compared with primary repair
- For primary repair, referral to a tertiary care center with a congenital surgeon and CHD cardiologist is optimal
- Optimal management of other coexisting medical conditions is crucial for prompt recovery
- Sensitivity to cosmetic concerns regarding the surgical incision is particularly important in this age group

---

Interventional/Device therapy

Catheter-based interventional therapy has undergone tremendous advancement in the last 2 decades. Most of the simple shunts such as atrial septal defect, patent ductus arteriosus, and selected ventricular septal defect can be repaired primarily by the transcatheter route. Coarctation, valvular, conduit, or baffle stenosis and branch pulmonary artery stenosis can be repaired percutaneously in many instances. Transcatheter pulmonary valve therapy is now approved for use in children and adults who have failing pulmonary valve conduits with promising initial results.[29–31] Arrhythmia is a frequent finding in postoperative patients during adolescence and adulthood. Serious arrhythmia may lead to heart failure, exercise intolerance, thromboembolic complications, or even sudden cardiac death. The risk of sudden cardiac death is higher in this group of patients compared with healthy adolescents. Silka and colleagues[32] reported 25 to 100 times greater risk of sudden cardiac death in a postoperative patient with CHD compared with age-matched controls with a higher risk for cyanotic CHD and after the second decade.

With advances in electrophysiology, a range of treatment options are now available including ablations and device therapy. Contact sports such as tackle football, judo, karate, and wrestling should be avoided in anyone with a device or a pacemaker. Additional restrictions or limitations may be specific to the underlying CHD and should be discussed with the cardiologist. Patients with implanted metallic devices may require magnetic resonance imaging (MRI), which requires knowledge of the current recommendations. The AHA and the American College of Radiology (ACR) have issued guidelines stating that a careful risk-benefit ratio must be established and that cardiac implantable devices remain a relative contraindication to MRI.[33] In 2011, the US Food and Drug Administration (FDA) approved the first cardiac pacemaker designed to be used safely, but conditionally, during MRI examinations.[34] Keeping detailed records of the implanted metallic devices in individual patients is helpful for those who may require MRI in the future.

Key message

- The risk of sudden cardiac death is high in teenage patients with CHD compared with healthy adolescents
- Careful and judicious use of intervention and device therapy might lower this risk to some extent
- A variety of cardiac interventional procedures and device therapy are now available
- Contact sports should be avoided by those with devices
- Pacemakers are relative contraindications to an MRI study
- Newer pacing systems have been specifically designed that can safely be used in the MRI environment

---

Noncardiac surgeries

Teenagers and adults with CHD undergoing noncardiac surgery may be at increased risk of complications associated with the procedure.[35] This risk varies by individual cardiac lesion and associated findings. The ACC/AHA 2008 guidelines for management of adults with CHD classify congenital cardiac lesions as high and moderate risk based on their perioperative risk during a noncardiac surgery.[9] The risk of complication is highest when the procedures involve the respiratory or neurologic system.[36] Careful preoperative planning is necessary involving the cardiologist, cardiac anesthesiologist, surgeon, and the PCP. The objective of a preoperative evaluation is to identify the major risk factors and then modify them in an attempt to reduce the surgical risk. A detailed history, including any previous experiences with anesthesia and surgery, is valuable and a thorough physical examination is warranted. Baseline laboratory parameters such as a complete blood count, coagulation profile including bleeding time, renal function tests, and liver function tests when indicated should be obtained. For female patients, a pregnancy test should be performed when applicable. Warner and colleagues[36] report major perioperative risk factors such as cyanosis, treatment of congestive heart failure (CHF), poor general health, pulmonary hypertension, and younger age. Preoperative phlebotomy in certain cyanotic patients with hematocrit more than 65% may be beneficial.[9,37] CHD patients undergoing surgery should receive antibiotics for prevention of infective endocarditis based on recommendations made by the cardiologist as suggested by the revised AHA guidelines.[38] Pacemaker interrogations should be performed before and after the surgical procedure. Pacemakers can be programmed to an asynchronous mode during the procedure to avoid interference from cautery devices.[39] Adequate fluid management before, during, and after the operation is crucial. Optimal mechanical ventilation, appropriate pain management, early mobilization, and pulmonary toilet are also important aspects of postoperative care. Patients should be restarted on cardiac medications at the earliest possible time. Patients on anticoagulation require substitution with unfractionated heparin depending on the underlying CHD, with prompt resumption when possible. In-line filters should be used for intravenous lines to decrease the risk of air embolism especially in patients with right to left shunts.

Key message
• There is increased risk of complications in patients with CHD during noncardiac surgery compared with healthy adolescents
• A team approach between primary provider, cardiologist, anesthesiologist, and surgeon with involvement of the patient is optimal
• Preoperative laboratory assessment and pregnancy test should be done when applicable
• Patients should receive endocarditis prophylaxis when indicated as per revised AHA guidelines
• Need for pacemaker interrogation should be assessed when applicable
• Oral anticoagulation should be substituted with unfractionated heparin based on the procedure and underlying CHD
• Cardiac medications should be restarted at the earliest

Psychosocial Issues

Adolescence is a vulnerable period in many different ways. During this time, teenagers develop self-esteem, self-identity, and autonomy, and hence their self-image. In patients with chronic illnesses such as CHD, the issues of adolescence such as puberty, autonomy, self-esteem, personal identity, sexuality, education, vocational training can be complicated because of their need to cope with their disease. Coping or living with CHD includes many psychosocial factors in addition to the ongoing cardiac surveillance, hospitalizations, medications, reinterventions, and many others. It is important that there is an understanding of the whole patient with CHD as implied by Kovacs and Verstappen.[40] The medical demands of a chronic illness may disturb the adolescent's self-image, self-esteem, and delay the completion of normal developmental tasks.[41,42] The Society of Adolescent Medicine emphasizes the importance of addressing the medical, psychosocial, and educational or vocational needs during the transition process for adolescents with chronic illness.[43] Many of these teens feel different from their peers because of their CHD and concerns about their body image play an important role in their social functioning.[44,45] Their social functioning seems to strongly correlate with their psychological functioning. Social factors likely to affect the quality of life most in the future are family, friends, education, or career.[46] Studies have shown that there is no relation between the severity of the cardiac defect and psychological adjustment or any other demographic factors.[47–53] Data regarding the incidence of emotional and behavioral issues during the teenage years with CHD is conflicting. It varies from reports of no significant psychological issues[54] to reports of increased incidence of anxiety, diminished self-esteem, depression, increased dependency, and poor social and emotional adjustment.[55–58] A meta-analysis of 11 studies showed increased risk of internalizing problems such as depression and anxiety and externalizing behavior issues such as aggression and hyperactivity compared with healthy adolescents.[51] Many studies report a higher likelihood of psychological issues in adults with CHD compared with their healthy peers.[48,53,59,60] Psychiatric disorders such as mood or anxiety disorder may be frequent; as many as 1 in 3 patients with CHD meet diagnostic criteria for a psychiatric disorder. Only a small number actually receive mental health treatment.[48,53,60] A single institution study published by Spijkerboer and colleagues[61] looked at psychological outcomes before 1980 and a decade later and reported no improvement in psychological outcomes with improving medical outcomes and surgical techniques. The adolescents with CHD are less likely to smoke, drink alcohol, or use illicit drugs and are less likely to be sexually active.[62,63] This might come as a good news because the negative implications of these high-risk behaviors particularly in this group are well known; however, it might highlight another problem: their social unacceptability, low self-esteem, fear of rejection, and fear of forming close relationships. Their social unacceptability is also reflected by the discrimination and bullying they experience from their peers and the reported feelings of anger, exclusion, and embarrassment.[59]

This highlights an important aspect of care for adolescents with CHD. Rapid progress is being made with the diagnosis and interventions for CHD, but are the psychosocial issues that come as a package with these patients being recognized and dealt with? Lip and colleagues[64] discuss the role of psychological interventions for this group. The clinicians providing care to this group of patients must be familiar with the effect and interplay of the various psychosocial factors in their lives. Primary providers are usually at the forefront and share the responsibility to recognize and manage these issues with the cardiologist, using all available resources.

Key message

- The development of self-identity, self-esteem, and self-image can be complicated in patients with chronic illness
- Coping with CHD may include several psychosocial factors in addition to the medical issues
- The Society of Adolescent Medicine emphasizes the importance of addressing the medical, psychosocial, and educational or vocational needs during the transition process for adolescents with chronic illness
- No relationship has been shown between the severity of the cardiac defect and psychological adjustment
- The primary provider and the cardiologist must be familiar with the various psychosocial issues and be able to recognize and manage these using all available resources

---

Neurodevelopmental issues

Children and adolescents with complex CHD are at increased risk for developmental disorders including learning difficulties, attention-deficit hyperactivity disorder, and delay in areas of language and fine and gross motor functions.[65–71] The complexity of the CHD is directly proportional to the prevalence and severity of the developmental issues.[72] Many genetic syndromes are associated with CHD and developmental issues.[73–80] Teenagers with developmental disabilities and CHD should receive anticipatory guidance at each clinic appointment during adolescence in a manner appropriate for the adolescent's cognitive ability and level of function.[15] It is possible that a developmental disorder may manifest itself for the first time during adolescence. As the educational curriculum advances and the expectations from a teen rises, some of the developmental disorders may now be unmasked. It is crucial to monitor the developmental progress of adolescents with CHD closely during teenage years. In a recent Scientific Statement put forth by the AHA, and approved by the American Academy of Pediatrics (AAP), periodic developmental surveillance, screening, evaluation, and reevaluation are recommended for children with CHD who are at increased risk for a developmental disorder.[69] A list of specific cardiac lesions at high risk for developmental issues and an algorithm for surveillance, screening, and management is included in this Scientific Statement. The use of such an algorithm may result in improved identification of developmental issues, allowing for appropriate therapies and education to improve their academic, behavioral, psychosocial, and adaptive functioning.[69] A systematic assessment for risk factors and age-specific developmental progress should be incorporated into the annual well-child visits. Based on this algorithm, adolescents suspected to have developmental issues during screening should be referred for further evaluation and care by a behavioral or mental health specialist, along with ongoing care by the PCP in the primary care medical home.[12,69]

Key message

- Children and adolescents with CHD are at increased risk for developmental disorders including learning difficulties, attention-deficit hyperactivity disorder, and delay in areas of language and fine and gross motor functions

- A teenager with CHD may exhibit signs of a developmental disorder for the first time during the teenage years

- The AHA Scientific Statement (2012) proposes an algorithm for health care providers involved in taking care of patients with CHD in an attempt to optimize the neurodevelopmental outcomes

- A systematic assessment of risk factors for developmental issues should be incorporated in the routine preventive visits for patients with CHD

Knowledge About Heart Disease

Educational intervention

Adolescents are encouraged to take charge of their health and life. Ongoing education is central to this process of transfer of responsibility from parents to the patients themselves. They should receive detailed information regarding their cardiac diagnoses and surgical repair with the help of a diagram or a heart model. They should be familiar with their medications, need for endocarditis prophylaxis, preferred lifestyle, and recommendations about contraception and child bearing.[81–83] The Alliance for Adult Research in Congenital Cardiology (AARC) investigators along with Adult Congenital Heart Association (ACHA) recently demonstrated the benefits of a focused educational intervention and an improvement in the knowledge gap of adult patients with CHD.[14] Because all educational topics cannot be discussed in 1 visit, Kovacs and Verstappen[40] suggest an educational checklist to be placed in the patient's chart so that all topics are covered at some point during adolescence. Parental education should emphasize the benefits of transition of responsibility[41,84] because it is not unusual to see parental overprotection.[48,85]

Key message

- Patients and families should be aware of their diagnosis and details of the repair and anticipated issues

- Need for lifelong care for patients with moderate and complex CHD should be emphasized by the PCP and cardiologist

- An educational check list can be placed in the chart and used to keep track of the various topics that require discussion during adolescence

- Parental education should occur with emphasis on transferring responsibility to the teenager

Exercise recommendation

Obesity is a major problem in the pediatric age group and the problem is further intensified in patients with CHD.[86,87] According to the Scientific Statement published by the AHA "exercise is an important component of quality of life (QOL) and health maintenance."[15] Physical activity is beneficial for overall good health including cardiovascular health and particularly in adolescents with CHD.[88] Good exercise habits developed in adolescence can help promote these benefits. Despite the potential benefits, exercise and activity levels are often not discussed by the cardiologist and primary provider. Patients with CHD may even be discouraged from exercise and may lead a sedentary lifestyle because of personal, parental, or school personnel fears.[89] To allay these fears, the recommended level of activity should be discussed and patients with CHD should be encouraged to carry out activities within that range. It is the responsibility of the PCP and the cardiologist to provide patients and families with a clear message regarding exercise. The AHA has published guidelines to assist specifically with the recommendations for sports participation in patients with CHD and those with genetic heart disease.[90,91] The Association for European Pediatric Cardiology recommends "a daily participation in 60 minutes or more of moderate-to-vigorous physical activity" for all children with CHD.[92]

Key message

- Health benefits of being active should be discussed with the teen during each visit
- Adolescents with CHD should be encouraged to stay active within a prescribed range of activities
- Patients should receive a clear message regarding their recommended level of activity
- The AHA has published guidelines for sports participation for patients with CHD

Endocarditis prophylaxis

Infective endocarditis (IE) is a rare occurrence. However, when it occurs, it can be life threatening. Certain cardiac conditions and repairs increase the risk for IE. In 2007, a writing group was appointed by the AHA with representation from American Dental Association, the Infectious Diseases Society of America, and the American Academy of Pediatrics and updated recommendations for antibiotic prophylaxis were published.[38] It is useful for health care providers to have access to this document and to be familiar with the major changes in the updated recommendations. Health care providers might encounter teenage patients inquiring about body piercing and tattoos, which are generally discouraged as they might increase the risk of IE.[93]

Key message

- Health care providers should be familiar with the revised recommendations for antibiotic prophylaxis and the specific recommendations for each patient with CHD

High-risk behaviors and sexuality

For healthy adolescents, the primary provider is responsible for guidance and education pertaining to sexuality, contraception, pregnancy, and reproduction. In adolescents with CHD, this might be best dealt with by a combined effort from the cardiologist and the PCP. The data regarding sexual and contraceptive practices of adolescents with CHD are limited.[8] It is known that nearly half of all healthy adolescents have engaged in sexual intercourse at least once during their teenage years. The average age of the first sexual activity is 17 years for girls and 16 years for boys.[94–96] Adolescents with CHD are less likely to be sexually active at a younger age,[62,63] which could be caused by psychosocial developmental delay[97] or uncertainties regarding their CHD.[98,99] However, of those 16- to 18-year olds with CHD who are sexually active, three-quarters of them are likely to take greater risks including more than 2 partners in a 3-month period, using drugs or alcohol before sex, and lack of contraception.[62] Among teens with CHD, there is a lower level of knowledge about sexuality, contraception, and reproduction with many misconceptions and fears.[98,99] Sexually transmitted diseases is a significant problem in this age group. There is a definite need for education, guidance, and counseling regarding safe sexual practices in all adolescents including those with CHD. The AHA recommends making health education material available to all preadolescents and their parents. They suggest obtaining a comprehensive history in all postpubertal patients inquiring about their knowledge of sexuality and other high-risk behaviors including drugs and alcohol.[15] All adolescents are encouraged to use a condom with a spermicide to protect against sexually transmitted diseases, hepatitis B, and human immunodeficiency virus.

Key message

- Adolescents with CHD are less likely to be sexually active at a younger age; however, they are more likely to take greater risks

- Sexually transmitted diseases are a significant problem in adolescents

- There is a definite need for education, guidance, and counseling regarding safe sexual practices among all adolescents particularly those with CHD

- A PCP can play an important role in counseling and guiding teenagers with CHD regarding high-risk behaviors and sexuality

- All adolescents should be encouraged to use a condom with a spermicide to protect against sexually transmitted diseases, hepatitis B, and human immunodeficiency virus

---

Contraception

Contraception use is erratic in this age group and data show that 50% of adolescent pregnancies occur within 6 months of the first sexual encounter.[96] Currently, there are several contraceptive options available to a healthy teenager. In teenagers with CHD, the choice of contraception should be individualized based on their primary cardiac defect, the type of surgical repair, residual defects, and functional status. A team approach between the PCP, cardiologist, and gynecologist may be beneficial. It is important to involve the patient and the family in this decision making. Contraceptive options include oral pills (combination of estrogen and progestin, progestin-only pills, injectable progesterone [Depo-Provera], implantable progesterone rod [Implanon]), intrauterine devices, and barrier methods. The World Health Organization has made recommendations regarding the use of combined hormonal contraceptives in women with CHD and this has been outlined by Silversides and colleagues[100] and reproduced by Sable and colleagues[15] in their Scientific Statement. Patients with simple, repaired CHD with no sequelae have no restrictions regarding contraception use. Patients with cyanosis, right to left shunt, and pulmonary vascular disease should avoid estrogen-based contraception because of the risk of thromboembolism. The presence of prosthetic conduits and valves are relative contraindication for oral contraceptives.[100] Sexually active teenagers should also be familiar with the emergency contraception options, which include either a combined estrogen-progestin pill (Yuzpe regimen) or a progestin-only pill (plan B).[101–103] Both regimens involve taking 2 doses of the pill 12 hours apart. The progestin-only pill is available without a prescription to women older than 17 years and may be the preferred method in teenagers with CHD who are at risk of thromboembolic complications. Permanent sterilization should be postponed until the patients are in an adult age range to ensure that they have the maturity to make this decision. Abstinence during adolescence is an option and these patients should be encouraged and supported for their decision.

Key message

- Patients with simple, repaired CHD with no sequelae have no restrictions regarding contraception use

- Patients with cyanosis, right to left shunt, and pulmonary vascular disease should avoid estrogen-based contraception because of the risk of thromboembolism

- Prosthetic conduits and valves are relative contraindication for oral contraceptives

- Progestin-only options should be used in patients at higher risk for thromboembolic complications

---

Pregnancy and reproduction

Pregnancy and child bearing during adolescence is a challenge from many different aspects including social, psychological, and medical.[104,105] Medical issues include poor compliance with prenatal care, anemia, pregnancy-induced hypertension, and preterm and low-birth-weight infants.[106] Specific to this population, there are maternal and fetal risks related to the CHD, residual defects, or medications. Medical termination of pregnancy is not risk free and is recommended only after careful consideration of all possibilities in specific cases by the cardiologist who knows the patient well. When a decision is made to continue the pregnancy, a collaborative approach including the cardiologist, obstetrician, PCP, and a social worker is required. The availability of a psychotherapist/counselor can be beneficial in some cases.

Key message

- Pregnant adolescents with CHD pose unique social, psychological, and medical challenges

- Medical issues common to all adolescents include poor compliance with prenatal care, anemia, pregnancy-induced hypertension, and preterm and low-birth-weight infants

- Specific to this population, there are potential maternal and fetal risks related to the CHD, residual defects, or medications

- A collaborative approach including the cardiologist, obstetrician, the PCP, and a social worker is optimal

---

Genetic counseling

Even though adolescents with CHD are not actively considering starting a family and child bearing, many of them have numerous questions, misconceptions, and fears about their sexuality and reproductive ability.[98,99] Some of the fears might include the risk of CHD in the offspring. This perceived risk might be more than the actual risk. Some cardiac defects occur in isolation (nonsyndromic), whereas others occur as a component of a genetic anomaly (syndromic). Up to 15% of newborns with CHD have a genetic basis, whereas in others the occurrence of CHD is multifactorial.[107] Bernier and Spaetgens[108] describe a checklist that can be used in adolescents with CHD to identify those who will benefit from genetic evaluation. This includes a targeted 3-generation family history including individuals with CHD, other malformation, pregnancy loss, or developmental delay.[15] Based on the results of the detailed assessment, the next step is genetic evaluation. Genetic evaluation may include newer genetic tests that may have been previously unavailable and may help better assess the risk of transmission of CHD to the offspring. (The genetic basis for cardiovascular malformation is discussed in detail by Miller and colleagues, elsewhere in this issue.)

Key message

- Cardiac defects can occur in isolation (nonsyndromic) or as a component of a genetic anomaly (syndromic)

- 15% of newborns with CHD have a genetic basis

- A checklist has been developed by Bernier and Spaetgens[108] that can be used in adolescents with CHD to identify those who will benefit from genetic evaluation

---

Career counseling and employment

There is a higher rate of unemployment among patients with CHD compared with healthy adults.[109] This difference is more pronounced when considering patients with complex CHD. There is evidence that structured career or employment advice increases the employment rate compared with no career or vocational counseling.[110] Therefore, adolescents with CHD should receive career and vocational counseling to assist them in making career choices such that they can combine personal interest with their physical limitations, if present.[111] It is recommended that such discussions take place between 13 and 15 years of age (early adolescent period) and a PCP may be able to initiate this in conjunction with the cardiologist. In 1986, the AHA classified occupational activities into 5 categories and made specific career recommendations based on the type of CHD.[112] After assessing the individual's occupational activity level, education capacity, and social ability, the highest level of education should be encouraged.[15] Higher level of education results in an increase in job participation.[113] Maintenance of full employment with early education and counseling may have a positive effect on health and quality of life.[114] All health care providers should be familiar with the various resources available at their state level for this purpose.

Key message

- There is a higher rate of unemployment among patients with CHD compared with healthy adults

- Career counseling during adolescence may improve the rate of employment

- Adolescents with CHD should receive career or vocational counseling to assist them in making career choices

- All health care providers should be familiar with the various resources available at their state level for this purpose

Insurability and disability

Among the general population, the highest rates of uninsured are among those between 19 and 26 years of age.[115,116] The uninsured young adult with a chronic condition is 8 times more likely to have unmet medical needs and 6 times more likely to have no access to routine care compared with a young adult who is insured.[117] It is difficult for this group of patients to obtain health or life insurance.[118,119] Hence, the AHA in their Scientific Statement recommends that health care professionals address the issue of insurability before a patient leaves their parent's policy or loses their eligibility for children's services.[15] The need for health care providers to be familiar with various informational resources in this regard is emphasized.

Key message

- There is a high rate of uninsured adults with a chronic condition
- The AHA recommends that the issue of insurability must be addressed before a patient leaves their parent's policy or loses their eligibility for children's services

---

End-of-life issues

There has been a steady decrease in overall mortality rates for CHD with a shift in the pattern away from infants toward the adults.[120] Those patients with moderate to severe complexity remain at increased risk for early mortality. It is likely that during the transition process, a patient with CHD will encounter a discussion about mortality for the first time. Reid and colleagues[121] have shown that adolescents between the ages of 16 and 20 years overestimate their life expectancy. There is a need to incorporate discussions about life expectancy and end-of-life issues during routine visits, allowing the adolescents to be involved actively in the decision making and in taking charge of their own health.[122] Adolescence is a time to formulate and strengthen self-identity, gain independence and define the future role in life.[123] The end-of-life discussion might place the health care provider and parents in an uncomfortable position.[124–127] However, data suggest that adolescents are prepared and willing to discuss these issues.[128–136] The AAP, the Institute of Medicine, and the World Health Organization recommend involving adolescents and young adults in care decisions and making them primary guardians of their personal health, because they are developmentally and emotionally ready for it.[136–138] It is also important to identify a medical power of attorney for patients with disabilities. Preparing advance care documents addresses their medical and palliative care preferences and helps to identify a legal decision maker.

Key message

- There is a shift in mortality pattern for CHD away from infants toward adults
- Patients with CHD, particularly those with moderate to severe complexity, remain at increased risk for early mortality
- There is a need to incorporate discussions about life expectancy and end-of-life issues during routine visits to allow adolescents to be actively involved in the decision making
- It has been shown that adolescents are prepared for such discussions

---

SUMMARY

Even after successful treatment, most patients with CHD require lifelong care. The importance of understanding the interplay of various medical and psychosocial factors in patients with CHD is underscored. There is a definite need for PCPs to take charge of their patients and provide guidance and support to the adolescents with CHD during the transition phase. There should be provision for career counseling and other forms of psychosocial interventions when indicated, in addition to the availability of optimal specialty care. A successful smooth transition from adolescence to adulthood in patients with CHD can be achieved with collaboration between the primary provider and the congenital cardiologist.

Some of the resources suggested by the AHA[15] that may be useful for this population are as follows:

1. For employment and insurance: http://www.hrtw.org

2. For insurability issues: www.achaheart.org (under information/resources)

3. For financial assistance: *Pocket Guide to Federal Help for Individuals With Disabilities*

REFERENCES

1. Lloyd-Jones D, Adams R, Carnethon M, et al. Heart disease and stroke statistics–2009 update: a report from the American Heart Association Statistics Committee and Stroke Statistics Subcommittee. Circulation 2009;119(3):480–6.
2. Botto LD, Correa A, Erickson JD. Racial and temporal variations in the prevalence of heart defects. Pediatrics 2001;107(3):E32.
3. Webb GD, Williams RG. Care of the adult with congenital heart disease: introduction. J Am Coll Cardiol 2001;37(5):1166.
4. Gatzoulis MA, Hechter S, Siu SC, et al. Outpatient clinics for adults with congenital heart disease: increasing workload and evolving patterns of referral. Heart 1999;81(1):57–61.
5. American Academy of Pediatrics, American Academy of Family Physicians, American College of Physicians-American Society of Internal Medicine. A consensus statement on health care transitions for young adults with special health care needs. Pediatrics 2002;110(6 Pt 2):1304–6.
6. Adolescent Health Transition Project. A resource for teens and young adults with special health care needs, chronic illness, physical or developmental disabilities. Washington State Department of Health and the Clinical Training Unit, University of Washington, Seattle (WA). Available at: http://depts.washington.edu/healthtr/. Accessed July 15th, 2013.
7. Foster E, Graham TP Jr, Driscoll DJ, et al. Task force 2: special health care needs of adults with congenital heart disease. J Am Coll Cardiol 2001;37(5):1176–83.
8. Luyckx K, Goossens E, Van Damme C, et al. Identity formation in adolescents with congenital cardiac disease: a forgotten issue in the transition to adulthood. Cardiol Young 2011;21(4):411–20.
9. Warnes CA, Williams RG, Bashore TM, et al. ACC/AHA 2008 guidelines for the management of adults with congenital heart disease: a report of the American College of Cardiology/American Heart Association Task Force on Practice

Guidelines (Writing Committee to develop guidelines on the management of adults with congenital heart disease). Circulation 2008;118(23):e714–833.

10. American Academy of Pediatrics Medical Home Initiatives for Children With Special Needs Project Advisory Committee. Policy statement: organizational principles to guide and define the child health care system and/or improve the health of all children. Pediatrics 2004;113(Suppl 5):1545–7.

11. Medical Home Initiatives for Children With Special Needs Project Advisory Committee. American Academy of Pediatrics. The medical home. Pediatrics 2002; 110(1 Pt 1):184–6.

12. Council on Children with Disabilities, Section on Developmental Behavioral Pediatrics, Bright Futures Steering Committee, Medical Home Initiatives for Children With Special Needs Project Advisory Committee. Identifying infants and young children with developmental disorders in the medical home: an algorithm for developmental surveillance and screening. Pediatrics 2006;118(1):405–20.

13. American Academy of Pediatrics Council on Children with Disabilities. Care coordination in the medical home: integrating health and related systems of care for children with special health care needs. Pediatrics 2005;116(5):1238–44.

14. Valente AM, Landzberg MJ, Gianola A, et al. Improving heart disease knowledge and research participation in adults with congenital heart disease (The Health, Education and Access Research Trial: HEART-ACHD). Int J Cardiol 2013. http://dx.doi.org/10.1016/j.ijcard.2013.04.004.

15. Sable C, Foster E, Uzark K, et al. Best practices in managing transition to adulthood for adolescents with congenital heart disease: the transition process and medical and psychosocial issues: a scientific statement from the American Heart Association. Circulation 2011;123(13):1454–85.

16. Gurvitz M, Valente AM, Broberg C, et al. Prevalence and predictors of gaps in care among adult congenital heart disease patients: HEART-ACHD (The Health, Education, and Access Research Trial). J Am Coll Cardiol 2013;61(21):2180–4.

17. Mackie AS, Ionescu-Ittu R, Therrien J, et al. Children and adults with congenital heart disease lost to follow-up: who and when? Circulation 2009;120(4):302–9.

18. Norris MD, Webb G, Drotar D, et al. Prevalence and patterns of retention in cardiac care in young adults with congenital heart disease. J Pediatr 2013;163(3): 902–4.e1.

19. Dearani JA, Connolly HM, Martinez R, et al. Caring for adults with congenital cardiac disease: successes and challenges for 2007 and beyond. Cardiol Young 2007;17(Suppl 2):87–96.

20. Dore A, de Guise P, Mercier LA. Transition of care to adult congenital heart centres: what do patients know about their heart condition? Can J Cardiol 2002; 18(2):141–6.

21. Wacker A, Kaemmerer H, Hollweck R, et al. Outcome of operated and unoperated adults with congenital cardiac disease lost to follow-up for more than five years. Am J Cardiol 2005;95(6):776–9.

22. Marelli AJ, Mackie AS, Ionescu-Ittu R, et al. Congenital heart disease in the general population: changing prevalence and age distribution. Circulation 2007; 115(2):163–72.

23. Reid GJ, Irvine MJ, McCrindle BW, et al. Prevalence and correlates of successful transfer from pediatric to adult health care among a cohort of young adults with complex congenital heart defects. Pediatrics 2004;113(3 Pt 1): e197–205.

24. Fernandes SM, Verstappen A, Ackerman K, et al. Parental knowledge regarding lifelong congenital cardiac care. Pediatrics 2011;128(6):e1489–95.

25. Yeung E, Kay J, Roosevelt GE, et al. Lapse of care as a predictor for morbidity in adults with congenital heart disease. Int J Cardiol 2008;125(1):62–5.
26. Dore A, Glancy DL, Stone S, et al. Cardiac surgery for grown-up congenital heart patients: survey of 307 consecutive operations from 1991 to 1994. Am J Cardiol 1997;80(7):906–13.
27. Monro JL, Alexiou C, Salmon AP, et al. Reoperations and survival after primary repair of congenital heart defects in children. J Thorac Cardiovasc Surg 2003; 126(2):511–20.
28. Mott AR, Fraser CD Jr, McKenzie ED, et al. Perioperative care of the adult with congenital heart disease in a free-standing tertiary pediatric facility. Pediatr Cardiol 2002;23(6):624–30.
29. Gillespie MJ, Rome JJ, Levi DS, et al. Melody valve implant within failed bioprosthetic valves in the pulmonary position: a multicenter experience. Circ Cardiovasc Interv 2012;5(6):862–70.
30. McElhinney DB, Hellenbrand WE, Zahn EM, et al. Short- and medium-term outcomes after transcatheter pulmonary valve placement in the expanded multicenter US melody valve trial. Circulation 2010;122(5):507–16.
31. Butera G, Milanesi O, Spadoni I, et al. Melody transcatheter pulmonary valve implantation. Results from the registry of the Italian Society of Pediatric Cardiology. Catheter Cardiovasc Interv 2013;81(2):310–6.
32. Silka MJ, Hardy BG, Menashe VD, et al. A population-based prospective evaluation of risk of sudden cardiac death after operation for common congenital heart defects. J Am Coll Cardiol 1998;32(1):245–51.
33. Levine GN, Gomes AS, Arai AE, et al. Safety of magnetic resonance imaging in patients with cardiovascular devices: an American Heart Association Scientific Statement from the Committee on Diagnostic and Interventional Cardiac Catheterization, Council on Clinical Cardiology, and the Council on Cardiovascular Radiology and Intervention: endorsed by the American College of Cardiology Foundation, the North American Society for Cardiac Imaging, and the Society for Cardiovascular Magnetic Resonance. Circulation 2007; 116(24):2878–91.
34. Mitka M. First MRI-safe pacemaker receives conditional approval from FDA. JAMA 2011;305(10):985–6.
35. Maxwell BG, Wong JK, Kin C, et al. Perioperative outcomes of major noncardiac surgery in adults with congenital heart disease. Anesthesiology 2013. [Epub ahead of print].
36. Warner MA, Lunn RJ, O'Leary PW, et al. Outcomes of noncardiac surgical procedures in children and adults with congenital heart disease. Mayo Perioperative Outcomes Group. Mayo Clin Proc 1998;73(8):728–34.
37. Territo MC, Rosove MH. Cyanotic congenital heart disease: hematologic management. J Am Coll Cardiol 1991;18(2):320–2.
38. Wilson W, Taubert KA, Gewitz M, et al. Prevention of infective endocarditis: guidelines from the American Heart Association: a guideline from the American Heart Association Rheumatic Fever, Endocarditis, and Kawasaki Disease Committee, Council on Cardiovascular Disease in the Young, and the Council on Clinical Cardiology, Council on Cardiovascular Surgery and Anesthesia, and the Quality of Care and Outcomes Research Interdisciplinary Working Group. Circulation 2007;116(15):1736–54.
39. Levine PA, Balady GJ, Lazar HL, et al. Electrocautery and pacemakers: management of the paced patient subject to electrocautery. Ann Thorac Surg 1986;41(3):313–7.

40. Kovacs AH, Verstappen A. The whole adult congenital heart disease patient. Prog Cardiovasc Dis 2011;53(4):247–53.
41. Tong EM, Kools S. Health care transitions for adolescents with congenital heart disease: patient and family perspectives. Nurs Clin North Am 2004;39(4): 727–40.
42. Kovacs AH, Silversides C, Saidi A, et al. The role of the psychologist in adult congenital heart disease. Cardiol Clin 2006;24(4):607–18, vi.
43. Blum RW, Garell D, Hodgman CH, et al. Transition from child-centered to adult health-care systems for adolescents with chronic conditions. A position paper of the Society for Adolescent Medicine. J Adolesc Health 1993;14(7):570–6.
44. Tong EM, Sparacino PS, Messias DK, et al. Growing up with congenital heart disease: the dilemmas of adolescents and young adults [see comment]. Cardiol Young 1998;8(3):303–9.
45. Claessens P, Moons P, de Casterle BD, et al. What does it mean to live with a congenital heart disease? A qualitative study on the lived experiences of adult patients. Eur J Cardiovasc Nurs 2005;4(1):3–10.
46. Moons P, Van Deyk K, Marquet K, et al. Individual quality of life in adults with congenital heart disease: a paradigm shift. Eur Heart J 2005;26(3):298–307.
47. Linde LM, Rasof B, Dunn OJ, et al. Attitudinal factors in congenital heart disease. Pediatrics 1966;38(1):92–101.
48. Brandhagen DJ, Feldt RH, Williams DE. Long-term psychologic implications of congenital heart disease: a 25-year follow-up. Mayo Clin Proc 1991;66(5):474–9.
49. DeMaso DR, Campis LK, Wypij D, et al. The impact of maternal perceptions and medical severity on the adjustment of children with congenital heart disease. J Pediatr Psychol 1991;16(2):137–49.
50. DeMaso DR, Lauretti A, Spieth L, et al. Psychosocial factors and quality of life in children and adolescents with implantable cardioverter-defibrillators. Am J Cardiol 2004;93(5):582–7.
51. Karsdorp PA, Everaerd W, Kindt M, et al. Psychological and cognitive functioning in children and adolescents with congenital heart disease: a meta-analysis. J Pediatr Psychol 2007;32(5):527–41.
52. Uzark K, Jones K, Slusher J, et al. Quality of life in children with heart disease as perceived by children and parents. Pediatrics 2008;121(5):e1060–7.
53. Kovacs AH, Saidi AS, Kuhl EA, et al. Depression and anxiety in adult congenital heart disease: predictors and prevalence. Int J Cardiol 2009;137(2):158–64.
54. Kellerman J, Zeltzer L, Ellenberg L, et al. Psychological effects of illness in adolescence. I. Anxiety, self-esteem, and perception of control. J Pediatr 1980;97(1):126–31.
55. Linde LM. Psychiatric aspects of congenital heart disease. Psychiatr Clin North Am 1982;5(2):399–406.
56. Utens EM, Verhulst FC, Meijboom FJ, et al. Behavioural and emotional problems in children and adolescents with congenital heart disease. Psychol Med 1993; 23(2):415–24.
57. Donovan E. The pediatric cardiologist and adolescents with congenital heart disease. Int J Cardiol 1985;9(4):493–5.
58. Spurkland I, Bjornstad PG, Lindberg H, et al. Mental health and psychosocial functioning in adolescents with congenital heart disease. A comparison between adolescents born with severe heart defect and atrial septal defect. Acta Paediatr 1993;82(1):71–6.
59. Horner T, Liberthson R, Jellinek MS. Psychosocial profile of adults with complex congenital heart disease. Mayo Clin Proc 2000;75(1):31–6.

60. Bromberg JI, Beasley PJ, D'Angelo EJ, et al. Depression and anxiety in adults with congenital heart disease: a pilot study. Heart Lung 2003;32(2):105–10.
61. Spijkerboer AW, Utens EM, Bogers AJ, et al. A historical comparison of long-term behavioral and emotional outcomes in children and adolescents after invasive treatment for congenital heart disease. J Pediatr Surg 2008;43(3):534–9.
62. Reid GJ, Siu SC, McCrindle BW, et al. Sexual behavior and reproductive concerns among adolescents and young adults with congenital heart disease. Int J Cardiol 2008;125(3):332–8.
63. Reid GJ, Webb GD, McCrindle BW, et al. Health behaviors among adolescents and young adults with congenital heart disease. Congenit Heart Dis 2008;3(1): 16–25.
64. Lip GY, Lane DA, Millane TA, et al. Psychological interventions for depression in adolescent and adult congenital heart disease. Cochrane Database Syst Rev 2003;(3):CD004394.
65. Brosig CL, Mussatto KA, Kuhn EM, et al. Neurodevelopmental outcome in preschool survivors of complex congenital heart disease: implications for clinical practice. J Pediatr Health Care 2007;21(1):3–12.
66. Miatton M, De Wolf D, Francois K, et al. Neuropsychological performance in school-aged children with surgically corrected congenital heart disease. J Pediatr 2007;151(1):73–8, 78.e1.
67. Hovels-Gurich HH, Konrad K, Skorzenski D, et al. Attentional dysfunction in children after corrective cardiac surgery in infancy. Ann Thorac Surg 2007;83(4): 1425–30.
68. Mahle WT, Clancy RR, Moss EM, et al. Neurodevelopmental outcome and lifestyle assessment in school-aged and adolescent children with hypoplastic left heart syndrome. Pediatrics 2000;105(5):1082–9.
69. Marino BS, Lipkin PH, Newburger JW, et al. Neurodevelopmental outcomes in children with congenital heart disease: evaluation and management: a scientific statement from the American Heart Association. Circulation 2012;126(9): 1143–72.
70. Wernovsky G, Stiles KM, Gauvreau K, et al. Cognitive development after the Fontan operation. Circulation 2000;102(8):883–9.
71. Schaefer C, von Rhein M, Knirsch W, et al. Neurodevelopmental outcome, psychological adjustment, and quality of life in adolescents with congenital heart disease. Dev Med Child Neurol 2013. http://dx.doi.org/10.1111/dmcn.12242.
72. Mahle WT, Wernovsky G. Long-term developmental outcome of children with complex congenital heart disease. Clin Perinatol 2001;28(1):235–47.
73. Byrne A, MacDonald J, Buckley S. Reading, language and memory skills: a comparative longitudinal study of children with Down syndrome and their mainstream peers. Br J Educ Psychol 2002;72(Pt 4):513–29.
74. Brugge KL, Nichols SL, Salmon DP, et al. Cognitive impairment in adults with Down's syndrome: similarities to early cognitive changes in Alzheimer's disease. Neurology 1994;44(2):232–8.
75. Moss EM, Batshaw ML, Solot CB, et al. Psychoeducational profile of the 22q11.2 microdeletion: a complex pattern. J Pediatr 1999;134(2):193–8.
76. Bearden CE, Woodin MF, Wang PP, et al. The neurocognitive phenotype of the 22q11.2 deletion syndrome: selective deficit in visual-spatial memory. J Clin Exp Neuropsychol 2001;23(4):447–64.
77. Swillen A, Fryns JP, Kleczkowska A, et al. Intelligence, behaviour and psychosocial development in Turner syndrome. A cross-sectional study of 50 pre-adolescent and adolescent girls (4-20 years). Genet Couns 1993;4(1):7–18.

78. Temple CM, Carney RA. Intellectual functioning of children with Turner syndrome: a comparison of behavioural phenotypes. Dev Med Child Neurol 1993;35(8):691–8.

79. Grossfeld PD, Mattina T, Lai Z, et al. The 11q terminal deletion disorder: a prospective study of 110 cases. Am J Med Genet A 2004;129A(1):51–61.

80. Raqbi F, Le Bihan C, Morisseau-Durand MP, et al. Early prognostic factors for intellectual outcome in CHARGE syndrome. Dev Med Child Neurol 2003; 45(7):483–8.

81. Knauth A, Verstappen A, Reiss J, et al. Transition and transfer from pediatric to adult care of the young adult with complex congenital heart disease. Cardiol Clin 2006;24(4):619–29, vi.

82. Saidi A, Kovacs AH. Developing a transition program from pediatric- to adult-focused cardiology care: practical considerations. Congenit Heart Dis 2009; 4(4):204–15.

83. Van Deyk K, Moons P, Gewillig M, et al. Educational and behavioral issues in transitioning from pediatric cardiology to adult-centered health care. Nurs Clin North Am 2004;39(4):755–68.

84. Hutchinson JW, Stafford EM. Changing parental opinions about teen privacy through education. Pediatrics 2005;116(4):966–71.

85. Gantt LT. Growing up heartsick: the experiences of young women with congenital heart disease. Health Care Women Int 1992;13(3):241–8.

86. Chen CW, Chen YC, Chen MY, et al. Health-promoting behavior of adolescents with congenital heart disease. J Adolesc Health 2007;41(6):602–9.

87. Chen CA, Wang JK, Lue HC, et al. A shift from underweight to overweight and obesity in Asian children and adolescents with congenital heart disease. Paediatr Perinat Epidemiol 2012;26(4):336–43.

88. Morrison ML, Sands AJ, McCusker CG, et al. Exercise training improves activity in adolescents with congenital heart disease. Heart 2013;99(15):1122–8.

89. Reybrouck T, Mertens L. Physical performance and physical activity in grown-up congenital heart disease. Eur J Cardiovasc Prev Rehabil 2005;12(5):498–502.

90. Mitchell JH, Haskell W, Snell P, et al. Task Force 8: classification of sports. J Am Coll Cardiol 2005;45(8):1364–7.

91. Graham TP Jr, Driscoll DJ, Gersony WM, et al. Task Force 2: congenital heart disease. J Am Coll Cardiol 2005;45(8):1326–33.

92. Takken T, Giardini A, Reybrouck T, et al. Recommendations for physical activity, recreation sport, and exercise training in paediatric patients with congenital heart disease: a report from the Exercise, Basic & Translational Research Section of the European Association of Cardiovascular Prevention and Rehabilitation, the European Congenital Heart and Lung Exercise Group, and the Association for European Paediatric Cardiology. Eur J Prev Cardiol 2012;19(5): 1034–65.

93. Lick SD, Edozie SN, Woodside KJ, et al. *Streptococcus viridans* endocarditis from tongue piercing. J Emerg Med 2005;29(1):57–9.

94. Abma JC, Martinez GM, Mosher WD, et al. Teenagers in the United States: sexual activity, contraceptive use, and childbearing, 2002. Vital Health Stat 23 2004;(24):1–48.

95. Klein JD. Adolescent pregnancy: current trends and issues. Pediatrics 2005; 116(1):281–6.

96. Dailard C. Recent findings from the "Add Health" survey: teens and sexual activity. Guttmacher Report Public Policy 2001;4:1–3. Available at: http:// wwwguttmacher.org/pubs/tgr/04/4/gr040401.html.

97. Kokkonen J, Paavilainen T. Social adaptation of young adults with congenital heart disease. Int J Cardiol 1992;36(1):23–9.
98. Canobbio MM. Health care issues facing adolescents with congenital heart disease. J Pediatr Nurs 2001;16(5):363–70.
99. Meschke LL, Bartholomae S, Zentall SR. Adolescent sexuality and parent-adolescent processes: promoting healthy teen choices. J Adolesc Health 2002;31(Suppl 6):264–79.
100. Silversides CK, Sermer M, Siu SC. Choosing the best contraceptive method for the adult with congenital heart disease. Curr Cardiol Rep 2009;11(4):298–305.
101. Randomised controlled trial of levonorgestrel versus the Yuzpe regimen of combined oral contraceptives for emergency contraception. Task Force on Postovulatory Methods of Fertility Regulation. Lancet 1998;352(9126):428–33.
102. Ho PC, Kwan MS. A prospective randomized comparison of levonorgestrel with the Yuzpe regimen in post-coital contraception. Hum Reprod 1993;8(3):389–92.
103. Grimes DA, Raymond EG. Emergency contraception. Ann Intern Med 2002;137(3):180–9.
104. Chandra PC, Schiavello HJ, Ravi B, et al. Pregnancy outcomes in urban teen-agers. Int J Gynaecol Obstet 2002;79(2):117–22.
105. Jolly MC, Sebire N, Harris J, et al. Obstetric risks of pregnancy in women less than 18 years old. Obstet Gynecol 2000;96(6):962–6.
106. Lao TT, Ho LF. The obstetric implications of teenage pregnancy. Hum Reprod 1997;12(10):2303–5.
107. Brown DL. Family history of congenital heart disease. In: Benson CB, Arger PH, Bluth EI, editors. Ultrasound on obstetrics and gynecology: a practical approach. New York: Thieme Medical Publishers; 2003. p. 155–66.
108. Bernier FP, Spaetgens R. The geneticist's role in adult congenital heart disease. Cardiol Clin 2006;24(4):557–69, v–vi.
109. Simko LC, McGinnis KA, Schembri J. Educational needs of adults with congenital heart disease. J Cardiovasc Nurs 2006;21(2):85–94.
110. Crossland DS, Jackson SP, Lyall R, et al. Employment and advice regarding careers for adults with congenital heart disease. Cardiol Young 2005;15(4):391–5.
111. McGrath KA, Truesdell SC. Employability and career counseling for adolescents and adults with congenital heart disease. Nurs Clin North Am 1994;29(2):319–30.
112. Gutgesell HP, Gessner IH, Vetter VL, et al. Recreational and occupational recommendations for young patients with heart disease. A statement for physicians by the Committee on Congenital Cardiac Defects of the Council on Cardiovascular Disease in the Young, American Heart Association. Circulation 1986;74(5):1195A–8A.
113. Kamphuis M, Vogels T, Ottenkamp J, et al. Employment in adults with congenital heart disease. Arch Pediatr Adolesc Med 2002;156(11):1143–8.
114. Campbell FA, Pungello EP, Miller-Johnson S, et al. The development of cognitive and academic abilities: growth curves from an early childhood educational experiment. Dev Psychol 2001;37(2):231–42.
115. Callahan ST, Cooper WO. Uninsurance and health care access among young adults in the United States. Pediatrics 2005;116(1):88–95.
116. Kriss JL, Collins SR, Mahato B, et al. Rite of passage? Why young adults become uninsured and how new policies can help, 2008 update. Issue Brief (Commonw Fund) 2008;38:1–24.
117. Callahan ST, Cooper WO. Access to health care for young adults with disabling chronic conditions. Arch Pediatr Adolesc Med 2006;160(2):178–82.

118. Uzark K, Jones K. Parenting stress and children with heart disease. J Pediatr Health Care 2003;17(4):163–8.
119. Lawoko S, Soares JJ. Quality of life among parents of children with congenital heart disease, parents of children with other diseases and parents of healthy children. Qual Life Res 2003;12(6):655–66.
120. Khairy P, Ionescu-Ittu R, Mackie AS, et al. Changing mortality in congenital heart disease. J Am Coll Cardiol 2010;56(14):1149–57.
121. Reid GJ, Webb GD, Barzel M, et al. Estimates of life expectancy by adolescents and young adults with congenital heart disease. J Am Coll Cardiol 2006;48(2):349–55.
122. Kovacs AH, Landzberg MJ, Goodlin SJ. Advance care planning and end-of-life management of adult patients with congenital heart disease. World J Pediatr Congenit Heart Surg 2013;4(1):62–9.
123. Facts for families (No. 58): normal adolescent development. American Academy of Child and Adolescent Psychiatry; 2011. Available at: http://www.aacap.org/AACAP/Families_and_Youth/Facts_for_Families/Facts_for_Families_Pages/Normal_Adolescent_Development_Part_II_58.aspx. Accessed July 15, 2013.
124. Feudtner C. Collaborative communication in pediatric palliative care: a foundation for problem-solving and decision-making. Pediatr Clin North Am 2007; 54(5):583–607, ix.
125. Morgan ER, Murphy SB. Care of children who are dying of cancer. N Engl J Med 2000;342(5):347–8.
126. Davies B, Sehring SA, Partridge JC, et al. Barriers to palliative care for children: perceptions of pediatric health care providers. Pediatrics 2008;121(2):282–8.
127. Steele R, Davies B. Impact on parents when a child has a progressive, life-threatening illness. Int J Palliat Nurs 2006;12(12):576–85.
128. Read K, Fernandez CV, Gao J, et al. Decision-making by adolescents and parents of children with cancer regarding health research participation. Pediatrics 2009;124(3):959–65.
129. McAliley LG, Hudson-Barr DC, Gunning RS, et al. The use of advance directives with adolescents. Pediatr Nurs 2000;26(5):471–80.
130. Lyon ME, McCabe MA, Patel KM, et al. What do adolescents want? An exploratory study regarding end-of-life decision-making. J Adolesc Health 2004;35(6):529.e1–6.
131. Wiener L, Ballard E, Brennan T, et al. How I wish to be remembered: the use of an advance care planning document in adolescent and young adult populations. J Palliat Med 2008;11(10):1309–13.
132. Lyon ME, Garvie PA, McCarter R, et al. Who will speak for me? Improving end-of-life decision-making for adolescents with HIV and their families. Pediatrics 2009;123(2):e199–206.
133. Hammes BJ, Klevan J, Kempf M, et al. Pediatric advance care planning. J Palliat Med 2005;8(4):766–73.
134. Hinds PS, Drew D, Oakes LL, et al. End-of-life care preferences of pediatric patients with cancer. J Clin Oncol 2005;23(36):9146–54.
135. Stevens MM, Dunsmore JC, Bennett DL, et al. Adolescents living with lifethreatening illnesses. In: Balk DE, Corr CA, editors. Adolescent encounters with death, bereavement and coping. New York: Springer; 2009. p. 115–40.
136. Field M, Behrman RE, editors. When children die: Improving palliative care and end of life care for children and their families. Washington, DC: National Academy Press; 2002.

137. American Academy of Pediatrics. Committee on Bioethics and Committee on Hospital Care. Palliative care for children. Pediatrics 2000;106(2 Pt 1):351–7.
138. McGrath PA. Development of the World Health Organization Guidelines on Cancer Pain Relief and Palliative Care in Children. J Pain Symptom Manage 1996; 12(2):87–92.

Index

Note: Page numbers of article titles are in **boldface** type.

A

ADHD. *See* Attention deficit hyperactivity disorder.
Aldosterone antagonists, for hypertension, 140–141
Alpha-antagonists, for hypertension, 140–141
Ambulatory blood pressure monitoring, 136–137
American Association for the Surgery of Trauma, organ injury scale of, 112
Amlodipine, for hypertension, 141
Amoxetine, for ADHD, 85–87
Amphetamine, for ADHD, 85–87
Aneurysm, aortic, 194–195
Angiotensin receptor blockers, for hypertension, 140–141
Angiotensin-converting enzyme inhibitors
    for dilated cardiomyopathy, 177
    for hypertension, 140–141
Anorexia nervosa, palpitations in, 74
Anticoagulation, for restrictive cardiomyopathy, 183
Antihypertensive agents, 139–142
Anxiety, sinus tachycardia in, 73–74
Aortic aneurysm and dissection, 194–195
Aortic systolic murmurs, 11
Aortic valve, bicuspid, 12
Aortopathy, family history of, 195
Arrhythmias
    in blunt cardiac injury, 117
    in electrocardiography, 49–51
Asthma, chest pain in, 20, 24
Atenolol, for hypertension, 141
Athlete's heart, 99–101
Atrial abnormalities, in electrocardiography, 48–49
Atrial premature contractions, palpitations in, 74–75
Atrial septal defects, 13
Atrioventricular block, 53–55
Attention deficit hyperactivity disorder, **81–90**
    causes of, 82
    challenges with, 88–89
    classification of, 82
    controversial issues in, 84
    diagnosis of, 82–83
    guidelines for, 84–85
    historical review of, 81–82
    in congenital heart disease, 213–214
    treatment of, 83–88

Pediatr Clin N Am 61 (2014) 229–239
http://dx.doi.org/10.1016/S0031-3955(13)00185-5
0031-3955/14/$ – see front matter © 2014 Elsevier Inc. All rights reserved.

Moving?

Make sure your subscription moves with you!

To notify us of your new address, find your **Clinics Account Number** (located on your mailing label above your name), and contact customer service at:

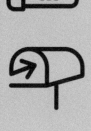

Email: journalscustomerservice-usa@elsevier.com

800-654-2452 (subscribers in the U.S. & Canada)
314-447-8871 (subscribers outside of the U.S. & Canada)

Fax number: 314-447-8029

Elsevier Health Sciences Division
Subscription Customer Service
3251 Riverport Lane
Maryland Heights, MO 63043

Printed and bound by CPI Group (UK) Ltd, Croydon, CR0 4YY

03/10/2024

01040412-0003